HEALING
AND
RECOVERY

David R. Hawkins, M.D., Ph.D.

HAY HOUSE, INC.
Carlsbad, California • New York City
London • Sydney • New Delhi

Previously published by Veritas Publishing (ISBN 978-0-9715007-8-5)

Library of Congress Control Number: 2013946875

Tradepaper ISBN: 978-1-4019-4499-5

17 16 15 14 13 12 11 10 9
1st Hay House edition, July 2015

Printed in the United States of America

SUSTAINABLE
FORESTRY
INITIATIVE
Certified Chain of Custody
Promoting Sustainable Forestry
www.sfiprogram.org
SFI-01268

SFI label applies to the text stock

HEALING
AND
RECOVERY

ALSO BY DAVID R. HAWKINS, M.D., PH.D.

Please visit:

Hay House USA: www.hayhouse.com®
Hay House Australia: www.hayhouse.com.au
Hay House UK: www.hayhouse.co.uk
Hay House India: www.hayhouse.co.in

DEDICATION

Dedicated to the Highest Good:
Physical, Mental, and Spiritual

TABLE OF CONTENTS

PREFACE

These are transcriptions of a series of popular lectures originally presented in a videotape format and now edited and updated for convenience in written form. They originated at the request of the original publisher of *A Course in Miracles* (The Foundation for Inner Peace), subsequent to a large joint meeting in the 1980s in Detroit, Michigan, of members of several self-help groups, including Alcoholics Anonymous, A Course in Miracles (ACIM), Attitudinal Healing Centers, and a number of clinicians and recovery groups.

Although the lectures have been adapted for written format, they remain close to the original presentations and include references to discoveries in consciousness research as well as clinical and spiritual premises. There is purposeful repetition of basic information as each lecture was complete within itself. A benefit of repetition is that the material becomes familiar and absorbed without putting forth mental effort or memorization. It is intrinsically simple, and the inherent truths become obvious and easy to assimilate. The information provided is of a general nature and is not meant to displace or replace personal medical advice by one's own health practitioner.

FOREWORD

Information tends to become compartmentalized, especially in academic versus clinical science and practice (Hawkins, 2006, "Paradigm Blindness"). These areas in turn become separated from spiritual principles and realities, which are subsequently also isolated from depth psychology, psychoanalysis, and group dynamics. Psychopharmacology research proceeds in its own development independently of all the above, as does advanced theoretical physics and the emergence of nonlinear dynamics and chaos theory. Each discipline developed within the limitations of its own parameters because there had been no context of sufficient dimension to include all of them until the development of the clinical science of consciousness research. This provided a common context of reference and an all-inclusive paradigm of reality via the now well-known "Map of the Scale of Consciousness" (Hawkins, 1995, *Power vs. Force*).

Traditional sciences were limited to the linear dimensions and primarily to the Newtonian concepts of cause and effect, included in the consciousness level of the 400s (see Map, pg. 16, Chapter 1), whereas experiential reality is nonlinear and subjective (and proceeds from level 500 and up). Phenomena are the consequence of the emergence of potentiality as actuality, a process whereby content is subject to overall context. Thus, healing is the result of not just clinical processes but also of overall biological potentialities that often do not materialize without the unseen power of spiritual alignment. Chemistry is within the predictable

Newtonian discipline of scientific (linear content) expectation, but health recovery is greatly facilitated by the unseen power of the spiritual dimensions of intentionality of consciousness itself (nonlinear context).

The clinical power and influential impact of spiritual context is overwhelmingly displayed by the millions of recoveries from medically hopeless illnesses as exhibited by worldwide membership in faith-based organizations of which Alcoholics Anonymous and A Course in Miracles (ACIM) are prime examples. Since the basic principles of faith-based recoveries are outside the paradigm of the reality of academic science, their importance was not studied or comprehended because academic science was concerned with just content and not context. The emergence of the Heisenberg Uncertainty Principle finally accorded respectability for the recognition of the reality and influence of the effect of consciousness itself. Thus, the power of intention came to be recognized as an important critical factor in catalyzing potentiality into actuality. (See Stapp's *Mindful Universe* for correlation of quantum theory, consciousness, and intention.

INTRODUCTION

The lectures on healing and recovery represent the integration and concordance of experience and information from multiple fields, including more than fifty years of clinical practice that encompasses diverse fields of healing, such as holistic health, psychiatry, psychology, psychoanalysis, psychopharmacology, medicine, and the application of spiritual principles as well as concepts and discoveries from the emerging clinical science of consciousness research.

The development of consciousness research was reported in multiple lecture series (Hawkins, 2002-2008) as well as in a series of books: *Qualitative and Quantitative Analysis and Calibration of the Levels of Human Consciousness* (Bell and Howell, 1995; Veritas Publishing, 1995); *Power vs. Force* (Veritas, 1995; Hay House, 2002); *The Eye of the I* (Veritas, 2001); *I: Reality and Subjectivity* (Veritas, 2003); *Truth vs. Falsehood* (Axial Publishing, 2005); *Transcending the Levels of Consciousness* (Veritas, 2007); *Discovery of the Presence of God: Devotional Nonduality* (Veritas, 2007); and *Reality, Spirituality, and Modern Man* (Axial, 2008). A collection of lecture slides and a comprehensive Index of Calibrations are also in preparation.

All the above give detailed descriptions as well as explanations of theory, along with the application of a simple, calibrated scale of levels of consciousness and Truth as exemplified by the Map of Consciousness on page 16. The fields of suffering calibrate below level 200, and the progressive levels of truth are above 200. Science is in the 400s; spiritual realities begin at 500

(Love) and progress upward to 540 (Unconditional Love), to 570 (saintly), and then to the levels of joy, the stages of Illumination, and, finally, Enlightenment.

The fields below level 200 potentiate illness; those above 200 support healing, including medical science, which calibrates in the 400s. The spiritual power of the consciousness levels of the 500s facilitates further recoveries that are not otherwise possible.

All illnesses are physical, mental, and spiritual, and the highest levels of recovery are the consequence of simultaneously addressing all three levels and seeing them as being of equal importance. Spiritual intention and contextualization increase the percentage of positive responses to strictly medical treatment. Innate to the human condition, however, are inherent limitations consequent to evolutionary design, some of which can be transcended and some of which cannot be. Therefore, hope and faith need to be accompanied by surrender to and acceptance of a Higher Will. As our research has validated, life cannot be destroyed; it can only change expression from the limited physical linear reality to the unlimited nonlinear spiritual reality.

MAP OF THE SCALE OF CONSCIOUSNESS

God-view	Self-view	Level	Log	Emotion	Process
Self	Is	Enlightenment	700-1,000	Ineffable	Pure Consciousness
All-being	Perfect	Peace	600	Bliss	Illumination
One	Complete	Joy	540	Serenity	Transfiguration
Loving	Benign	Love	500	Reverence	Revelation
Wise	Meaningful	Reason	400	Understanding	Abstraction
Merciful	Harmonious	Acceptance	350	Forgiveness	Transcendence
Inspiring	Hopeful	Willingness	310	Optimism	Intention
Enabling	Satisfactory	Neutrality	250	Trust	Release
Permitting	Feasible	Courage	200	Affirmation	Empowerment

▲

LEVELS OF TRUTH

LEVELS OF FALSEHOOD

▼

God-view	Self-view	Level	Log	Emotion	Process
Indifferent	Demanding	Pride	175	Scorn	Inflation
Vengeful	Antagonistic	Anger	150	Hate	Aggression
Denying	Disappointing	Desire	125	Craving	Enslavement
Punitive	Frightening	Fear	100	Anxiety	Withdrawal
Uncaring	Tragic	Grief	75	Regret	Despondency
Condemning	Hopeless	Apathy, hatred	50	Despair	Abdication
Vindictive	Evil	Guilt	30	Blame	Destruction
Despising	Hateful	Shame	20	Humiliation	Elimination

16

CHAPTER 1

A Map of Consciousness

We will present the concept of utilizing a conscious-ness approach to a variety of man's problems, such as stress, alcoholism, various diseases, depression, fear, and major loss, to name a few. In discussing these chal-lenges, reference will be repeatedly made to the Map of Consciousness. It is referred to frequently to explain the relationship between body, mind, and spirit, which is so important to comprehend in relation to self-healing.

To understand the value of the Map of Consciousness itself without reference to a particular problem, we will describe its implications and useful-ness in its application to all human problems. It is an exponential model (to the base 10) that evolved out of a composite of decades of research in a variety of fields. It documents the first time that these energy fields have ever been calibrated.

When referring to consciousness, we are describ-ing those energy fields. Shown on the Map are general fields of consciousness that have been calibrated as to the power of the field and its direction, as indicated by the arrows. Those below the level of Courage at 200 go downward, and those above Courage go upward. There is significance in the direction of the energy fields. Those that are in a negative direction do not support life and could be called 'anti-life'. Those that are in the positive direction of Truth support and nurture life. At the top of the Map, we approach an alignment with Truth and see that the energy fields become more powerful as their numerical calibrations increase.

The calibration of the fields starts at zero, and what

the world calls Enlightenment calibrates from 600 to 1,000. Enlightenment means that one has transcended duality and identification with the small, personal self. Within the Map, these levels are what a person generally means when they talk about 'me' or 'myself'. They represent the ego, which is the self with a small 's', in contrast to Self with a capital 'S' at the top of the Map.

To the right of the list of energy fields are the emotions associated with each specific level. Farther to the right is the process that is going on in consciousness. The left side of the Map shows the view that one has of God and of life at each level of consciousness.

The average person (if they calibrate over 200) can verify these numbers by using the simple system of muscle testing (fully described in Appendix B). Someone can test you by pressing down on your arm while they say, "Fear is over 50? Over 60? Over 70? Over 80? Over 90? Over 100?" At 100, the arm will go weak. These calibrations have been verified worldwide by many people for decades and are pragmatically very useful clinically as well as for research. Starting at the bottom of the Map are the energy fields called Shame at 20 and Guilt at 30. The emotion that accompanies these levels is self-hatred, and the process going on in consciousness is one of self-destruction. The view of the world associated with this energy field is that of sin and suffering. Therefore, the God of such a world would have to be the potential, ultimate destroyer who is even angry with mankind and would throw their eternal souls into hell forever. With such a perception of God, one does not really need a devil, so there is no devil listed under 'God-view' because that is really the demonic depiction of God. For many people on the planet, death comes as a matter of passive suicide because of unconscious guilt and self-hatred. (This is mentioned later, especially in relation to addictions.) Suicide can take the forms of not caring for oneself, not getting out of the way of the bus, rolling the car over, an accidental drug overdose, high-risk behaviors, and more.

Apathy calibrates at 50 and also has a negative energy field. The emotions of Apathy are hopelessness, despair, despondency, and depression, which are the result of the loss of energy. Apathy leads to viewing the world as hopeless, and the God of a hopeless condition of mankind would be dead or nonexistent. There are many skeptics, atheists, and philosophers who unconsciously justify any particular position that negates Reality and try to rationalize it, defend it, and make it sound sensible (see *Truth vs. Falsehood*). The ideas that God is dead and that man and the condition of life are hopeless invalidate the value of life and are therefore destructive.

Apathy is like an old lady rocking back and forth in her rocking chair, staring hopelessly out the window after receiving an erroneous telegram that her son was killed in the war. A large portion of the world lives in a state of apathy, including whole countries and subcontinents, where the people stare blankly because there is no hope and no chance. About one-third of the world lives at the bottom three states of Fear, Grief, and Apathy. The woman rocking back and forth has also had adverse changes occur in her brain. We could add a column to the Map that says 'Brain Chemistry' because this energy field of Apathy results in a shift of neurotrans-mitters, creating a clinical state called 'hopelessness'. (See Brain Function and Physiology diagram at the end of this chapter.)

If the woman in the rocking chair were to start crying and expressing emotion, then she would be improving and moving up to an energy field called Grief, which is characterized emotionally by regret and feelings of loss and despondence. The process going on in consciousness is dispirited. Grief is the loss of the energy of life, spirit, and the will to live. When the will to live is lost, then the energy from the universe is lost, leading to depression. People in Grief see a sad world and a God who ignores them.

Fear is the next energy field, which is also negative, but it calibrates at 100 and therefore contains a lot more energy. One can run a great distance with fear. Fear runs a great part of the world and plays a very important part in everyone's life. The advertising industry plays off our fears to sell us products. Grief has to do with the past, but fear, as we ordinarily experience it, is of the future. Fear is emotionally experienced in everyday life by the average person as worry, anxiety, or panic. The process going on in consciousness is that of deflation. For example, the animal shrinks when it is frightened.

Remember in grade school when the teacher called on somebody for an answer, everyone would shrink and hide behind the person in front of them? Fear is a shrinkingness and a fear of the future, yet it has a lot of energy. If we know what to be afraid of, the energy of fear can really be beneficial as caution.

The lower states on the Map actually represent the failure to face the energy field above them. The way out of depression is to look at the fear that is underlying the depression and notice how it usually takes the form of "I have lost the source of my happiness." All these levels below Courage have a negative energy field stemming from the same thought—that happiness comes from outside oneself. Putting one's survival on something outside oneself therefore results in states of powerlessness, victimhood, and weakness by virtue of having projected the source of one's power outside of oneself.

Underlying depression is the fear that one has lost something, because grief has to do with loss. Getting a person to face that fear and handle it rapidly overcomes the depression. Later, we will look at how consciousness views fear and will present the specific technique of how to let go of resisting the energy field of fear by letting it run out so that depression subsequently disappears.

The energy field above fear is Desire, which calibrates at 125. It is still a negative energy field, which one experiences in ordinary life as 'wanting'. There are the general feelings of wantingness and cravingness, which are part of the field of addictions and can become obsessions and compulsions. The process going on in consciousness is entrapment. One is run by what one desires, and the source of happiness is seen as external. Advertising takes advantage of this by creating a desire via an unconscious connection; it is a symbolization with something archetypal in the unconscious mind that creates a desire.

Desire can run an entire lifetime. It can be the motivation to become successful or famous, to have a lot of money, to be a celebrity, or to acquire whatever one thinks is going to bring happiness, including a special relationship. Wantingness and cravingness are often insatiable as they originate from an energy field that can never really be satisfied. It is an ongoing, continuous energy field that keeps creating more desire. However, the energy field can be used positively as motivation and intention towards fulfillment of potential and inner goals. Failure to internalize goals leads to frustration and resentment.

Anger, which calibrates at 150, is accompanied by a large amount of energy. If the angry person knows how to utilize that anger constructively instead of destructively, the energy of anger can then lead to progress. Through television, people in the third-world countries began to see what other people had, which fired up their desire, led to frustration and anger, and culminated in that energy being utilized to create entire social movements, changes in the legislature, and constructive changes in society. Thus, anger can be utilized to energize resolve and determination.

The anger we witness or experience in daily life is usually in the form of resentment. At a more severe level, it may lead to hatred, grievances, grudges, and eventually even to murder or war. The process going on in consciousness is one of expansion; for example, when an animal is angry, it swells up. When the cat gets angry, its tail swells up to almost twice its normal size, and the cat tries to look imposing. The biological purpose of expansion is to intimidate one's apparent enemy. The energy of anger can be utilized positively to pursue something better for oneself and thus move up to Pride.

Pride calibrates at 175, which denotes far more energy than the levels below it. However, Pride still has a negative direction. We have heard that "pride goeth before a fall." There are many famous examples in history indicating that pride is a very vulnerable position (e.g., hubris). Pride can be useful in that it has much more energy than the lower levels of consciousness. It expresses itself in daily life as arrogance, contempt, and sarcasm. The downside of it is really denial, and the problem is that the process in consciousness is one of inflation.

We say that a person in Pride has a swelled head, is too big for his britches, is unteachable, cannot hear, or has a closed mind. This level of consciousness leads to a polarized position of opinion that puts the person constantly on the defensive for being 'right', so the world must be wrong. The energy is dissipated in end-less defensiveness.

A reason for pride relates to an underlying fear. Once the person faces the fear, they can let go of pride. These negative fields tend to reinforce each other; seldom do they occur alone. One predominates, but all are really feeding into each other so that one has grief over one's anger; one has anger over one's pride; one has fear over one's grief, and so on. They all tend to rein-force each other, so an emotional upset is usually com-posed of a combination of all these negative energy fields. The techniques and realizations necessary to overcome the negative energy fields are described in detail in *Transcending the Levels of Consciousness*.

By being willing to surrender the ego's narcissistic emotional payoffs of the negative energy fields, one then progresses to the first level of true power, called Courage, at calibration level 200. Something crucial now happens at this level because it has an enormous amount of power. It is obvious that Courage settled the United States of America. Courage created all the great industries and was the basis for man's getting to the moon. The Marines start at the level of Pride but really move up to the more stable level of Courage. Why? It is not so much in the increment of the twenty-five-point increase, although that is sizeable. The critical element is that the energy field is now positive because the person values truth rather than falsehood, and integrity instead of temporary gain.

Above level 200, one is no longer the victim because the energy field is now positive. One might say that this field is like an antenna, and below the level of Courage, the antenna is tuned to the negative, thus pulling adversity into the energy field.

At level 200, energy goes positive, so the field stops pulling negativity from the universe to itself. A person is now in a different condition as well. One is able to face, cope with, and handle things, and, for the first time, able to be appropriate.

At the level of Courage, people still experience the lesser negative feelings, but they now have the power to handle those energies. The critical process is one of empowerment. A person becomes re-empowered by telling the truth. This is obviously critical in the recovery from all illnesses. It is very visibly so in the millions of recoveries of members of Alcoholics Anonymous, where Step 1 and all the basic steps are admissions of the truth.

When people admit they are powerless over something, instead of going weak with the muscle test, they suddenly go strong. When they get rid of the arrogance of pride, they may still have other negative feelings. Persons at the level of Courage who plan to ask their boss for a raise may still have knots in their stomach, be angry, and even feel hopeless about getting one. They might even be arrogant, but now, at the level of Courage, they have enough power to handle all that and be appropriate. They are then able to face it, cope with it, and function in an effective way in the world.

The next major level is that of Neutral at 250, where the energy field is positive and even more aligned with Truth. The emotion of Neutral is self-trust. For example, it is 'okay' if one gets the job and 'okay' if one does not. The process going on in consciousness is detachment. One is not attached to any particular outcome and is no longer a victim. The person now has a great deal more power and is not dominated by aversions or cravings. The upside of this can be the okayness of life; the downside of 'unattached' can be detached or flat. At Neutral, one is no longer suffering painful emotions and now feels free. One is therefore in a far more powerful state. The way that person sees the world as okay considers God as granting freedom. The advantage of the level of Neutral is that one has let go of resisting things and therefore has a lot more power, but then one has to introduce a new energy to move up to the next level of Willingness.

Willingness, at 310, is far more powerful. The emotion of it is accompanied by the thoughts of 'yes', saying yes to life, to join, to agree, to commit, and to align with because there is now the introduction of intention. A person at the level of Neutral, when asked if they would like to go to a movie tonight, would say, "Well, it's okay if we go, and it's okay if we don't." The response lacks enthusiasm and aliveness and is still a long way from abundance, but it is certainly far more comfortable than being attached and in fear, grief, apathy, or anger. The one who becomes willing brings aliveness and intention to say yes, to commit, and to agree. Real power begins with Willingness because one has let go of resistance.

The next field above that is called Acceptance, at 350. It is a very powerful energy field, one of being capable, adequate, and confident. There is the beginning of transformation in consciousness. Transformation has to do with the person's re-owning that they are the source of their own happiness, and that the power is within them. A person on this level is the one whom a big corporation depends on because they are realistic and can admit their upside and downside. They are not dominated by pride, which means denial, so they can allow for their weaknesses and shortcomings. An executive on this level can say, "You know, I don't do very well with that guy in Argentina. It would be better if you send Jake; I'm sure he would get along better." The executive can indicate where he is limited, accept how the world works, avoid getting into 'right and wrong' about it, and therefore deal with it effectively. The transformation comes from re-owning one's power.

A person on this level knows that no matter where they are, they will create a circumstance that will bring happiness. Rick Warren's *The Purpose Driven Life* represents this level, as do benevolent public-service organizations.

The utilization of opportunities occurring at this level can turn lemons into lemonade, which comes from a position or way of being and the re-owning of one's own power. To do so leads to a general way of being easygoing, and the people at this level do not ruffle easily. Constant re-owning of one's power and recycling the energy back into the universe (e.g., through selfless service) moves a person up to the energy field of Reason at 400.

Reason, logic, and the intellect are the prime evolutionary characteristics of the human species. They are the product of intelligence that is capable of symbolic thinking and abstraction. This level is also representative of disciplined structure that is in accord with the observable world and its processes. Thus, emotions, including desires and aversions, are subordinated as less relevant in comparison to impersonal facts.

The use of reason transcends the limitations of narcissistic/emotional distortion that is characteristic of childishness and the personal emotionality of pervasive likes, dislikes, and endless wants. The silencing of the clamor of emotionality allows for cool calculation and dominance of processing by facts and confirmable data. Thus emerges the capacity for assimilation, recognition, classification, and comprehension of the significance and meaning of vast amounts of information by virtue of abstract symbols and their interrelationships.

Intellect and reason are necessary to interpret meaning, value, and significance, which are subserved by the term 'philosophy' and its offshoots of metaphysics, epistemology, ontology, theology, and science. The history of the evolution of the intellect is imparted by *The Great Books of the Western World* from which we see that the evolution of the intellect reached its zenith during the classical period of ancient Greece. It resurged again much later as the appearance and dominance of an historical Reformation out of which emerged modern science. Philosophical dereliction is termed 'rhetoric', which reflects nonintegrous manipulation of reason as demonstrated by the decline of the level of philosophy in academia of recent decades and the emergence of the theories of relativism (cal. 190) and their consequent social discord (see Chapter 12, *Truth vs. Falsehood*).

At its purest level, reason and the intellect represent increased reality testing and nonemotional respect for truth and the means of its discernment. This can evolve even more as the love of Truth for its own sake. This eventually leads to a paradigm jump at consciousness level 500 (Love). Whereas reason is linear and objective, Love is a different dimension as it is nonlinear and subjective. Thus, it is said that reason is of the mind (the brain), whereas Love is of the being (the heart).

At its emergence, love is selective and conditional, but as it evolves, it progressively becomes a lifestyle and a way of relating to all life. Love emanates from within the Self and is an expression of happiness. Love nurtures and supports life and is the beginning of a revelation. Brain neurotransmitters change, beginning with the release of endorphins, which opens up millions of banks of neurons that up to this time have been waiting for this energy field to activate them. Scientists are currently researching the whole field of endorphins (e.g., oxytocin is associated with concern for others and socialization).

Unconditional Love at calibration level 540 is the energy field of healing and also that of the twelve-step groups. There is a rise in the intensity of the energy field of aliveness, so it is preferable to be around that kind of people because they make us feel more alive by giving out energy to the field itself.

At the bottom levels of consciousness are situations of lose-lose. People lose, and those who become associated with them lose. This point of view is one of losing, so the person says, "Everywhere I look, there is a closed door. If I go this way, I'll lose." They see life as a losing proposition. The people in the middle calibration range look at life as win-lose. Their pridefulness and the polarization of angriness cause them to see the world as one of competition, conflict, and win-lose. "If I win, then you lose." They have endless unconscious fears of retaliation because they look at success as vanquishing and expect retaliation. "If we beat somebody in this game, we cannot really win because, after all, he has friends that may come looking for us some day, so we can never relax."

The people at 500 conceptualize and hold life as a win-win situation. When they win, everybody wins—the family, the company—so the more money the company makes, the better for the employees. Companies seek people in the 500s; they do not have to look for jobs, invitations, or relationships because employers want to hire them. They call and say, "Wouldn't you like to work for us? Wouldn't you like to be vice president of marketing for our company?" Employers and others seek out those persons at the higher levels.

Correlation of Levels of Consciousness and Societal Problems

Level of Consciousness	Rate of Unemployment	Rate of Poverty	Happiness Rate "Life is OK"	Rate of Criminality
600+	0%	0.0%	100%	0.0%
500-600	0%	0.0%	98%	0.5%
400-500	2%	0.5%	70%	2.0%
300-400	7%	1.0%	50%	5.0%
200-300	8%	1.5%	40%	9.0%
100-200	50%	22.0%	15%	50.0%
50-100	75%	40.0%	2%	91.0%
<50	97%	65.0%	0%	98.0%

As we move up towards 540, inner joy, quiet, and inner knowingness begin to take place. Within this energy field, we connect with something that is rock-like and ever present. This is the beginning of the trans-figuration of consciousness, the beginning of an inner serenity, and the opening of compassion. At 560, there is Ecstasy—an exquisite, inner knowingness and trans-figuration of consciousness that lead to states of illumi-nation (sainthood is at level 570) as it gets closer to the 600s.

The energy field of Compassion is one that can be elected. We can make a commitment to lovingness as a way of being, so this requires no belief in God or any theological spiritual system. It is a commitment to lovingness that nurtures and supports life in all its expressions. It sees Divinity in all things as it moves up to an even higher level where it begins to see the perfection of all life.

Compassion is a way of knowing and looking into the hearts of others. Due to the release of endorphins at this level of revelation and transfiguration, there comes an awareness that the separation between oneself as an individual and another self as an individual starts to break down. It is almost like the beginning of a oneness of the heart, a knowingness—not a thinkingness, but a way of being.

The level of revelation in the high 500s then opens the way to transfiguration and compassion that lead to ecstasy and the states close to 600. These are states of bliss and the beginning of states of illumination and enlightenment. They are often accompanied by feelings of Light. For example, the room lit up when Bill Wilson of AA had his spiritual experience. He said the room was lit by the Infinite Presence (cal. 575). That was the beginning of the approach to the energy field of 600. The Radiance suffused out into the world as the worldwide, great Twelve-Step movement through which Alcoholics Anonymous has brought about the recovery of millions of people.

The energy field called Bliss, at 600, is very important in relation to addictions because the field transforms a person's life. The person who falls into *samadhi* (deep meditation) by accident goes into a transcendental state when they reach 600 or higher. Usually that person's life is changed thereafter. People who have near-death occurrences experience those fields over 600, including their own higher Self. Those levels go on up to Infinity and are the realm of various world-famous spiritual teachers.

The energy field of Krishna, the Christ, and the Buddha is 1,000, and the field progresses on up to Infinity. The people at those levels have such enormous power that we call them avatars. As an Avatar, in the three years of his ministry, Jesus Christ totally transformed the consciousness of all mankind for thousands of years to come. He transformed lives on the horizontal as well as the vertical planes, which are fields of enormous power.

The lower energy fields are like clouds covering the sun. As we remove the clouds, we experience the sun, which is always shining. In the chapter about addictions, we make a very precise point that it is not the removal of the clouds that causes the sun to shine, which is what the addicted person begins to think. People who get addicted to anything think that A causes B causes C. The removal of this left-brain type of thinking and linear causality is the whole purpose of spiritual work, which is the removal of the clouds so that one experiences the shining forth of the Self.

Energy fields are so powerful that they dominate our perception. They are really portals out of which we see the world. We often hear that this is really just a world of mirrors, and that all we experience is our own energy field reflected back upon us as perception and experiencing. We will look at perception, the view of the world, and the view of life as it comes out of these various energy fields.

As we said in the beginning, guilt (cal. 30)—that field of self-hatred and destructive energy—sees a world of sin and suffering. Therefore, that person walking down the street looks around and sees only suffering. When they open the newspaper, they also see the endless suffering of mankind.

The people who are in the energy field of hopelessness and despair (cal. 50) literally see a hopeless world. When they open the newspaper, they notice the hopeless condition of mankind, the endless wars, poverty, and crime. They actually experience perceptually, visually, auditorily—through all the senses—a world of hopelessness. The God of a hopeless world is dead.

The persons in a dispirited state of grief, regret, loss, and despondency come from the loss of the will to live. They walk down the street and see a sad world. This is actually experienced. We know that when we are in a sad state and walk down the street, we see the children and old people and think," How sad." We look at the buildings, see mankind's condition when we open the newspaper, and think how sad life is. Our own energy field is coloring everything else. It is as if we put on colored glasses and then experience everything as being colored by this energy field.

People dominated by fear perceive this as a world of danger, a threatening, frightening world that is in constant jeopardy. When walking down the street in that energy field, they see danger all around them. They see threats and muggers everywhere; they think there is a rapist under the bed; and when they open the newspaper, they see the frightening conditions of life with its jeopardy and danger. They live inside their house, lock their car in their own garage, and then lock the garage that is attached to the house, which is locked and inside a fence, which is also locked. (Fear can be transformed into a more positive expression as caution.)

Having more police really does not help because where will the police be when one's house is robbed? Of course, they are going to be at the other end of town, so that does not help. Trying to change the world does not assuage the fear energy because it is really coming from within one's own energy field.

The field above Fear is that of Desiringness (cal. 125), which represents a frustrating world of endless wantingness. The people dominated by this field are said to have a 'solar plexus' fixation, so they walk down the street seeing all the things they want. They see the car they want; the beauty they want; the status, positions, and buildings they want. They are frustrated because their endless desires and cravings and more and more millions of dollars do not bring happiness. The fact of having fifty million dollars does not help because the desiring and wanting for more power are insatiable.

The person in these energy fields cannot be satisfied and becomes frustrated and angry. The angry person then sees a competitive world, a world of conflict and war, of 'me against you'. This person looks out in the woods and thinks the tall trees are competing with the small trees for sunlight. This is the matrix of the political/social view of cultural perpetrator/victim. This concept is projected onto a field where no such thing as competition is even happening. This person lives in a world of endless possibility of war and conflict and sees everything as competition, not as cooperation.

People who are fixated at the level of Pride would see this as a world of social ranking, so when walking down the street, they would notice the Gucci shoes, name tags, clothing labels, status, the kind of car they would want, or the house they would like to live in. Everything is classified in terms of status, and they are preoccupied with a social-image positionality.

When one reaches the level of Truth and Courage (cal. 200), the world now appears to be a place of opportunity. It is an exciting, challenging place with opportunities for growth and expansion. That person opens the newspaper and sees the endless opportunities for man to grow, to meet those challenges and even go beyond them, and to learn in the process. That person is excited about life.

At the level of Neutral (cal. 250), life and the world is 'okay' due to one's being nonattached. Everything just becomes okay. One moves into an easygoing view of the world and begins to say, "Well, that's human nature. That's the way it is. It's serving some kind of ultimate purpose."

The people who move on up to the level of Willingness (cal. 310) experience the world as friendly. They walk down the street, see endless friendliness, and think the universe is friendly no matter what they have. The world is harmonious, benign, and supportive.

The persons who have moved on up to the level of Acceptance (cal. 350) really begin to experience the harmony of life and discover synchronicity and how everything just sort of flows together. They experience a world of cooperation because they are holding cooperation as their own energy field. This helps them to move up to Enthusiasm (cal. 390), and into Lovingness (cal. 500) and the experience of endless loving support and the endless presence of that loving energy in the universe.

The states of Illumination (cal. 600 and up) reveal the incredible beauty and perfection of life, the absolute perfection of Creation, the actual experience of the Divine essence and nature of all life, and the incredible beauty of all its expressions. It is not just aesthetic beauty, which is pleasing to the senses, but the intrinsic beauty of Creation. When one walks down an alley, which, to the eye of the unenlightened would look ugly, one experiences the incredible perfection and beauty of the aliveness of life and begins to see all life as unfolding. One does not see imperfection but process. That person sees the entire universe as the unfoldment of that perfection.

Correlated with each of these various energy fields are the concordant view and depictions of Divinity. For example, the person in apathy and hopelessness experiences God as uncaring or nonexistent. The person who is in this energy field sometimes says, "I believe in God, but I feel he wouldn't have anything to do with me because I am just a worm and worthless. I am so worthless that God just ignores me."

The person who lives in fear projects a punitive, frightening, terrifying image of God. The person who lives in frustration feels separated from God. That is the God who constantly withholds from them that which would allow them to be happy; therefore, God is non-supportive. The person in anger expects a retaliatory, punishing God, and because these things go together, this is the God who is really demonic, the God who really hates us and threatens to throw us into hell. He is the ultimate destroyer, the punisher, the God who is revengeful and jealous. It is an anthropomorphic depiction of a God who is fitfully jealous, 'hates sinners', and is given to emotional extremes of destructiveness.

When we get up to the level of Pride, there are two directions to take because of the arrogance of the inflated ego. The atheist is on one side and the zealot, bigot, and unbalanced extremist is on the other.

As we move up to Courage, which is the level of Truth, God can primarily be a question mark. For the first time, because we are now approaching the level of Truth, we can then have an open mind and say, "Actually, I really don't know about God. It's only hearsay that comes from all I've read and heard, and all that religion teaches. It is really other people's experiences in other times and places. On the witness stand, frankly, I would have to say I don't know anything about God," so there is the question mark. The spiritual seeker really begins at this level. The person says, "I, of my own self, would like to know what is the truth of this." The person is then free to move into the God of one's own inner experience and understanding.

At the level of Neutral, one begins to experience a world of okayness and God as freedom. One begins to discover that there is no punitive, hateful, negative God at all because one has moved out of those energy fields. Instead, there is a God of absolute, infinite freedom allowing one to expand, explore, become, and fulfill one's potential.

At the friendly level of Willingness, one begins to experience God as something that is perhaps helpful, promising, hopeful, and now positive. Down at the bottom of the Map, it was negative, but at this level, it opens to candidness and freedom and now begins to look optimistic. The person on this level experiences life as harmonious and realizes that God is all merciful. The person in lovingness then begins to experience the God of unconditional love and the ever presence of the love of God as the source of one's happiness and life.

As we move into joy and the awareness of beauty and perfection as the divine essence of all things within the oneness and unity of God, we move up to the top of the Map, with God as Beingness, Isness, Reality, Truth, and the Eternal Source of Existence.

There is now a context that will give a background and a way to see one's spiritual work and progress from a different perspective. We can see healing from a different viewpoint and also how to approach that great enigma called the ego. The energy fields of compassion are at 540 and up; the people here are forgiving and benign.

Students of spiritual work are often those who are perfecting the levels of the 400s, where they have acquired a dedicated learningness and knowledge about spiritual matters. They then put the principles into practice in order to reach the 500s. Some join A Course in Miracles or Twelve-Step groups and are concerned with perfecting the capacity to love. They move up to transcending what the world calls the ego and lose attraction to money, wealth, power, sexuality, and worldly success.

To repeat: the bottom of the Map is the world of havingness. It is what one has that counts, and status comes from that. At the bottom, people want to know what others have and rate them accordingly. In the middle of the Map is the world of doingness. Here, people want to know what others do in the world. What is their position and function? Havingness is no longer impressive.

At the lower levels, possessions are desired and esteemed, but with progress in the evolution of consciousness, they are no longer so impressive because everybody knows that if someone works seven days a week at two jobs, they can have all they want, so havingness no longer has status. As one moves towards the top of the Map, it is not what one has or does but what one is. People seek that person out now for what they have become, which is the truth they have owned about themselves. We seek out those people because of what they are and do not even care what they have. I have known people like that for many years and never actually knew what they did occupationally.

Utilizing this knowledge, we have an understanding of many things. The way to heal the small self is to reject taking a polarized, right/wrong position, which makes it our enemy, and instead view life with loving compassion and see the intrinsic innocence of the child. We first see the innocence of the child's consciousness and then the programming that is superimposed. It is because of the child's lovingness and trustingness that it is so programmable, and we begin to see the innocence even within those who seem most hateful. Out of compassion to see into the hearts of things, one finds the intrinsic innocence within the ego that then gets healed through that compassion and love. We can love our humanness and that of others, and instead of condemning it, we now say, "I see the seeming validity of that at that time."

For example, instead of being ashamed of anger and hatred, we say to ourselves, "Well, being angry was inevitable at that time," because a person who has never hated will not move up to Love since they have never cared that much about life. If one does not care enough about life to have gotten angry and actually hated, then they would be down at the level of Apathy.

When we look at our humanness from the viewpoint of forgiveness and compassion, we can then love it and hold it within our greatness. We look at our smallness like we look at the child and begin to heal it through understanding and compassion. When we do this, we are putting forth a very powerful energy field that is healing. When we look at ourselves from compassion and lovingness, we begin to heal. We also now know that what we forgive in others is forgiven within ourselves and disappears from our perception of the world.

Our perception of the world begins to shift, and we begin to experience a world that is totally different. It is like putting on a different pair of colored glasses— the world is not the same, and we can experience it in a totally different manner.

The purpose of the Map of Consciousness is to

create a context from which to view and experience the world and see that it presents whole new avenues that begin to open up automatically. Our intention, which is the capacity to heal ourselves as well as others, is now facilitated. It is the fulfillment of our own potential as we see ourselves move forward in our own realization of the truth.

From the Brain Function and Physiology chart (next page), we can see the profound influence of the levels of consciousness on brain physiology and concomitant neurotransmitters. Important is that from calibration level 200 and up, there is a release of endorphins, which is accompanied by feelings of pleasure and happiness. Below consciousness level 200, there is a predominance of adrenaline and animal-instinct survival responses. In contrast, consciousness levels over 200 are termed 'welfare emotions', which are benign and signify the emergence, and eventually the dominance, of spiritual energies.

BRAIN FUNCTION AND PHYSIOLOGY

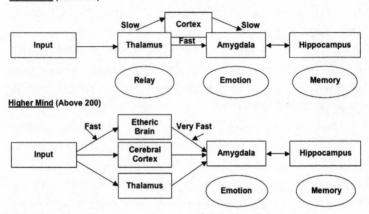

Below 200	**Above 200**
Left-brain dominance	Right-brain dominance
Linear	Non-linear
Stress—Adrenaline	Peace—Endorphins
Fight or flight	Positive emotion
Alarm—Resistance—Exhaustion (Selye—Cannon: Fight/Flight)	Support thymus
▼ Killer cells and immunity	▲ Killer cells
Thymus stress	▲ Immunity
Disrupt acupuncture meridian	Healing
Disease	Balanced acupuncture system
Negative muscle response	Positive muscle response
▼ Neurotransmitters—Serotonin
Track to emotions twice as fast as through prefrontal cortex to emotions	Track to emotions slower than from prefrontal and etheric cortexes
Pupil dilates	Pupil constricts

Importance:

Spiritual endeavor and intention change the brain function and the body's physiology and establish a specific area for spiritual information in the right-brain prefrontal cortex and its concordant etheric (energy) brain.

CHAPTER 2

Assisting Healing

In the previous chapter, we explored the utilization of knowledge that arises from studying the nature of consciousness itself and its applications to mankind's problems, especially in the areas of suffering. Now we will explore the origin of illness and the letting go of it.

This will not be about philosophies or theories; instead, it will concern what can be clinically verified in our own personal experiences—that which is true because we can validate it. This is the basis of clinical science—the ability to repeatedly duplicate and verify an observation within our own personal experience and apply it to our individual problems to see if it works. Essentially, we are expressing empirical pragmatism. We will believe what we can prove to be true through our own experience.

It is important to again explore the relationship between body, mind, and spirit. It is a useful model that is experientially real. What is the nature of spirit? Is that just a concept, a metaphysical extraction, a philosophical position, or is it a confirmable reality? What is the exact nature of body, mind, and spirit?

In order to facilitate healing, it is essential to understand the relationship between the body, the mind, and the spirit. It is important to know that the body has no capacity to experience itself; it is insentient. The arm cannot experience its armness nor can the leg experience its legness. Instead, we experience the sensations of the body and where it is in space. Sensations, curiously enough, also have no capacity to experience themselves. They have to be experienced in something that is greater, which is mind. The experience of the sensations and what they report about the body is actually experienced within the mind.

As surprising as it may seem, the mind cannot experience itself. A thought cannot experience its own thoughtness; a feeling cannot experience its own feelingness; memory cannot experience its own memoryness. They all have to be experienced in something greater than the mind. The principle is that each thing is experienced from an energy field that is less restricted and less limited; each is always experienced in something that is greater. Therefore, mind is experienced because of the energy field of consciousness itself. Consciousness is formless, infinite, and analogous to a movie screen upon which we experience the movement of the movie. It is because of consciousness that we experience what is in mind. That is the basis of anesthesia in that when we remove consciousness, there is no experience of either the mind or the body.

Consciousness itself is experienced in the infinite energy field called awareness. Because of awareness, we know what is going on in consciousness. Because of consciousness, we know what is going on in mind. Because of mind, we know what the senses are reporting about the body. Thus, we can see that what we really are is several levels removed from the body, making it rather clear that we are not the body. We are that which is aware within that infinite field of consciousness. This is very important to realize, and in meditation, it is relatively simple to verify the truth that one is that which is aware of all these levels of reality.

We will focus on the actual techniques that assist healing, including how they occur and how to apply them. We will also focus on the basic principles, such as how the source of illness is often unconscious guilt plus a specific belief system that is aggravated by suppressed emotions. I will describe how I used these techniques and understandings to heal myself of more than twenty chronic, intractable illnesses that had been totally refractory, or resistant, to traditional medical treatment.

With a step-by-step approach, we will see how illness is also a result of programming via the collective consciousness (and how not to buy into it), and how it comes about as a result of belief systems. We will learn that one can recover from illnesses within the parameters of karmic inheritance. There is no order of difficulty, no matter how severe the illness may sound. We will learn how to energize the self-healer that is present via Nature in all of us, and we will look at the phenomenon of multiple personalities, which demonstrates the truth of much of the following information.

Science and psychiatry are studying the clinical condition of multiple personalities with increasing interest because it explains so many different phenomena. In this condition, more than one personality expresses itself through the body. Clinically, one personality may have multiple illnesses, such as asthma, allergies, gout, and many others, but when that personality leaves and the other personality comes in, the second one may well have none of those illnesses whatsoever. That personality says, "I don't believe in any of those things. I am not subject to them." As a result, we will look at the power of the mind over body.

A basic principle of recovery is that we are subject to what we hold in mind, which may, however, be unconscious (out of awareness). We will refer to the Map of Consciousness to make this understandable rather than sound mystical or puzzling in our expressions. It is helpful to remember that the direction of the energy fields indicates whether it is a negative field with a destructive influence or a positive field. Knowing this will enable us to feel confident that we are operating from something that is reasonable, confirmable, and understandable.

Sharing my personal experiences demonstrates the basic truths being presented here. You already know these things intuitively, but in making them conscious, you can use them as therapeutic tools, such as how to prevent being programmed by a negative belief system, or how not to buy into a thought system. The mind is so powerful that what it believes tends to manifest.

An interesting study appeared in the January 1987 issue of *Brain-Mind Bulletin* entitled "Expectancies: What You See Is What They Give You." Research by Princeton University showed that self-fulfilling prophecy is just that, and what we actively believe tends to manifest in our behavior and in that of others. This is what they call a "creative social reality," a serious issue that affects everything from stock prices to the arms race, not to mention everyday interactions (and, additionally, the details of one's personal health).

We will proceed from the premise that all phenomena are experienced in consciousness and address the level of consciousness itself and its expression in mind.

We will go to the level of cause instead of the level of effect. The body is at the effect of what is held in mind. If we want to know what we are holding in mind, all we have to do is look at what is going on in the body and observe its behavior, which tells us what we believe. If we look back into our memory, we often will not be able to recall that we had any such belief system, or that we thought it applied to us. The fact that it is in our life tells us that it must have been there somewhere in the personal or collective unconscious.

The most common example of this occurs in people who are allergic and say, "Well, I didn't have any belief in allergies. I didn't bring this into my life consciously." Yet, if we go back into their childhoods, almost invariably we find that the belief system and allergies occurred very early in life, usually at ages two or three. The little child picks up a remark by someone in the family such as, "Allergies run in our family." The minute the child's mind hears this, buys it, and, of course, believes it, it becomes an operative program.

A lot of the phenomena we see expressing in the body of the adult were picked up very early in life from a chance remark heard on television, or something misunderstood in a book, or a remark that a teacher made. These things constitute suggestive programming and common belief systems and become conscious when we begin to work on them.

We are subject to what we hold in mind, so what does that mean? What is the nature of illness itself? We see, first of all, it is that of pain and suffering. Consequently, it is obvious and merely common sense that illness is an expression of pain and suffering. When we look at the Map of Consciousness, pain and suffering are located at the lower energy levels, with the energy field in a negative direction, meaning that it has an adverse effect on our life. Then we have to look into the nature of guilt, the unconscious guilt, and how it expresses itself.

The thought patterns in the mind are belief systems. Guilt stems from judgmentalism and negative opinions. Negative feelings tend to go together, so all the negative feelings then contribute to illness, including pride, anger, desire, fear, grief, apathy, and guilt. We know that when we test a person's muscle strength, if they hold anything in mind below the energy level of Courage, such as prideful or angry thoughts, wantingness or cravingness, a fearful thought, some grief, apathy, or a guilty thought, the muscle goes weak. Other feelings, such as regret, loss, hopelessness, despair, self-hatred, worry, anxiety, grievances, and any kind of arrogance or contempt also result in a person's instantly going weak with muscle-strength testing. (The pupils also dilate.)

The muscle weakness and pupil dilation represent desynchronization of the cerebral hemispheres and an instant weakening of the body's energy field. It also indicates something that is deleterious to life. Through this method, we can prove to anyone that any negative thought or feeling desynchronizes the body's acupuncture energy system, which is more responsive than the central nervous system and far more rapid than the autonomic sympathetic nervous system.

The body's acupuncture energy system, via the twelve main meridians of the body, instantly responds to anything that is negative because all the energy fields below the level of Courage at 200 represent that which is not the truth. That then brings in the whole energy field and thought system of being a victim. As a sick person, we view ourself as a victim of the disease. Therefore, it is important to realize that there is the illness, and there is the person who has the illness. We then understand that the person who has that illness needs to change in order for it to disappear. We are going to learn about recovering from a specific illness, including how to handle the actual event on the physical, psychological, emotional, and mental levels, and how we must change as a being so that healing becomes automatic.

The Map of Consciousness shows that all the negative emotions facilitate illness, and all the positive emotions tend to cure illness. Once we get above the level of Courage, a level that we cross by telling the truth about things, we become detached, which opens a space for us to become a willing, accepting, and loving person. On the calibrated scale, Love occurs at 500 and Healing appears at 540. What kind of lovingness brings about an almost automatic healing within the body? It is unconditional love, that which is nonjudgmental, forgiving, and aligned with understanding and compassion. Love sees, nurtures and supports all of life and honors its sacredness, and of itself creates a healing energy field that calibrates at 540.

How do we become the kind of person in whom healing begins to occur automatically because of the level and general nature of our consciousness? At the same time, how do we facilitate the healing of a specific illness?

In viewing the specifics of an illness, we will talk about certain mechanics of consciousness and how to use some of the techniques presented here and in later chapters. We have to begin by letting go of resisting the sensations that we are experiencing and stop labeling them. For example, we cannot experience a 'duodenal ulcer' or 'asthma'. They are labels, mental constructs, elaborate programs, and belief systems. We cannot experience 'asthma', but what do we experience? This is where the technique of radical truth comes up.

We go into the inner experience of the exact sensations and let go of resisting them. In effect, we will eventually disappear them through aligning with them by welcoming the inner experiences of the sensations. At the same time, within mind we cancel any labels. We stop calling it an 'ulcer' and instead go into the inner sensation of it. The inner sensation may be a pressure or a burning. Even the words 'burning' and 'pressure' are labels and names. We cancel those and again go into the core, the absolute essential, of what we are physically experiencing, and then let go of resisting that experience.

The actual healing of the physicality of the illness is letting go of resisting the inner physical experience of it without any mental label. At the same time, in fact, we begin to cancel the mental label and replace it with the truth. We cancel by affirming, "I no longer believe in that. I am an infinite being, and I am not subject to that. I am only subject to what I hold in mind."

What does it mean to be "an infinite being and not subject to that"? It means we are only limited by our belief systems, and if we let them go, what takes their place? If form is removed from consciousness, what is left? The formless is left, and the inner experience of it is infinite, without boundaries, without beginning or end. The formless is the essential nature of consciousness itself and is unlimited. If we place a limitation or introject form, then we subject ourself to what we are holding in mind. To replace it, we consciously cancel it by saying, "I cancel any belief in duodenal ulcers," or asthma, or whatever the illness might be. We then say, "I'm subject only to that which I hold in mind. I am an infinite being, and in truth, I am not subject to that. And that is a fact."

When we muscle test that statement, we find it to be true. If we test a person and they say, "Cancel. I am not subject to that. I am an infinite being and subject only to what I hold in mind," we will see that they instantly go strong, indicating that this is a statement of the truth. Consequently, when we replace that which is false with that which is true, healing occurs.

What is the effect on our energy field in consciousness? Falsity by its nature puts us below the level of 200 and throws us into a negative energy field, which, in and of itself, brings about illness. The minute we tell the truth, the energy field at the level of Courage (meaning to tell the truth that we are an 'infinite being and subject only to what is held in mind') instantly puts us above the line at level 200).

The willingness to accept this truth lifts us up to a position to choose appreciation of the body instead of the 'make wrong' of the body; the lovingness of our life instead of the 'make wrong' of our life; the lovingness of the being that we are instead of the criticism of it.

We find that we have to let go of criticism, 'attack' thoughts, critical thoughts, and judgmental thoughts. We have to let go of putting ourselves in the position of being right and making other people wrong because the level of 'right and wrong' is at the energy level of about 180, which is that of negative thought forms. In other words, it has a deleterious effect on our health and life energy. If we are willing to let go of our illness, then we have to be willing to let go of the attitude that brought about the illness because disease is an expression of one's attitude and habitual way of looking at things.

The specifics of healing a particular illness consist of (1) letting go of resisting the sensory experience of it, (2) no longer putting names or labels on it, and (3) using no words at all. Welcome experiencing what you are experiencing in a very radical way and at the same time (4) cancel the thought form and belief system, and (5) choose the energy field of Love, which heals.

If we look at the basic physics of the energies involved, we can see why fear at calibration level 100 is overpowered by Love at 500 because these are exponential powers. Therefore, the power of Love is represented by 10^{500}, whereas Fear is only 10^{100}, a very big difference.

To put oneself in an energy field of 540 is to automatically heal oneself. A loving thought then heals, and a negative thought creates illness. Choosing to become a loving person results in the release of endorphins by the brain, which has a profound effect on the body's health and happiness (see Brain Physiology Chart, pg. 42). Happiness arises from the willingness to let go of that which is negative and to allow love to replace it in consciousness because the essential nature of consciousness, unless it has been impaired, is lovingness. We see this in the young child who is only innocence, and lovingness is the expression of the essence of human nature. It is as if the child has not yet been programmed to go into fear, doubt, or limitation.

It is essential to capture that essential expression of lovingness in order to help any illness within us, as well as to let go of the negativity of the belief system. How do we pick up the negative belief systems? We pick them up through television and well-intentioned people. Their intention is to prevent these illnesses in us by educating us about them. Instead, we find that the mind is now programmed to accept a specific belief system. Unconscious guilt then comes up and utilizes that belief system, which causes an impairment of energy flowing through the energy fields that run down through the twelve meridians of the acupuncture energy system.

For example, every time someone goes below level 200 (Courage), we find upon testing them that their energy system is imbalanced. Characteristically, most people will 'blow out' one particular acupuncture meridian rather than another. For example, every time they have negative thoughts or feelings consequent to a negative belief system, they may impair the heart meridian. As the years go by, every time they have a resentment, go into self-pity, or criticize someone else, it disrupts the energy and flows down the heart meridian. This depletes the life energy of the heart, and the continual repetition begins to alter its physiology in very delicate ways. It begins to express itself through irregularities in the autonomic nervous system, which operates in the functioning of the body organs.

As a result, there begins an impairment of the physiology of the heart itself, including the lining of the arteries. As the years go by, the habitual disruption of the heart meridian brings impairment on the physical level, which is an expression of what has been held in mind. That is the basic premise—the body expresses what is held in mind, not vice versa. The body expresses a person's habitual way of thinking.

The mechanics of negativity short-circuit the acupuncture system and the autonomic nervous system. This in turn alters and impairs the sensitive electrical and chemical processes that are going on in the cells, resulting in pathological changes within the anatomy and dysfunction that results in a coronary attack, heart disease, or heart failure. The heart failure comes about partly as a result of years of negative mental attitudes. The mind would like to blame it on cholesterol, stress, one's lifestyle, genetics, what goes on in the family, and so on. These are all merely explanations, excuses, and rationalizations to try to make intelligible that which is not clearly defined.

When looking at the exact mechanics, we see that what we hold in mind begins to manifest on the physical plane because it is the mind that has the power. Even a relatively neutral thought can have major consequences. For example, one has the thought, "I think I will go to Hawaii." That one thought now energizes one's finances and determines what one is going to do over the next six months to get ready for the trip. The thought held in mind now determines what one does with their money, their entire behavior, the packing, and moving their body thousands of miles through the air. That one thought influences the next six months of one's life.

We can see how powerful the mind is, and one of the difficulties to overcome in self-healing is the willingness to accept the great power of the mind. We cannot let a negative thought go unchallenged. One cannot say, "I have diabetes" and let that go unchallenged. That is a belief system so powerful that just believing "I have diabetes" is sufficient to potentiate the disease. Instead, one has to cancel it and say, "I am a person who once thought that, but I am only subject to what I hold in mind. I am an infinite being, and I am not subject to that." One releases any symptoms and cancels them. One replaces them with the truth, and in doing that, one moves above the line in the specifics of a given illness. Later, when I give an account of how I used this system to get rid of many illnesses within myself, perhaps these principles will become more apparent.

Because I had such a list of illnesses, I had to write them all down in order to remember them because half of them have been forgotten even though all of them lasted for many, many years. For example, I had a duodenal ulcer that was intractable. I was on all the traditional medicinal treatments and had psychoanalysis and a whole variety of things that began in medical school. Twenty years later, I still had the ulcer, and not only that, it was a different kind of ulcer that was making holes in other parts of my duodenum. It was threatening to perforate and hemorrhage, and it was creating recurrent attacks of pancreatitis. I also had colitis along with hemorrhage diverticulitis. In fact, the diverticulitis was so bad that I landed in the hospital several times and had to have transfusions. I almost hemorrhaged to death with it.

In addition, I had migraine headaches that were intractable. Psychoanalysis had helped to some degree, and I had seen neurologists and famous world experts, but there was really no help for the migraines, which were ostensibly associated with many allergies. I was also sensitive to inhalants in the atmosphere. I could not walk into a place that had been exterminated within the previous couple of weeks because I could detect one part in one million in the spray and would react with a migraine headache.

In addition, I also had Raynaud's disease, which was impairing the blood flow to my extremities, and I had threatening insipient gangrene of the fingertips, circulatory impairment of the hands and feet, and was cold all the time. On top of all that, I had gout and a high uric acid level. Of course, I was on a diet for that. I had gouty arthritis and carried a cane and medication in the back of my car. Can you imagine carrying a cane in the back of your car because when gout comes on, it happens very suddenly with pain that is very paralyzing? That cane was in my car for many years.

At the same time, I had severe hypoglycemia. I could not eat sugar, sweets, or starches. So, in addition to all the allergies, the ulcer, diverticulitis, other gastrointestinal problems, pancreatitis, and occasional gallbladder attacks, there were actually very few things I could eat. When I occasionally went to a restaurant, the only thing I could safely eat was lettuce in a salad. I could not eat the tomatoes because the seeds might aggravate the diverticulitis, which had required hospitalization and blood transfusions in the past. I was also fifty pounds overweight. (I will later describe how I handled that problem.)

From one end to the other, things were wrong with the gastrointestinal tract; the circulatory system; the digestive system; the hormonal balance; the blood chemistries, including elevated blood cholesterol and uric acid levels; and migraine headaches. All these things indicated stress and pressure within the central nervous system and impairment of the autonomic nervous system. Additionally, I had a pilonidal cystic tumor, which normally would require surgery, but it slowly disappeared spontaneously.

Later, I went into severe heart failure from undiagnosed Grave's disease (hyperthyroidism) for which surgery or radiation was prescribed, but I refused. Chest x-rays revealed a tumor in the apex of the right lung. The lung was biopsied, resulting in its collapse and pneumothorax (the collection of air or gas in the space surrounding the lungs). The biopsy revealed that the lesion was a form of aviary (bird) tuberculosis (noncommunicable to humans). I refused to take the recommended $10,000-per-month's worth of five antibiotics, which had a low cure rate anyway. The lung lesion slowly disappeared with no physical treatment. The heart failure cleared up, as did the pneumothorax. The thyroid function eventually returned to normal without surgery or radiation. In addition to the above, the left thumb was amputated while I was doing carpentry work and was repaired in surgery without anesthesia, as was a recurrent right inguinal hernia, also without anesthesia. The chronic recurrent, intractable duodenal ulcers disappeared after three acupuncture treatments.

All the above illnesses and surgeries were processed and handled as described by letting go of resisting in every instant, canceling the belief systems, and totally surrendering to Divine Will. All healing was accomplished without narcotics or anesthesia. The whole series of illnesses was consequent to karmic proclivities that were surfaced by intense inner spiritual work, which speeded up their emergence initially but later facilitated their seemingly miraculous healing and disappearance.

Mental systems had to be questioned to find out what was going on because it was obvious that a person with so many illnesses could hardly be said to be free of conflict. I began to study my perfectionism and see how this tendency, which allowed me to forgive others but did not allow me to forgive myself, was creating an intolerance of my own humanness. As you can see, to be intolerant and condemn and attack all these things within oneself produces unconscious guilt about one's own human limitations.

The origin of this mental proclivity began in childhood in the form of moral scrupulosity and fear of sin. I had to move to a willingness to accept, love, and forgive my own humanness, acknowledge that it was only human to have imperfect feelings, and to let go of attacking myself for being human. Therefore, I had to look into the essence of seeing what is the inner core and essence of one's humanness. This took me to the awareness of the intrinsic innocence within consciousness itself. I then had to look at the nature of consciousness. How does the child, in its innocence and lack of negativity, end up with so many programs within the mind to create all these illnesses?

We can find the answer when we look at the nature of innocence and track what happens to it in the child. The child's innocence might also be compared to the hardware of a computer. The hardware is innocent, and it is the software that goes through the hardware, creating the output. However, the hardware is not affected by the software itself. We look at the child and see the innocence of its consciousness. How does all the negative programming come in to the innocent child? It comes in because of innocence; the child believes anything it is told.

It is out of its lovingness and trust of its parents, its teachers, and the world of television, commercials, and society that the child becomes programmed. The innocence of the child becomes progressively less apparent because it is now displaying all the programs it has picked up out of that primary innocence. It starts to believe the prejudices of its parents and playmates, such as little sly remarks like, "We don't play with certain kinds of people." What buys that negative program? It is the innocence of the child, which remains within our consciousness throughout our life. It is always going on. It is out of that innocence that we buy into error, but the inner innocence itself is unsullied. We have to go back into the recognition of that inner innocence in order to forgive ourselves as well as others.

That inner innocence allows us to learn anything new. The innocence of the child never changes; in fact, it is the innocence of the child within you that is reading these words this very second. It never changes; it is that same trusting, believing, and 'hoping to hear the truth and be open to it' innocence that continues. Even if you do not believe what you are reading now, it is because some opposite program within your mind says, "Don't trust." And it was your innocence that bought the program of "Don't trust anybody."

Even the mistrusting person is doing so out of trust. They are trusting the truth of that statement. Maybe one day their father said, "Don't trust anybody out there," and it was their innocence that bought the distrust. Yet the innocence itself is unsullied and untouched because it never changes. It is the inherent nature of consciousness itself. It is the hardware of the computer, and no matter how many negative thoughts were heard, the programs that are played through the mind do not affect the hardware, leaving it untouched, unsullied, pristine, and pure. That inner pristine purity is still within all of us.

That bring us to compassion because we now see how we picked up programs as we grew up in youth or adolescence. For example, we do not want to admit that we have negative thoughts, feelings, or even fear, or that we have desire or feelings of loss, regret, or hopelessness. These are not acceptable. The self-hatred and guilt then accumulate from the constant rejection of our own humanness. As a result, we have to move to a better, healing way of being with ourself. It is easy to do by merely choosing to be compassionate and forgiving.

The decision came to me to be that way about myself, the same as I was about others, because if I am that way about myself, then automatically I am that way about others. That which I forgive in others I automatically forgive in myself because all I am seeing out there is myself projected into the world.

With the undoing of all this negativity and the replacement of the low negative energies by a positive energy, we begin to experience the world, ourselves, and our relationship to life in a different way. We begin to experience an inner joyfulness as a result of our willingness to let go of condemning ourself and others. This then becomes a habit and the way we are in the world. Intention to be a source of healing to ourself and others sets up a context.

What does context mean? Intention sets up context. Our intention to be this kind of person then sets up the whole energy of our consciousness and aligns it so that we begin to see things that way. In other words, there is an actual alteration of perception. We literally begin to see the world through forgiving, healing, and compassionate eyes. We are not talking about sympathy, which is in the lower energy fields; we are talking about a lovingness as an inner decision to be that kind of human being towards ourself and others. There is the willingness to let go of being critical, along with our moralizing 'right and wrong' attitude that occurs when we polarize ourselves with others by saying, "My position is right and your position is wrong."

Because the body expresses what the mind believes, this decision then begins to affect the body. We can track down the mechanics of that with muscle testing. When we hold a loving thought in mind or picture somebody in a loving way, our arm is strong when someone tests its resistance. When we hold an unloving thought in mind, the arm will instantly go weak because the body is immediately reflecting what the mind believes.

As we move into the decision to be forgiving and compassionate, to be that which supports and nurtures life instead of condemning it or moralistically putting it down and getting into a 'make wrong' scenario, and as we become willing to let go of the 'make wrong', we let go of attacking ourself for being ill. Some people who are involved in spiritual work or metaphysical studies will compound the problem by making themselves wrong because they have a physical illness. It is helpful to have the willingness to accept whatever is being expressed on the physical level, to look within our own consciousness to see what is being brought to our attention, and to see that whatever is occurring in our life is happening in order to come up to be healed.

Instead of being ashamed that we are a spiritual seeker with a physical illness, we instead become thankful and say, "Aha! Something is coming up to be healed." We want that capacity to bring up the various things to be healed; thus, it is a sign of progress, not of falling back. We can be happy that we have a chance to heal these things that, paradoxically, are actually brought up by major or rapid spiritual progress (i.e., karma). Most of the great mystics of history had records of many physical illnesses (e.g., see "Mystics" in *Encyclopaedia Britannica*).

An illness is merely our consciousness calling attention to something that needs to be looked at. There is something about which we are feeling guilty, fearful, or other negative emotion. There is a belief system we are holding that has to be let go of and cancelled. There is something that has to be forgiven, and something within us that has to be loved, so we thank whatever it is for bringing it to our awareness. We say, "Thank you, ulcer. I see. You forced me to look at the way in which I was condemning myself and not loving myself. Thank you, hypoglycemia, for showing me how much I have been living in fear." We thank all our illnesses because they have brought us to that willingness and acceptance to move into the field of lovingness and the joy of realizing now, out of compassion, that this is how the body brings about self-healing.

The pain serves a purpose, and we now hold it in a different way. We are going to make lemonade out of lemons. Instead of going into self-pity or resentment about an illness, instead of 'poor me' or being a victim, we say, "What is that trying to tell me? What is it that I'm supposed to learn?" We get interested in learning about the nature of consciousness and finding out what is underlying the illness so we can heal it through a greater understanding.

The first tools we need are willingness and an open mind—the willingness to say that the mind is looking at something which it is being asked to view so it can be healed. The healing of the body comes about with the healing of the mind. All the physical illnesses, which I eventually let go of, finally healed of their own nature as a result of healing the thought forms in mind. All the healings resulted from the willingness to let go of the condemnation of self and others, to let go of criticalness, self-pity, resentment, and all the negative energies at the levels below 200, including regret, worry, anxiety, grievances, self-contempt, and self hatred. It was the letting go of those things that shifted the energy field to one that brought about the healing. I kept working with it, canceling the belief systems of hypoglycemia and gout. As each belief system would come up, I would cancel it and say, "I no longer believe in that. I am no longer subject to that. It is the result of a belief system, and I have the power to cancel it." Thus, we begin to own that we have the power to refuse, reject, and deny. "I have the power to refuse that. I don't have to buy into that."

Because these belief systems are so prevalent in our culture, we naïvely think that they must have a certain reality or else everybody would not believe them. The only reality they have is on the level of a thought form. The fact that there is agreement about a certain thought form does not give it a reality. It only means that there is an agreement about it. Therefore, I can refuse to buy into the collective belief systems about all these various diseases, and I watch as those programs come in. I refuse to believe in all the well-intentioned educational programs about all these diseases—hypoglycemia, gout, heart disease, cholesterol, etc. As each illness is devised, we become subject to it. We are subject to what we believe in mind.

If we think eating eggs is going to raise our cholesterol, and we think raising our cholesterol is going to give us heart trouble, then eating eggs does raise our cholesterol, and the cholesterol does give us heart trouble because of the power of the mind. Mind is so powerful that it creates the thought form which manifests on the physical plane, thus becoming a physical reality.

We can see that self-healing then really depends on the reversal of the usual belief systems of causality. What we hold in mind manifests on the physical level; it is not the other way around. Eating the cholesterol did not give us the heart problem; it was the belief that eating a lot of cholesterol gives us heart trouble. That is a very critical point to grasp. The belief system elucidates the entire disease picture.

If we don't believe it, the illnesses disappear from the body. At the same time, we are letting go of the sources of unconscious guilt and stopping the reinforcement of the illnesses that comes from labeling and propagating them, thereby bringing about a fulfillment of our own self-prophecies and watchfulness.

We cannot allow the mind to come up with a belief system without challenging it. If the mind unconsciously has been working against us, and we have been unaware of how much power it has, we can turn it around and use that power on our own behalf. The same power that undid us can now work for us when we consciously utilize the power of mind. Now, when the thought comes up, "I have hypoglycemia," I stop it, I cancel it, and I say the truth: "I am no longer subject to that. I am an innocent being. I am no longer subject to that."

Hypoglycemia is a good example because it took me a considerable amount of time to undo that one. After all, I had given lectures about it for many years. It was operative clinically within me as an actual physical reality. I did a lot of work on nutrition, especially on its relationship to addiction, and to alcoholism in particular. It was a very important issue. I was a firm believer in it when I came to the understanding and realization that my firm belief in it was then operating within my body, which was expressing my mind's belief in hypoglycemia. Therefore, I had to keep canceling it repeatedly and stating the truth about it. Eventually, the condition of severe hypoglycemia disappeared, and the abnormal blood sugars corrected themselves. After many years with this disease, I finally let go of the belief system of hypoglycemia and recovered from it. It took about two years of using the technique.

The various illnesses disappeared within differing periods of time. Some of them disappeared within a matter of days; some even disappeared within an hour. Others took months, and the hypoglycemia took the longest, other than a blocked Eustachian tube that took two years. (I forgot to include that on my list of illnesses.) I never gained weight and no longer had any hypoglycemic symptoms; it just no longer existed in my life.

There is the principle of watchfulness. Because the mind is so powerful, we cannot let it get away with a negative belief system even once. Every time the thought, "I'm allergic" comes up, it has to be instantly challenged and cancelled. One powerful thought, as you can see, is sufficient to create it on the physical plane, so we cannot be sloppy about this work. We have to watch it carefully within ourself.

There is really no order of difficulty in the healing of these various illnesses. This means that what the world considers to be a severe disease is just as easy to let go of as a minor illness.

Among friends, co-workers, acquaintances, patients, and other people I have worked with, there is a group of people who have recovered from many serious illnesses totally and completely. They were given up as hopeless, as almost dead, and yet those people who have become my friends are extremely alive and well, with no traces of their illnesses at all. It does not make any difference because the truth is the truth, and that which is false is false. It does not depend on the form of falsehood; all that is false is false, just as all that is true is true. If your mind can create it, then your mind can cancel it. We thereby begin to use the power of the mind on our own behalf.

The process of self-healing is handled on the level of the specific by letting go of our resistance to experiencing it and then canceling the thought forms. The healing is going on in general, more powerful ways due to our willingness to let go of all criticism and attack, along with beginning to love the humanness in ourself and others, and the reawakening of our awareness of its innocence.

What about the third level, that of traditional medical treatment? What part does it play in this kind of self-healing? Traditional medical treatments now surprisingly become very effective. As we let go of our guiltiness, which came about through our lack of compassion for our own humanness, medical measures that were once fruitless now begin to be effective. In other words, during all the illnesses I had, such as migraine headaches, ulcers, and diverticulitis, I received traditional medical treatment for twenty years or more. I was on the diets, medications, antispasmodics, and antacids, and I did all the traditional medical things, but they were not working; however, they perhaps kept things from getting worse. After all, I did not have my stomach or colon removed, so the treatments were working, but they were working against all the negative programming going on within the mind.

When we start to let go of all the negative programs, all the previously relatively ineffective medical treatments now become effective. In my case, the antispasmodic that once barely kept the symptoms under control then totally relieved the symptoms. A healing came about. The antispasmodic, the antacids, and the diet that was considered necessary (in addition to acupuncture treatments) then brought about a healing of the ulcer; the medications were very powerfully effective. The medications for relieving the allergies then worked wondrously well. We found that the need for the medication dwindled off. The need for all these ameliorative measures finally disappeared, and I resumed eating a normal diet. You might imagine the kind of diet I had had to live on, with an elevated cholesterol level, hypoglycemia, diverticulitis, an active ulcer, migraine, and most of all, the allergies.

I remember walking into a restaurant and looking at the menu. The only thing I could eat was the salad and the spinach because the seeds in the other foods would aggravate the diverticulitis, and the acids would aggravate the ulcer. I could not eat tomatoes or anything of that nature, and of course, nothing containing sugar. I could not eat pasta, any of the bakery offerings, the desserts, or the meats; I had to avoid them because of the elevated uric acid levels of gout. Frankly, there were very few things left on this planet for me to eat.

As those things relieved themselves, however, I then found that diet was also a belief system. That is the downside of holistic health—the belief system that all these things are injurious to us. They are injurious to us because we are holding in mind that they are. No such thing exists in the world of the 'real'. As a result, I am not on a low-sugar, low-cholesterol, low-fat diet. My cholesterol and blood sugar are normal. I am on a regular diet and never get a gout attack. All those things turned out to be corollary to the belief systems.

If we have a belief system about gout, then we will have all that goes with it, including the beliefs about the various meats that supposedly bring it on, such as pickled herring, which I love (and now eat almost daily). I used to have gout so severely that if I ate just a small amount of liver pâté on a cracker, it would bring on a gout attack.

I always tell the story of how one day I cooked a frying pan full of liver and kidneys for my kitty, thinking she would love them. Instead she stuck her nose up and would not eat them. There was a big pan of them, and they smelled delicious as they were cooking with onions and a little bit of bacon. I even put a little catnip in some of it, but Kitty just was not interested. All of a sudden, I saw that my whole dietary limitation was just a crazy belief system that I was holding in mind, and I said, "I am an infinite being. I am not subject to this. I mean this is absurd." So I sat down and ate almost the whole pan of kidney and liver, and needless to say, I did not have a gout attack nor have I ever had one since. I just canceled it as a belief system. It was a joke—a sad joke, but still a joke. We are subject only to what we hold in mind-consciously or unconsciously.

When we re-own the source of our power and stop

giving it away to the world, we find that the cause of gout is not in kidneys and liver; it is not in stress; it is not in uric acid levels or purine metabolism. It has to do with what we hold in mind. When we re-own and stop denying the power of our own mind, we begin to realize that we are the source of either health or illness. What do I mean when I say, "I am the source?" I mean my consciousness, my infinite being.

Let us now consider the energy fields that explain how this works. What are the intrinsic physics, the energy fields, and the levels? Instead of owning ourselves at a level below the level of Truth at 200 and putting power that is a lie out into the world, we begin to re-own the truth about ourselves. Our willingness to look into this brings about the experience and realization of the truth of it. That is the experiential purity of what we are discussing. We, ourselves, can reduplicate the truth of this through our own experimentation. We are our own individual self.

As we re-own ourselves as the source and move up in the levels of consciousness, we begin to realize that we are subject to anything that we hold in mind, and that the belief systems and thought forms we bought into have been the source or 'cause' of what we have been experiencing. The world has no power to create any such thing. Does a piece of kidney have power in it? Of course not. Do our minds have the power to create illnesses? Yes, indeed.

Now we will begin to undo the syndrome of the 'bubble' person. What happens to the bubble person? Its innocent, childlike mind enthusiastically buys the whole idea of holistic health and nutrition, for example.

It begins to read all the literature. Well, let me tell you that if we continue to read that literature long enough, we will find that everything in our world, everything in our experience, everything in our environment, and everything in this universe will kill us. That is the message we will get. Magnesium will kill us; calcium will kill us. The energy given off by rugs, paint, and everything in the air will kill us. If we walk by somebody who is smoking a cigarette—"Aha! I'm going to get lung cancer." We unwittingly buy into all these powerfully negative thought systems. However, we can begin to cancel them, one by one. I did it.

I had a friend who said eggs would kill me. Goodbye, eggs. Cholesterol will kill me. Good-bye, cholesterol. Water will kill me; dairy products will kill me; meat will kill me. Well, eat fruit. Okay. And fruit is full of pesticides. Holy smokes! I was into fruit. Fruit did not last long at all because the minute I got the pesticide story, goodbye, fruit. Then I went to vegetables. Oh, oh! Vegetables are full of it, too. They spray all those fields in California, and fish contains mercury. What is left to eat?

We become increasingly paranoid. We do not become increasingly healthy; we become increasingly paranoid, and all my 'brown-bag' friends are dead! Brown-bag friends—those are people who used to belong to one of the medical societies that really got going on this. A brown-bag person is one who has bought into so much of this in the world that now they can eat only one or two kinds of natural organic rice or grains. There are only a few things left on the planet that they can safely eat, and they carry them around in a brown bag.

A bubble person goes to a banquet event where everybody is eating food full of what he considers to be nothing but poison. They are "killing themselves with the steak and the pesticides on the peas, fruit, and lettuce." While, in his view, they are killing themselves, he eats out of his brown bag. He sits in the back corner at a table filled with brown-bag people. (This was an actual scene at a big banquet.) He fasts a lot, does a lot of running and other 'healthy' things, and, of course, he is dead now. Why is he dead, this man who ran every day and lived this health? He died because he became a bubble person with the paranoid view of the world that began to close in on him. He could not breathe the air with trust. He could not even enjoy the carpets because they were probably giving off something to which he was allergic, such as fiber particles that caused him to choke. Other things, such as the fumes emanating from the paints or insulation, or smoke particles from a cigarette that were going to give him cancer, caused his life to become smaller and smaller.

What happens in this type of situation is the progressive denial of the truth about ourselves, along with progressively giving away the power of our being to the power of causality in the world, which is actually powerless. This is the reversal of truth. By progressively reversing the truth, we become increasingly vulnerable and a victim. We end up with the total paranoia of the bubble person with 'environmental allergies' who can live only within a protective bubble of purified air.

All this is going on in consciousness, in mind. It is not going on anywhere in reality. It is by buying back the truth of the power of our own decision that we can cancel the whole syndrome. We are not subject to 'that'. We are infinite beings who are subject only to what we hold in mind. We have the power of canceling the belief systems. We have the power to refuse to buy into the negativity of the collective belief systems and to say 'no' to them.

We also have the power to say 'no' to belief systems that come from our family. Really major allergies ran in my family. My grandmother was allergic, as were my mother and sister. Everybody had hay fever and sensitivity to ragweed, dust, hay, and horses. As a consequence, I had all of those allergies also, with swollen, itchy eyes, and all the rest of the symptoms. We all lived on antihistamines. In addition, I was severely allergic to poison ivy and ended up in the hospital with generalized severe poison ivy dermatitis. It did not respond to any treatment except for a brown salve obtained from a Native American medicine woman from the Wisconsin Dells tribe.

Years later, I participated in A Course in Miracles and was surprised to discover I no longer got migraine headaches from pesticides. I walked right into a house that had just been sprayed, and all of a sudden, I 'knew' I was no longer subject to belief systems.

After this amazing discovery, I awoke one day to the realization that I was no longer subject to poison ivy, either, so I went outside, picked some, planted some in a pottery jar, and played with it. It was miraculous! I carried it around to show family and friends. They thought I had gone 'over the edge', so to speak, but after that, my life changed and the negative belief systems fell away, one after the other. I subsequently also let go of the excess weight (fifty pounds) and felt a greater safety overall about physical life. To realize that we have power over our own lives brings a reduction in overall anxiety and a renewed sense of well-being and aliveness.

All illness is physical, mental, and spiritual, and therefore it is best to utilize all modalities to assist recovery. There are also unknown factors that influence recovery, such as karmic proclivities. Thus, some illnesses may persist, awaiting further inner discovery or the evolution of one's personal level of consciousness whereby the source of the illness is revealed. Therefore, spiritual work should proceed for its own sake and recovery surrendered to God. Successful treatment is one thing; healing is of a different dimension because the vast sources have been discovered and brought to light.

How can one know if humility and surrender are complete? They are complete when one is indifferent to whether a healing occurs or not. That is the result of surrender to God at great depth and relinquishment of the desire to control or change the way things are.

Practicality: Caveat

It is always advisable to have medical diagnoses confirmed by a second opinion. Major errors are not uncommon, and I myself had several major misdiagnoses that were potentially fatal if not detected. The cause of severe heart failure as being due to Graves disease (hyperthyroidism) was totally misdiagnosed earlier. Prostatic obstruction did not require surgery but instead merely cessation of the use of nasal decongestants.

CHAPTER 3

Stress

Having been a physician and psychiatrist for over fifty years, I have worked in the fields of psychoanalysis, psychotherapy, group therapy, and the psychodynamics of the various schools. In addition, there were years of research in the field of nutrition and its relationship to brain chemistry, mental illness, and emotions, which resulted in the textbook, *Orthomolecular Psychiatry* (co-authored by Nobel Prize winner Linus Pauling). I have also extensively researched and used alternative healing modalities that were found to be beneficial.

For the last thirty-five years, I have been doing research into the nature of consciousness itself and the application of that knowledge to an understanding of spirituality. Inherent in this is the relationship between body, mind, and spirit and what that really means. Is that something scientific that we can clinically verify, or is that some kind of fantasy?

There is a lot of emphasis today on the subject of stress and its prevention, along with its implications for physical, emotional, and psychological health and how it impacts industry and the business world. There is a greater awareness of stress in our culture and what this disorder implies. We are going to look closely at the relationships between the body and its response to stress, and the mind and how it relates to spirit.

Stress results from a point of view—from what we hold in mind—and from our attitudes and beliefs. Emotional stress originates primarily from within ourselves and not just from the world. There is no such thing as escaping stress because its source is within us and not located within the world as commonly believed. Thus, we will be reversing the way the mind usually looks at cause and effect. By observation, one can see that 'cause' is not in the world nor is 'effect' in the mind, but vice versa. The level of power, the level of 'cause', is held in mind, bringing about one's experience of what happens in the world. Our folklore intuitively knows this because it says, "One man's meat is another man's poison." That quotation contains the secret of what we are talking about. The power is not in the event or in something 'out there'. The power of creating our experience of all events in life lies within each of us. Thus, it is by re-owning our power that we can learn how to prevent stress.

There are methods of precluding stress instead of treating its aftermath. The so-called stress-reduction programs that are commonly available in our society today are really methods of handling the effects of stress once it has already occurred, such as in relaxation programs designed to relieve the tension within the body. One might say that the horse is already out of the barn. There are ways to offset this so that the tension never arises in the body and thus precludes the necessity of the various ways of handling stress based on the medical model.

Some time ago, I received a brochure entitled "Stress and Heart Disease," which presented an entire belief program. The article promoted the idea that stress is something 'out there', that it is really something that is inherent in life, and that the result of stress is going to affect the heart, with all its symbolic mean-

ing to us. The various articles in the pamphlet dealt
with heart disease and the consequences of stress coming about through our physiology and manifesting
within the body. Because all things are experienced
within consciousness, it is essential to look again at the
relationship between body, mind, and spirit.

We are going to discuss things that we can verify
through our own experience, along with verifiable
clinical experience derived from the viewpoint of the
clinical scientist who believes only what can be clinically repeated and verified through inner experience.

A characteristic of the body is that it is insentient,
that is, the body has no capacity to experience itself.
This means that the arm, in and of itself, cannot experience its own existence or 'armness'. It cannot even
experience that it 'is', much less where it is, how big it
is, or what it is doing. How do we know what is going
on with the body? We know solely because of the senses.
We do not experience the body itself, but instead, the
senses' report of the body. We also note that the senses
themselves have no capacity to experience themselves. For instance, in the ear, the vibrations going
through the auditory nerve and stimulating the tym-
panic membrane have no way to experience themselves as sound.

Where does the experience of the body take place?
It registers in the brain, but then awareness occurs in
something greater than the brain itself, in what we call
'mind'. It is because of the energy field of the mind that
we experience the brain and the body. Mind itself, very
curiously, also lacks the capacity to experience itself.
This is an amazing thought until we look into it. We see

that a thought, of and by itself, has no capacity to experience its own 'thoughtness'. A memory has no capacity in and of itself to experience its own 'memoryness'. Similarly, a fantasy about the future has no such capacity either. The imagination, the emotions—all that goes on in mind—are only experienced because of that greater and larger energy field than mind called consciousness. It is an energy field that is more diffuse, formless, and capable of experiencing change as well as any phenomena. It is only because of consciousness itself that we are aware of what is going on in mind, and it is because of mind that we are aware of what is going on with sensations. Because of sensations, we are aware of what is going on with the physical body.

Curiously, however, even consciousness itself cannot report what is going on within itself except for a greater field that is infinite and without dimension called the experiential knowingness of subjective awareness. Because of that quality of awareness that accompanies existence and beingness, we are capable of awareness. Out of awareness comes the knowingness of what goes on within consciousness. Consciousness reports what is going on within mind, and mind reports what goes on with sensations about the body. Thus, we can see that what we are, in its highest and greatest sense, refers to the capacity for subjective awareness.

It is solely within consciousness itself that all experience is being experienced. Therefore, to directly address the source and place of experiencing will lead to the capabilities of precluding the sources of stress.

As described in Chapter 1, the Map of

Consciousness is a numerical model based on energy
fields and levels of consciousness. The energy fields are
calibrated as to their relative power, labeled according
to common human experience, and thereby readily
and easily understood. At the very bottom of the chart,
for example, is 'Guilt', which, in its form of self-hatred,
is a destructive, negative emotion. From the position of
Guilt, the world is seen as a place of suffering.
Guiltiness has an energy field of 30. The lower states
are close to Death, which calibrates at zero. With Death
at zero, achieving a consciousness high enough to
become enlightened calibrates at 600 and over.

Guilt, apathy, grief, fear, desire, anger, and pride are
all negative energy fields that have adverse or destructive effects and therefore have a low calibration number. For instance, Apathy at 50 has much less energy
than Fear, which calibrates at 100. Fear at 100 has much
less energy than that of Courage, which calibrates at
200. Desire at 125 has less energy than the state called
Neutral (at 250), or being detached.

Calibration of the energy fields can be replicated by
using very common techniques, such as simple muscle
testing, that verify the relative energies and directions
of the fields. These fields calibrate lower when one
holds in mind a thought that is angry, a thought about
something one regrets or is sad about, or a thought
about something one fears. When the arm of the person having such a thought is tested, it will instantly
become weak. The cerebral hemispheres become
desynchronized, the acupuncture energy system goes
out of alignment, and the person instantly loses power
and energy.

At the level of Courage, where truth is told, the energy field moves upwards to that which is positive and supports and reinforces life. It is the energy of aliveness and is aligned with integrity and honesty.

When we calibrate the great teachers of wisdom who have walked this earth, we find that they are at the level of 600 and above. The great avatars, the great saviors of mankind, and the great mystics and saints are in the energy fields of the 700s on up to 1,000. It could be said that truth begins at energy field 200 and expands upward into an ever-increasing lovingness and alignment with Truth. Interestingly, health follows the same pattern.

The farther up we go in our energy fields, the healthier our bodies automatically become until, finally, there is joy in the aliveness and exquisite pleasure of the body. At level 540, the energy field of Unconditional Love and healing, the body begins to heal its own diseases, depending on inherent propensities as well as limitations (e.g., karma, both individual and human).

In relation to stress, it is essential to look at the pre-existing conditions within a person's consciousness that set them up to experience life in a stressful way. It is obvious that a person who has identified with the attitudes of a lower energy field experiences a world that is perceived as negative. A person who identifies with the lower energy field of hopelessness and despair is going to experience the world as hopeless, and all of life's experiences are going to be colored by that expectation.

At the level of Grief, people are full of regret, concerned with loss in the past, and see this as a sad world. If there were a God, he would be a God who doesn't love us, doesn't care for us, and ignores us.

In the energy field of Fear, there is the appearance of a suppressed energy that has been held throughout life as fearfulness. There is preoccupation with anxiety and constant worry about the future. The world looks like a frightening place, and a person at that level experiences everything in the form of fright. The God of such a world would be considered to be fearsome (punitive).

The person who is always desirous and wanting experiences this as a frustrating world. The angry person is prone to conflict and war. The prideful person is vulnerable to perceived challenges and therefore assumes a defensive posture. We will discuss the Map of Consciousness in greater detail to learn how we are automatically set up for stress.

One begins to suspect from the statement "One man's meat is another man's poison" that the set-up for stress comes from one's own inner values, belief systems, and positions about life. These stem from the programs that are being held operative within one's consciousness. One starts to look for the source of stress not in the world, but in what is being held in consciousness that assigns stress to the experience of a given event. Following are some examples, available to all of us, that show how some attitudes and ways of being with life set us up for the experience of stress.

There was an elderly lady, for instance, who used to visit her married daughter who lived in the middle of one hundred acres of woods out in the country, thirty miles from New York City. There was only stillness; in fact, the only sounds that one could hear were the rustling of the leaves and the songs of the birds.

The older woman had lived all of her life in New York City, on the lower East Side. She hated to make the visit to the country, and when she did, stayed as briefly as possible. Two or three days were all that she could stand. The peace and silence would drive her 'crazy', and she could not wait to return to the city where she would sigh with relief. Her apartment faced the street, and from her open window, she could talk to anybody, hear the hustle and bustle of the city, and feel secure— all in the midst of the lower East side (her 'mother-land'), despite all the noise and muggings. She was in a situation that another person might consider stressful.

A lot of people might consider that part of the city scary indeed. What she experienced as security— being there in the throngs of people, with the sounds of garbage cans and garbage trucks making a racket at 5 AM, was reassuring to her. In contrast, peace and silence in the middle of one hundred acres of woods were stressful.

We can look at a comparable example of Devil's Island, the French penal colony. The French govern-ment, out of social protest, closed much of the prison and allowed the prisoners to run loose on the island. They released them from the animal and torture cages and allowed them the freedom of the island and to walk around at will. What did the prisoners do? Much to the surprise of the authorities, they went back to their cages to sleep at night. They felt frightened, lonely, and insecure even though, for the first time in all the years, they had the freedom they so vociferously had demanded and died for during that time. The sense of security came from the feeling of being back in the cages.

To most people, a jail cell would be the maximum threat. No greater horror could be imagined. Yet, what have other people done in a prison cell? They have written prize-winning novels and staggering pieces of literature. Things written in jail cells and prisons have changed the course of the history of mankind, for better or worse. Adolf Hitler wrote *Mein Kampf* while in prison.

Another interesting example, in contrast to Devil's Island, is exemplified by the famous movie, *Lost Horizon*. If you remember, in that movie Ronald Coleman and the other passengers of a plane made an emergency landing in the Himalayas. They went through a pass and came upon Shangri-La, which represents an almost heavenly condition. Its energy field (540-600) is very high and is a place of unconditional love and unending peace. Although the character played by Coleman was ready for the experience, benefiting greatly and expanding his own consciousness, the other passengers reacted to it differently. It was interesting to watch six different people with six different reactions. A couple of them were not quite ready for the experience and reacted to it as a stress due to its newness and strangeness. Others felt stress for a while but then adjusted to it and accepted the sort of heavenly condition in their lives. In contrast, others were acutely disturbed by it.

The person playing Ronald Coleman's brother in the movie became agitated and almost paranoid. He demanded to return to the 'real world'. All these people exhibited a reaction not to where they were but to their individual positions. Their experiencing was not about the environment but about their own levels of consciousness.

One time I was leaving Ecuador and at the time, there were only two planes a week that flew out of Quito. I arrived for the Thursday flight, having made reservations many months in advance, but when I checked in, the first thing I was told was that my name was not on the list. Then I was told that the plane was not leaving on Thursday of that week; it was leaving on Saturday. For some reason, it just seemed to be humorous and even hilarious. Somehow, being in the culture of Ecuador at an altitude of 10,000 feet and above, the fact that the plane was going to leave three days late was viewed as not really important. Nobody got upset about it, and interestingly, the clock in the airport that hung from the middle of the ceiling had stopped working many years previously, and nobody had bothered to fix it.

There was no frustration in coming from the attitude of acceptance, so there was no stress. There was an easygoing social attitude in which precision in the material world was not considered to be important. Human values were of greater importance. In this case, because of human value, even the convenience of the crew was more important than the departure day, and nobody seemed to mind. The setting, the expectation, and the cultural attitude in Quito were not even experienced as stressful. If that had happened in a different social setting, such as LaGuardia Airport, for example, and the Thursday flight was not leaving until Saturday, it would have been experienced as stressful.

As a matter of fact, when I arrived for the Saturday departure scheduled at 11:45 AM, there was some kind of delay. It was the only plane on the runway and the plane just sat there. Suddenly it was noon, the time when everything shuts down for a siesta, so not only did the Thursday plane not leave until Saturday, it didn't leave at 11:45 AM; instead, it left at 3 PM. The plane just sat on the runway while everybody took a siesta. When it was over, everyone gathered their belongings, got on the plane, and away we went. No one was upset; everyone was totally relaxed and at ease. So it really is possible to be at peace with a three-day delay in a flight schedule.

Within these experiences is the key to the understanding of stress, because when we talk about stress, we are really talking about the experience of what is stressful within our own consciousness. To consider the body as part of a stress response means that the body is only responding to what is held in mind. By altering what we hold in mind—our expectations, our way of being with life—we can preclude the development of stress. We did not have to go to a relaxation program to handle the stress of the plane's being three days late. We did not have to go to some kind of coronary exercise program to protect our hearts from stress—there wasn't any stress. Consequently, the real approach to stress is to prevent it in the first place—to preclude it by understanding how and where it arises.

Our first understanding is that the source of what we experience as stress is within ourselves; it does not exist 'out there' in the world. It does not exist in plane schedules or prison cells; it exists only within our own consciousness.

As we examine the Map of the fields of consciousness more closely, our awareness of this subject will advance rather rapidly because it is easy to understand. It is something we already know; it is just necessary to bring it into our awareness.

The energy fields at the bottom of the Map are adverse or destructive to life and can be called stress because of their intrinsic nature, which indicates a stressful direction. When we move to Neutral, we go in a positive direction to that which is not stressful. At consciousness level 540, all things are experienced in their beauty and perfection, in the oneness of life, and in unconditional love and lovingness.

On the Map, to the right of these energy fields that are calibrated as to their relative power, we see the emotions that arise from those positions or ways of being with life. For example, we can see that people who are at the level of Guilt experience the emotions of blame and self-hatred. They experience life as destructive and see a world of suffering. The person who holds the position of Apathy about life experiences the emotion of hopelessness. They see life and their world as hopeless. They are in despair, and there is a loss of energy. The God of such a world is dead.

If enough energy is poured into a person in the state of apathy, they can move up to Grief, a stage in which they can express emotion. It has a certain biological purpose, and the expression of grief, such as the crying of a child, brings up the emotion. Those who are in that energy field are looking to the past and see their lives filled with regret and loss. They become dispirited and experience this as a sad world, feeling that the God of this world is ignoring them. In contrast, the person who is in the suppressed energy field of Fear looks at life with intense worry and anxiety and experiences life as frightening. Regret stems from clinging to the past, and fear results from living in the future.

What is life? It includes a view of the world and a view of ourself and others, as well as expectations of Divinity. What is life, in and of itself? Is it arising out of the event? We then see that these fields of energy are really portholes. They are ways in which we see the world. It is the color of the glasses we put on. If we put on gray glasses coming from Grief, then everything looks sad. A person walking down the street who is dominated by this energy field sees everything on the street as hopeless. He looks at man and man's condition or opens the newspaper, and he sees hopelessness; man's condition is hopeless. As he walks down the street, he looks at the elderly people or the children and sees how hopeless their condition is; they are going to have to grow up in a world of hopelessness.

The person who is sad walks down the street and literally experiences their perception of sadness. When they open the newspaper, they see all there is to be sad about in the world and the sadness of man's condition. They see the trash on the street. They look at the elderly people and think how sad aging is. They feel sorry for the children and think how sad is the world they are going to have to grow up in. They know the pain of life. They are holding so much pain that the pity expresses itself now—how sad for these children.

Those who are in the energy field of Fear see, experience, and create in their world the conditions of that which is fearful. They read the newspaper and see how fearful this world is—killings, murders, muggings, war, and bombings. They walk down the street and see everything as frightening. They see the chances for accidents and how people can twist their ankles on the curb. They think there should be warning signs everywhere. The people who see this as a frightening world put double locks on everything. They double lock their car within their own double-locked garages within their own double-locked yard in an area that has never had a robbery.

The fear comes from within and projects a frightening appearance out to the world. If we have fear-colored glasses, everything looks like fear, and if we search for God, we see a fearful God. The God of a frightening world is one to fear.

A person may move into a higher energy field of desiring this and wanting that, which occurs via social education. People at the bottom of the Map who are aligned with hopelessness, such as those in the Third World countries or segments of lower socioeconomic groups in our society, began to see what other people have when television became available. This created desire, which is felt in the emotional field as wanting and craving and is also expressed fully in the addictions. The process occurring in consciousness is that of entrapment. Because someone wants or begins to desire something, they then experience this world as frustrating. The stress they experience is that of endless frustration.

Wantingness can result in a person who is never satisfied, and no matter what they get, they always want something more. If they do not experience fulfill- ment of their wishes, this brings up more wishes and results in an endless desire for control. They see this as a very frustrating world, and as they walk down the street, they see all the things they want—the cars, the appurtenances, and the addresses. As they open the newspaper, they see more things they want. They want to change the world; they want to 'get'. This endless addiction to 'gettingness' creates endless stress that comes from within the self. The problem is the endless desire for something.

When people, out of their frustration, move up to Anger, they then begin to experience an angry world. They are full of resentment and are boiling over with hatred, blame, and grievance. With a person like this, the suppressed energy of anger is now ready to spill forth in any event. They see the world as competitive. Because of the angry glasses this person wears, when they open the newspaper, their stomach turns with wrath, indignation, and anger over the events that are reported.

If they walk down the street, they see many things to be angry about—the condition of the street signs and the street in general, including the newspapers that are strewn all over. Looking at children and old folks makes them think about their situations and makes them angry. They live in a world of injustice, indignation, and competition. If they own a used-car lot and someone down the street opens one, they look at it as competition and think they are going to lose as a result. Because these people live in a win-lose world, their stomachs are always tense. They have not moved up to a higher level of harmony and cooperation; as a result, they don't realize that the more used-car lots on the street, the better business will be for everyone.

To a person at the level of anger, the world becomes a threatening place. The God of that kind of universe would be the God of war. Out of their anger, these people with a chip on their shoulders become war-like and ready for combat. Their anger is ready to burst forth. The world is very stressful then because of the suppressed anger. If someone were to bump their fender in a parking lot, up would come the anger, the cursing, and the threat of a lawsuit. They are preoccupied with revenge and 'getting even' with enemies.

If a person moves up to the level of Pride, there is more energy available, along with negative, destructive emotions. Although pride is often thought of as constructive, innately it is actually destructive because pride is denial. Its expression is really one of arrogance and contempt because the process occurring in consciousness is that of inflation.

Prideful people are then very polarized and defensive in their positions and become like those who are angry. Their position is 'right', and they live in a world of right and wrong, of win or lose. Therefore, stress is always occurring within that person because they see all relationships, interactions, and transactions in terms of win-lose, which is about the importance of perceived status and has to do with ownership. When these persons read the newspaper, they are seeing the status of all that is involved, along with the status of the people being written about. They walk down the street and primarily see symbols of status—the labels on clothes and the addresses. All these things about life now become status, and these people become interested in who others are from a status viewpoint.

All these are obviously vulnerable positions of the victim mentality, because all the positions below the level of truth project the source of happiness as being outside oneself. Holding to these positions results in giving one's power away. Doing so says that the sources of meaning, happiness, and value are something outside oneself; they are somewhere 'out there'. These positions come from lack. "If it is out there, it is something I have to get. If it is something I have to get, it means I lack it, or that something could stand in my way of getting it."

To live in that kind of world is to always live in danger and under threat because something outside of oneself can block the attainment of something or take it away. It is the world of victimhood because people have given away their power to the world.

It is often said that the sources of happiness and stress are 'out there', and thus the hope for releasing stress is by 'changing the world'. Stress does not exist in the world. Instead, it is an inner experience within consciousness itself. There really is no way one can basically change the world to relieve stress. What, then, can be done?

We can begin to own the truth about it and have the courage to look at the facts. The minute we do this, we change the energy fields. As we move to Neutral, we move into a more positive space. Now there is the will-ingness to face, cope, and handle the situation, thereby bringing re-empowerment. That means reclaiming our power and living closer to the truth.

The person who is at the level of Courage sees a world of challenge, growth, and opportunity. It is an exciting, fun world, a place wherein one is glad to be alive. That person opens the newspaper and sees all the tremendous opportunities for mankind to move into and solve and resolve problems. One sees all kinds of problem-solving techniques in their own mind that they wish to try. The world then becomes exciting, one of opportunity and growth in which one begins to ask, "Where can I fit in? Where can I start expressing myself and experiencing some of these opportunities?" The kind of God one experiences in this world of opportu-nity is a God of open-mindedness. The open mind now begins to change that which is stressful. What is stress-ful at the level of Pride perhaps becomes an object of curiosity and an opportunity for growth to the person at the level of Courage.

Moving up to the next level called Neutral, the energy field calibrates at 250 and has much more power than the positions below, and the power is now being used in a constructive direction. It is as though at the lower levels, the antenna is first tuned to the negative; then it moves to neutral, and finally, to the positive. One then begins to experience life in a positive direction because one is the experiencer. The experience is not out there; it is within one's own consciousness. If a per-son is willing to let go of a lot of their positionalities, they no longer need to be defensive, which is a result of pridefulness, importance, and the need to always be 'right'.

The positions of the atheist, the bigot, or the zealot lead to conflict. These are based on the prideful belief that "my position is 'right'; therefore, your position is 'wrong'." With the willingness to surrender that, the person becomes somewhat unattached. People begin to transcend their vulnerability to the world, and the process occurring in consciousness releases them. The world begins to look okay, and the God of such a world is now the God of freedom.

How is that 'okayness' expressed? A person at this level, when on the way to a job interview, thinks, "If I get this job, it will be great, and if I do not, that is okay, too, because there are other job opportunities I would really like to look at." As a result, that person is not stuck because they have not based their survival on any one particular thing.

As we move into Willingness, we add intention to the process of consciousness. It means a 'yesness', a joining, an alignment, and an agreement with life, and such a person begins to see the world as friendly. When these people at the level of Willingness walk down the street, the God of that kind of world appears promising and hopeful. Now their experience of the newspaper is one of opening it up and seeing all the evidence of man's cooperation and struggle to solve his own problems. What another perceives as destruction, they see as merely the process, or the working out, of the balance of forces. When they walk down the street, they begin to see a friendlier world and now see people as friendly. Their perception has changed, and now 'old' people who no longer have to 'make it' in the world are frequently seen as more open to friendliness. It is now simple to walk up to most older people and instantly strike up a conversation.

Those at the level of Willingness no longer look at others with a paranoid distrust or size up people to see where they stand in a prideful world. They begin to see strangers and older people as friendly, as well as the friendliness of young children, and find that it is easy to strike up a relationship with them.

As we move up into Acceptance, we then begin to accept that we are the source of our own experience of life. The person who has reached this level of awareness has taken back the power over their own life and realizes that no matter where they are put, they are going to somehow make do. If they were put on a desert island, a year later, they would have built a tree house and would be carving coconuts.

If they were put in a jail cell, they would write a novel or maybe even sit cross-legged and go into meditation. Others often choose to become jailhouse lawyers and even get law degrees. The power to create the experience of life is within. These people have reclaimed their own power. Consequently, the God of that kind of world and universe of experience is now perceived as promising, hopeful, and merciful, and as a God no longer to be feared. These people now feel adequate and confident.

Companies want to hire that kind of person to go out after the big contracts. That person is able to accept the ups and downs in the realities of life as well as their own limitations. A person dominated by pride is unable to accept limitation. When a company says, "We would like you to go to Venezuela and close a deal," the person at the level of Acceptance feels adequate and confident and can say, "You know, I really do not do very well with that company, and I do not get along with that particular man. I would do much better in Belgium. I can sell twice as much there. Why don't you let Jim go down to Venezuela?"

There is the willingness to accept how the world works and to avoid going into indignation. Even the IRS has its own way of being in the world. One avoids 'right and wrong' and just accepts that is how it is in this world and goes along with it. (Acceptance is different from passivity.) The beginning of the transformation of consciousness is the realization that we are the source of our experiences, and therefore, the world begins to look more positive, harmonious, hopeful, and benign.

Empowerment moves a person up to the next energy field of Love. What do we mean by love? It is not the sentimental emotionalism that emanates from attachment or what Hollywood depicts as love. That emotionalism coming out of a possessive ownership of the other person, the back-and-forth control and the power struggles that occur, the words of a song that say, "If you leave me, I will kill myself" are not the elements of Love. These are all the consequences of an attachment rather than real love.

Unconditional Love is a way of being with life that nurtures, supports, and, of its own nature, is forgiving. It is the beginning of the revelation of some of the truths of life because, within the brain, there is a release of endorphins. (See Brain Function and Physiology chart in Chapter 1.) Endorphins allow a certain inner state to occur, a way of being with one's self and one's body in the world. Consequently, the world starts to appear to be lovable. Such a person now walks down the street feeling somewhat mellow. They see the lovingness that really occurs underneath the apparent trivialities of life and holds all of mankind together. The person is moving into a higher energy field.

To see life as harmonious and loving reduces stress, making this person less vulnerable because they are aligned with forgivingness. The intention of this field that one chooses is called lovingness, which is experienced as being loving towards all things at all times, as loving mankind and being nurturing towards one's self.

There is a difference in how people view themselves in contrast to the harshness of the perfectionist who is always at the level of stress with human nature. The person who is unforgiving, with a tendency to judge and condemn, carries self-hatred and guilt, and for that person to just breathe in and out causes a state of stress. If they get up late, they already hate themselves for getting up late. The stress stems from perfectionism, inflexibility, and the propensity for self-condemnation, and it is internally generated. The open-minded persons who start to be easier with themselves also start to be accepting of their own humanness. Forgiveness supports the mental attitude of the readiness to allow for the humanness of others, which also allows for one's own humanness.

With progressive inner spiritual work, one moves up to an even higher energy field of joyfulness, which approaches the beginning awareness of the reality that one really is the experiencer, not the experience. One is then not at the effect of the world but instead realizes that one determines the way it is experienced.

Out of inner serenity arises compassion for all of life. Awareness of its incredible beauty and perfection increases, along with experiencing the oneness and unity of it. Then the more evolved person opens the newspaper and sees and experiences the totality of man's lovingness. Despite the limitations of humanness, that which is making all the articles appear in the newspaper is the expression of the onward movement and evolution of man's consciousness. When an evolved person walks down the same street, they experience only the incredible beauty of it, the beauty of life in all its magnificent expressions. One can then see a rose in the middle of its perfect unfoldingness. The less-evolved person would look at the half-unfolded rose and say, "I don't want that, that's an imperfect rose." The evolved person sees perfection in the evolution of life itself and sees that half-unfolded rose in the same way. They then simply project forward in time and see the unfoldingness, the incredible beauty, and its precision and become aware of the inner sacredness of all life.

As we talk about these energy fields as levels of consciousness, it is obvious that they determine how we experience life. They determine what kind of a God we think exists in the universe as well as the kinds of emotions we express. All of this expression is a process going on within consciousness itself. It is now clear that there is nothing 'out there' that has the power to create stress, and that we ourselves are the creators of stress by our positionalities and attitudes.

It becomes obvious that the open-minded, easygoing person does not experience severe stress when somebody backs into their car's fender in the parking lot. What happens (as you may have experienced yourself) depends on whether you are in a 'good mood'. What is stressful in one mood is not stressful in another. Often the person whose fender was just bumped is very upset. A peaceful person is concerned about the upset person and tells them, "You know, there is nothing to be upset about; it's only a fender. We both have insurance. It's no big deal. In reality, it's a little nuisance in that you have to take your car to the body shop to get it fixed, but it's really no big deal." The evolved person desires to heal the upset that arose in the field of consciousness.

It is not events that send one into self-pity or anger about an unjust world where people back into a fender. The wish to punch the guy in the nose arises from so much anger within oneself. The detached person would just handle the event with no particular feeling. One's concern about the feelings of others and the desire to support life by relieving another's anxiety and fear arises from what one has become. It does not exist in the world. The dented fender, therefore, has no power over one's life. There is no 'cause' of emotions except from within. To see this fact results in empowerment, autonomy, and release from the illusion of victimhood.

Inner peace automatically arises out of our willingness to give up certain positionalities, such as judging others and making them 'wrong'. Willingness stems from a forgiving, understanding position. Judgmentalism does not really solve anything but instead adds to the problem. Making others wrong results in a world of lose-lose. This is a world where we lose and the company loses. It is stressful by virtue of the superimposed context. It is stressful in the very way that it is set up because even if we win, we still go through the anxiety of possibly losing, so that even in winning, we do not really win.

We know about people, for example, who say that they want to have a lot of money. What happens to them when they suddenly win a lot of money? Some interesting research has been done on people who have won millions of dollars in the big lotteries. In follow-up studies of lottery winners, it was found that within five years, the degree of happiness of the people in this group was dismal. The rates of suicide, divorce, sickness, and drug addiction had risen spectacularly among these people who ostensibly had gotten the very thing they had wanted. The reason they played the lottery was to win.

In the win-lose game, to win, in itself, means to defeat others who lose. To defeat others brings up guilt. As a result, one cannot even be happy in winning because in a win-lose context, one wins and others are defeated, which results in guilt. In competition, there are unconscious fears, for example, fear of the opponent. There is the fear that the sudden acquisition of money may mean that friends will be out to get the money. This can result in reactions leading to a depressed, paranoid attitude. At the lowest level of consciousness, everyone loses because it is a hopeless, dismal world. Stress automatically comes out of a win-lose position.

Positions of great success and power in the world automatically come to those who think in terms of win-win because they set up within their own minds a way of being in the world and a way for others to be in their life that is mutually beneficial. What kind of stress does the person experience who sets up everything as win-win? That person wins if a friend comes over to their house, and they win if the friend does not. If they visit, what is held in mind is how much one is going to enjoy their friendship and presence. At the same time, one knows that if their friend cannot make it, that is okay, too. As a result, the other person wins either way, also. If they come over for dinner, we are delighted with their presence. If they do not come for dinner, we have given them the free time to do something that we know will enhance their life.

To hold all of our expectations in business as a win-win situation results in success, which we experience as an enhancement of life. The better a company does, the better the employees do. The more a company does, the more it gives to the world. The better the product available to the world, the better the world supports the company. The more it supports the company, the more the company can support the economy. The more the employees are supported, the more they can support their families. The more the company supports the families, the more the families support the company.

The way to become a success is to make our boss a success. Instead of going into competition with him (meaning someone has to lose), making our boss a success moves him up the ladder and creates space for us to move up as well. When coming from a competitive position with the intent to defeat the boss, there arises unconscious anxiety, distress, and the fear of retaliation.

The willingness to surrender the adversarial position and become more easygoing lessens the experience of stress. The easygoing person at the level of Acceptance is able to accept human nature and the world as they are and is ready for any alternatives that arise.

A lot of people go into a state of fear at the prospect of being visited by the IRS. They assume an adversarial position that brings up all kinds of stress. As stated previously, stress does not exist in the outer world but only in our attitude about it. One year, the computer selected me for an audit. "Well," I thought, "here's a chance to find out how well I have been doing." I sort of looked at the prospect happily. I thought, "Here's a chance to find out if I am doing things correctly, and if not, what I can do about it."

I spent a couple of weeks preparing for the audit. I purchased fancy notebooks, inserted the specific pages into celluloid sheets that the accountant said the IRS would be interested in, and labeled everything. When the agent arrived, coffee was ready, and I treated him like an honored guest. I escorted him into the library, gave him the best desk, the best coffee, and the best cup and saucer, not for the purpose of 'buttering him up', but out of respect for his position because I could see how painful it must be to be a tax auditor.

My heart went out to this guy, and I really wanted his day to be a good day. He was actually very pleased, and as the day went on, I had my way of looking at things, and he had his way of looking at things. We had a friendly conversation and did a sort of swap. He had a great day. By making his day a great day, I also had an enjoyable day. He said, "You know, I really hate to leave at three o'clock in the afternoon, but frankly, we are all done." The IRS people are really very friendly, very helpful, and very positive in their attitudes because that is how it is being held in consciousness.

To become easygoing is to get out of the habit of seeing danger. The easygoing person who is really confident and adequate is able to accept the downside of or the possibility of the downside of human nature and therefore does not have to deny it. It is preparing for the 'what ifs' in life, creating an opportunity to handle the other side and the opportunities that may arise. An easy way to discover the source of stress is to take a book along when driving to work through heavy traffic. This converts the delays into a pleasant and welcome opportunity. There is the capacity within us to create an enjoyable experience when waiting in traffic because there is time to read, catch up on things, and really enjoy life.

What does it mean when we go into a neighborhood and see a zoning sign that says, "No children or pets"? It means that people who live in the neighborhood have the idea that children and pets are stressful. There are other people who would consider the lack of children or pets to be stressful. Some people have the television on, the radio playing, and the lights on;

there is a lot of action in their lives. To other people, that would be very stressful. Some people like silence and never turn on the television or radio because the constant 'noise' in the background interferes with their concentration.

Stress can also arise from that which is unexpected. The open-minded person sees many alternatives of what could happen in a situation and plans in advance how to handle the unexpected before it occurs. If one considers the downside of a situation in advance, for example, "What if the contract falls through," or "What if the person I am to meet on the street corner doesn't show up," and plans an alternative action if the unexpected does occur, then stress is minimized or does not occur at all.

The "Law of Initial Value" states that the effect one sees is not in the stimulus but has to do with the set-up of the organism, the preexisting condition. The response is not on just the intensity of the stimulus but on the position of the organism with which it is interacting. For example, in pharmacology, it would be senseless to ask what is the effect of twenty-five milligrams of the tranquilizer Thorazene. The effect of twenty-five milligrams of Thorazene would depend on the preexisting condition of the patient. If the patient was somewhat dull and in Apathy, twenty-five milligrams of Thorazene would be very, very sedating. If the patient was in a highly agitated state, twenty-five milligrams of Thorazene might have no effect. If the person was in a state of mild anxiety, twenty-five milligrams of Thorazene might be quite effective. The patient's present condition, which includes the amount of suppressed energy they are holding, their attitudes, and their belief systems, determines the effect of the same stimulus.

Some people say loud music drives them crazy. In contrast, consider teenagers who put on earphones, turn the volume way up, and go into a state of delight. Is loud music stressful or not? The basic principle is that we experience stress when we do not want a specific stimulus or situation. Consequently, when one is in the mood for loud music, it is pleasant and contributes to the state of joy and aliveness. In contrast, if one were tired or exhausted after a hard day at the office, the same loud music would be experienced as stressful. Desire determines whether or not a stimulus is stressful.

Stress is resisting what we do not want, and not stressed is getting what we do want. The problem is within ourself. The solution is to merely shift our attitude by choosing lovingness towards life, which includes an energy field called humor that contains the capacity to laugh at ourselves and at the nature of life itself, and to love and laugh at the comedy of it all. That is the value of the great humorists who also tend to be long lived.

Disturbed people are like Don Quixote—fighting their own projections in the world. The comedy of it all is the basis of humor, laughing at those qualities of life, holding them from a position that exposes the paradox, because humor is in seeing the paradox. It is by inner decision whether life is experienced as joyful, harmonious, and easygoing, or experienced as an enemy. We begin to admire instead of envy people who are capable and easygoing, which means acceptance and being adequate. To feel adequate and solid results from realizing ourself as the source of how life is experienced.

We can be the boss, and if the janitor does not show up, it does not really matter to a serious degree. The truth is that we are the quality which experiences experience within our own consciousness. Happiness results from the experience of our own existence and enjoying our own inner aliveness.

When we stop identifying with the events 'out there' and giving them power over our lives, then we experience an inner serenity as a consequence of having transcended the world.

CHAPTER 4

Health

The subject of health occupies the minds of a large part of the population. As a physician, psychiatrist, and spiritual researcher, my interests have been focused on the area of health and self-healing. Importantly, in the relationship between body, mind, and spirit, it has been found that the body has no way of experiencing itself; the body is experienced in mind only. The body expresses that which is held in mind. The mind cannot experience itself, either; it has to be experienced from an even greater energy field, which is called consciousness. A human being progresses from dense linear form to an ever-expanding and increasing nonlinear formlessness. One ends up with the experiencing of experience itself—that field called awareness.

The relationship between body, mind, and spirit is very important when considering the subject of health. Consciousness itself has to be understood because all experiencing is going on solely within consciousness. It has been discovered that, due to the power of the energy fields, healing comes out of attitudes and belief systems that are held in mind. Therefore, to a large degree, health is an expression of levels of consciousness.

To make this more understandable to the logical mind, the integrated Map of Consciousness is based on the mathematical relationship between the energy fields that resulted from calibrating the energy fields of the essence of literally thousands of things, including attitudes, feelings, perception, and beliefs.

From this model, in which the relative power of energy fields is calibrated, it can be seen that Apathy, which calibrates at 40, has much less power than that of Fear, which calibrates at 100. Fear, on the other hand, has much less power than that of Courage, which calibrates at 200.

Not only do these energy fields have different levels of power relative to each other, we can also see that the energy fields go in a certain direction. At the level of Courage, the scale progresses upward beyond the energy field of 200 to those of Neutral, Willingness, Acceptance, and Love. These fields give energy as well as nurture and support life and truth, thus increasing aliveness. At the bottom of the Map of Consciousness (below 200) are the levels that do not represent truth in the human. Truth really begins to prevail at consciousness level 200.

If we start at the bottom of the chart and move up to the level of 600, we leave the fields of duality and illusion. We leave behind identification with the small self, or that which is called the ego, and move into the fields of Enlightenment. The energy fields of the great enlightened beings—the great spiritual masters and avatars—start in the 600s and continue up to level 1,000.

Health means aliveness, which is an expression of an energy field. The body expresses and is subject to what is held in mind, and therefore, the greater the amount of negativity held in mind, the greater the effect of the negative energy field on the body's physical health. In contrast, the greater the positive energy that is being held in mind, the more powerfully positive is the energy field of life. This knowledge provides a tool to determine whether or not something supports health and the expression of life.

At the bottom of the Map are the energy fields that contribute to illness, and above level 200 are the energy fields that support life. Each of these fields correlates with an emotion. That which is anti-life has the negative emotions of self-hatred, hopelessness, despair, regret, depression, worry, anxiety, cravingness, resentment, hatred, and arrogance. These negative emotions accompany ill health. The process occurring in consciousness can be seen arising from the emotional states of destruction, loss of energy and spirit, deflation, entrapment, overexpansion, overinflation, and loss of power.

Spiritually, the kind of world that a person experiences from these negative mental states is one of sin and suffering, hopelessness, sadness, fright, frustration, competition, and status. They see the negative conceptualizations of God that come out of a lower energy field. God can be denied, or conversely, negatively depicted as the ultimate enemy of man—the God who is punitive and even throws man into hell forever; the God who ignores man through unlovingness; or the God who is retaliatory. These depictions emerge from an energy field that has a negative direction along with a negative emotion and a destructive process occurring in consciousness. The negative views of God correlate with lower levels of consciousness (below calibration level 200).

Health can be viewed as the expression of unopposed aliveness resulting from the removal of its obstacles, including all that is negative. Health results from transcending limitations and feelings of separation. Since we have the power of refusal, we can refuse things in our life that are negative.

If our mind can become programmed in a negative direction, we can choose to program it in a positive direction as well. Health is an expression of self-esteem. Just how does one learn to love one's real self? How is the body experienced, and how is one's relationship to that body? There is a sublime state called 'nonexperiencing the body' in which the body is barely experienced as even existing. It is something one catches out of the corner of the eye and not central to experiencing at all. It means letting go of identifying oneself as physicality.

At the bottom of the Map of Consciousness, there is identification of ourself as being the body, but as we move up higher in consciousness, this lessens and lessens until identification with the body is transcended, and we move to the realization of the Self as spirit.

It is necessary to look at the relationship between mind and body because of its great importance in the field of health and something that really is not clearly understood. A basic principle that is demonstrated clinically is that *we are subject only to what we hold in mind*. This is a principle of healing and health, with two sides to the coin—one side being illness and the other being health. They are the opposite sides of the coin of the same understanding that heals and brings about health—that we are subject to what we hold in mind.

A good clinical example is that of multiple personalities; another example is hypnosis. Under hypnosis, a suggestion can be given to a patient that they are allergic to the roses on the desk, and that when they get up, they will get hives, a rash, and start sneezing. Then amnesia is created for the suggestion. When the person wakes up from the trance, all of a sudden, they start to wheeze, get hives, and develop a rash. The body is responding to what the mind believes. With hypnosis, the symptoms can be induced, along with most any illness, by convincing the patient that the program is true, and then amnesia can be created for memory of the programming process. This illustrates how an illness comes out of a program or belief system, which, in ordinary life, is often unconscious.

In the laboratory, this occurs as a psychological experiment. It is important to remember, however, that in everyday life, people have been programmed (hypnotized) thousands of times. This occurs when sitting in a trance in front of a television. There is no conscious memory of the process; the program went in, and the person is now subject to it for the rest of their life.

Because of childhood amnesia, many people cannot remember what happened to them before the age of five years, and some people have very little or even no memory of anything from their entire childhood. Even in people with good memories of childhood, there are vast areas of vacant forgottenness. In those areas are the many programs that are now expressing in various forms of ill health, such as catch phrases like "Heart disease runs in our family."

"Being overweight runs in the family," "Allergies run in our family," or "Everybody in our family has hay fever."

These thoughts become a program that goes into the mind, and we can see that it is the same as though the person were hypnotized. Until that program is brought to the conscious mind and cancelled, it remains operative within the unconscious mind (e.g., a chill or a draft causes colds).

Another example of the power of mind over body is in the cases of so-called multiple personality. These have been gaining increasing attention within the field of psychiatry and are found to be far more common than was previously believed. The consciousness of one personality is adopted by the patient and operative within that body for varying periods of time; it could be minutes, hours, days, weeks, or even years. While that second personality is operative, the patient is subject to all the belief systems held by that personality. If that personality happens to believe it has an ulcer, a weight problem, allergies, diverticulitis, colitis, back trouble-whatever it believes-while it is operative in the body, those physical abnormalities are actually brought into existence.

The reverse side of this occurs when that personality leaves, which sometimes comes about through intoxication or shifts in emotionality or life circumstances, and then the other personality enters the body. Because the other personality has no such beliefs, the body promptly heals itself of all those illnesses.

Why does the mind have such power over the body? We will consider the physics involved, which will make it easily understood. The energy of the physical body calibrates at about 200, as does the earth itself. The energy field of the mind is stronger and often calibrates up to 499. The 400s are in the energy field of the intellect, reason, logic, mind, and what the mind believes. Therefore, if a thought is held in mind that says strawberry seeds, caraway seeds, or any kinds of seeds give me diverticulitis, then the power of that thought coming out of the energy fields of perhaps 300 to 400 overpowers the body at the energy field of 200. The body is overpowered by the influence of the pattern of the belief.

All thought has form, so the form in the personal or collective unconscious, or in the collective or social consciousness, is present in great detail. If we buy into a thought or go into agreement with it, the effect is to bring it into our own consciousness, which then expresses itself within the body. The body will do what the mind believes. The healing of the body and the achievement of health are accomplished not just by addressing the body directly, but also by addressing the mind and moving into the field of consciousness. If the body is expressing that which is held in consciousness, then it is necessary to look at what that is.

Often we are not aware of what is being held in consciousness, in which case it would be called 'being unconscious'. There may be no recall of ever having had such a thought, but the body expresses what must be. It is like an x-ray telling us what is being held in mind since it is presenting itself in the body. For example, a person develops clinical diabetes and says, "I don't remember anything ever being said about that in my family. No one in my family has diabetes. I don't see where it could have arisen in my mind." We know that somewhere in the collective unconscious is the belief of diabetes and all that goes with it. If we do individual research with the patient long enough, we will uncover the origin of the program, which confirms that the program exists. If the person thinks they are subject to an illness, then the belief system also has to be healed. It is necessary to heal where the origin of the illness began.

Health is the result of positive mental attitudes. It originates in the field of consciousness and reflects a level of consciousness that expresses itself on the lower physical plane. An expression of health originates from the fields above Neutral—out of Willingness, and out of lovingness, inner joyfulness, and an inner state of peace. That which is mental calibrates in the 400s, and that which is of Love is at 500 and above. Spirit dominates at level 500 and becomes increasingly consciously aware that it is Spirit. Therefore, the intellect is not man's highest faculty, contrary to the age of reason as expressed in other learned works or by those intellectuals who believe that the intellect is man's highest attribute. The intellect is only in the 400s. There is the nonlinear energy field called consciousness, which is beyond mind, logic, and reason and transcends mentalization, revealing a whole different paradigm and way of being.

If we understand illness, then we will also understand its reverse, which is health. In illness, there is always unconscious guilt (calibrates as true), a statement reaffirmed by research. There are whole systems of how to let go of unconscious guilt through the process of the willingness to forgive, to let go of criticism and judgment, to let go of right and wrong as an

orientation towards life, to move towards forgivingness, and through the desire to understand life out of
compassion. This resolution of negativity requires
recontextualization of perception as exemplified by
the transformative effect of doing the workbook of A
Course in Miracles.

We find that illness requires several components,
including unconscious guilt and a mental belief system.
The mind has to hold a certain belief for the person to
accept that they are subject to it. It is as though unconscious guilt looks for something to justify itself. Often a
certain illness gets notoriety on television because a
celebrity shares their experience of it. That is followed
by an epidemic of that illness because of suggestion.
The mind buys into the program, the belief system, and
the specificity of a particular disease. Unconscious
guilt gives it power by expression through the autonomic nervous system and the hormonal balance
through all the stress mechanisms within the body, and
through the acupuncture energy system.

With positive attitudes, the acupuncture energy system is balanced, and the energy flow of health and life
moves directly down through all the energy channels,
stimulating all the organs of the body. With a negative
thought, the energy flow through one of the twelve
main meridians is interrupted and, if done repeatedly,
disease comes about in the affected organ. Negative
emotions potentiate a disease process. Unconscious
guilt gives it energy, and the form the illness takes is a
consequence of mental mechanisms because the body
expresses what is believed.

We also have to look at how experience is actually

experienced. The body itself is insentient, as curious as that may seem. It has no capacity to experience itself. The next level of experience comes through sensations, from the senses of the body, so we do not experience the body; instead, we experience the sensations of the body. Senses themselves have no innate capacity to experience themselves. They are experienced in mind. The senses report what is going on with the body, so we are several levels removed. Mind itself is unable to experience its own experience. It has to be in a greater, larger energy field than itself, and in this case, it is the energy field of consciousness. Because of consciousness, we are aware of what is going on in mind. Mind then tells us via the senses what is going on in the body. We can see that perception is several levels removed from the physical body. Consciousness itself requires something greater than itself, called awareness. Awareness allows us to know what is going on in consciousness and reports what is happening within mind. Mind in turn reports what is happening about the body via the senses.

That which we call 'myself' is many levels removed from the physical body. It is necessary to understand that fact because we then see that the mind has power over the body. We can appreciate the physics of the energy fields of the 400s, and see that, just by their sheer power, they are greater than the energy of the physical body. The physical body (calibration level 200) does what the mind tells it to do. Therefore, if the mind says, "I have this disease," the body complies.

We can thus see the importance of not buying into programs, all of which are really limitations of the truth. We can see the importance of consciously canceling the limiting programs and instead saying something that is the truth. The truth is, "I am an infinite being not subject to that." So, when people hear something such as, "Eggs are full of cholesterol, and cholesterol gives you heart disease," they accept the thought as the truth and buy into the belief system that the cholesterol in eggs will raise their blood cholesterol. Their bodies simply agree and raise the blood cholesterol when eggs are eaten.

One time I had a very high cholesterol level and began to cancel the belief system. I repeatedly said, "I am an infinite being; I am not subject to that. I am only subject to what I hold in mind. This does not apply to me, and I hereby cancel it and refuse it." If the mind can program you with a negative belief system, it can also reverse itself, can it not? Therefore, we begin telling ourself that the belief system has no effect on us, that it is only a belief system, and that we do not have to buy into it or go into agreement with it.

When we go into agreement with a belief system, we give it the power of the collective energy of that belief. When we refuse it, we then release ourselves from the collective energy of the belief system and count ourselves out. One attitude is to not buy into agreement with negative belief systems that have to do with our health. This is very important when it comes to epidemic suggestion and hysteria. The programming that comes in is aided and abetted by an emotional program.

Much is still heard about AIDS, for example, which is accompanied by constant repetition in the media that play on fear—fear about this, anger about that, and, of course, the guilt about this. What better dis-ease to bring up all of man's feelings of sinfulness and guilt, especially about one's sexuality, which is so common in all cultures, not just ours? Of course, it then takes on a negative energy when the coin is turned over and becomes the lowest. What better area in which to create an epidemic to ensure the belief in it? There is the unconscious guilt, not to mention the conscious guilt about one's sexuality, the sadness about it, the grief over it, and the fear about the dis-ease itself. All this contributes to setting the stage for a mental belief system in an energy field of the 400s. There is also the negative energy field of fear, which is the energy field of the 100s, plus the guilt of calibra-tion level 30. This is the exact set-up for disease because the mind chooses that with which it is impressed and uses that as a form of expression.

In the case of the cholesterol experiment, I can-celed the thought every time it came up. After a short time, the cholesterol level decreased, and now I can eat three eggs for breakfast every morning, lots of cheese, even other high-cholesterol foods, yet my cholesterol is low and sometimes even below normal for my age.

The body will do exactly what the mind believes, but there is a credibility problem here. The person asks, "How could just my belief in that make it happen with-in my life?" It is due to the nature of the unconscious, which creates the opportunity for that to occur. There is the person who is 'accident prone' because that belief has taken hold in their mind. Unconsciously, the person just manages to get their body in the right place at the right time in order to get hit by the fender of a car, or slip down the stairs, or get hit on the head. There is no need to worry about it because the mind will find a way. People just slip into a sort of hypnotic trance and expose themselves to the correct opportunities to make that program manifest in their lives (e.g., extreme sports, climbing Mt. Everest, etc.).

There have been many experiments with a cold virus, for instance, in which one hundred volunteer subjects were exposed to very heavy doses of a cold virus. Interestingly, not everyone ended up with a cold, just a certain percentage. In other words, if the power were in the virus itself rather than within consciousness, all one hundred would have gotten a cold because the virus is so potent. What happens is that maybe only sixty-five percent will get it because one-third of the subjects do not believe in it. There is sufficient doubt within the mind, along with insufficient unconscious guilt. It is not acceptable to the person to express it in that form, so nothing is universal.

The same thing can be seen with healing. Pneumonia or bird influenza does not occur in one hundred percent of exposed people, just in a certain percentage of them. Comparably, only a certain percentage of people will respond to any medical treatment. The difference is because those who do respond are not dominated by unconscious guilt. Also, a negative belief system is not operative because the particular illness does not fit any specific thought form they have bought into, so both sides of it—the sickness and the healing—are reflecting the energy that is put into a certain belief system.

Health is the willingness to let go of buying into negativity. Why would a person buy into negativity in the first place? Why are some people so receptive to programming? There are people who become fearful every time they open a magazine that reports about a current illness, which relates to the amount of fear and guilt they already carry within them. The amount of fear is really consequent to the amount of unconscious guilt. It is as though the vulnerable person is attracted by fear, and when they hear of an illness, they become mentally programmed enough to make it happen in their lives.

Health requires the willingness to adopt mental attitudes that are positive and constructive and to let go of the negative ones. The willingness to take an easygoing and forgiving attitude towards life is also beneficial, along with the unwillingness to buy into negative programming. It takes the willingness to own the power of the mind. We give our power away when we go into denial and blame an illness on something 'out there'.

The energy fields below level 200 potentiate becoming a victim. Below 200, people have given their power away and placed it on something outside themselves. At the lower levels, people have told themselves unconsciously that the source of their happiness and survival arises from something outside themselves.

When people move up into the levels of truth above 200, the energy fields are now positive, and we can see that they are re-owning their power. They now say, "I, and I alone, have the power to create happiness and opportunity in my life. It is coming from within me." They also own that health is something which comes from within and no longer believe they are the helpless victims of disease.

In reality, we are not the victims of viruses, accidents, cholesterol, or imbalanced uric acid levels. When we re-own our own power, we say, "It's my mind that has been creating that. My mind believes that eating liver and kidneys is going to give me a high uric acid level that is going to give me gout. My mind is so powerful that if I believe such a thing to be true, it will make it happen." It takes a high level of awareness to accept that the mind has that much power. "Do you mean to tell me that if I believe that eating sugar and sweets is going to give me hypoglycemia, it will?" Yes, indeed, it will.

In going back to the physics involved, it is helpful to remember that the body's energy field of 200 is weak compared to the belief systems of the 400s. The beliefs that sugar and sweets will cause hypoglycemia, diabetes, or being overweight are sufficient to bring it about. The explanations then given are denials of the truth and rationalizations to justify being a victim. When we say that it is scientifically proven, it is still just an explanation. The real science of it is the mechanism. The description of the mechanism of how this occurs on the physical plane is still only a description of the mechanism, not of cause.

Cause is on the level of mind; effect is on the level of body, not the other way around. Merely reversing that understanding provides the whole key to health and healing. Health then comes out of a positive mental attitude, which we have heard many times, so much so that many people are annoyed by it because it implies that if they have a sickness, they do not have a positive mental attitude.

What is meant by mental attitude and the part that it plays in health and freedom from sickness and suffering? Primary in the unhealthy person is unconscious guilt. The cure for that is the willingness to be forgiving, even to the point of taking a course in forgiveness, if necessary, such as A Course in Miracles, or participating in Twelve-Step recovery groups, which are specifically designed to enable one to train the mind to let go of the tendency to criticize, attack, and judge others. These are replaced by the willingness to let go of judgmentalism. Since the mechanism is unconscious, the person may not see that when the mind is being critical and judgmental of others, it is also critical and judgmental of one's own self.

Unconscious guilt contributes to the negative energy that expresses itself adversely through the autonomic nervous system and the acupuncture energy system. However, simultaneously, there is the power of refusal, the power to deny the belief system. To own back one's power requires realizing that it is the mind itself that is the cause of the illness. This truth requires the willingness to give up the position of victim and to re-own one's own power, which is necessary for health and contributes to overall spiritual growth and development. The only requirements are the motivation to move out of the negative energy patterns and the willingness to face the truth about ourselves and choose to move into a positive energy field. This can actually be done rather rapidly.

The key is the willingness to look at it and say, "Well, I don't really believe this, but it is said that my mind has the power to create an illness within my body, so I'm willing to look at that because I have an open mind." As we open our mind and are willing to agree, our intention aligns and we begin to move into accepting what we discover. We begin to find that moving into lovingness has a curative and healing effect. How is that accomplished? The willingness to forgive can move us into the willingness to be compassionate. Having compassion means the willingness to see the innocence within all things, which coincides with the willingness to forgive. Out of compassion and intention arise the power and capacity to really see into the hearts of others and discover the innocence of the child.

Within each and everyone is that intrinsic innocence that never dies, no matter how long we live; it is intrinsic to the nature of consciousness itself. The innocence of the child is what bought the mistake or the negative program in the first place. It is helpful to be aware that the intrinsic innocence of the child is still present in everyone. It is the innocence that watches television and naïvely buys into the negative programming due to its lack of discernment. The innocence of the child has no warning within it, nothing that says, "This is a world that is out to program you with as much negativity as you are willing to buy." In fact, that world gets well paid to do so because advertising is often based on appealing to the negative energy fields. All of our fears, desires, and pridefulness are represented below the level of 200. It takes the willingness to be aware that within us is our innocence, and that that innocence needs to be protected.

When we look at 'self-care', which is the capacity to love one's self, we find it now means taking responsibility to protect ourselves from the consequences of that innocence and the willingness to undo mistakes that the mind picked up as a result. We can then handle looking at ourselves and healing that which we find within us if we accept the awareness of the intrinsic innocence of our consciousness. We see that it was the innocence that was programmed. We then take responsibility for that and say, "In my innocence, I bought all that; I didn't know any better. I thought that the right thing to do was to be judgmental, to condemn people, and to judge them as right or wrong. Now I see that all that has made me sick, so I'm going to let it go." The people who were willing to look into this and go through the processes already described had complete, full recoveries from their illnesses.

The capacity to be forgiving is within us, along with the capacity for compassion. Out of it comes a general attitude about the way in which we look at ourselves. From our bigness, from our greatness, we look at our humanness through forgiving eyes and begin to forgive ourselves as well as others for all the things that were limitations and denials of the truth. All the things in the energy fields below 200 are denials of the truth; all those above 200 are the acceptance of that which is true and positive. Because the body reflects what the mind believes, and the mind reflects our spiritual position, spirit has the greatest power of all. Therefore, our spiritual position literally determines whether we have a healthy physical body or not.

Once we are willing to accept the power of mind, we have to be attentive, persevering, and not let mind get away with expressing negativity. We have to stop it as soon as we become aware of it. We begin to develop an awareness of negativity and recognize it for what it is. We let go of false humility and start questioning such remarks as, "Well, you know, I'm not very bright," or "My handwriting is poor," or "I gain weight eating the same amount of food that thin people eat." The minute we become aware of ourselves saying or thinking these limiting, self-defeating, self-attacking thoughts, we have to stop and cancel them.

The handwriting is poor because there is a belief system that we have poor handwriting, so we then reverse the whole programming of the mind as far as cause and effect. We are returning to a principle that we can demonstrate through our own experience. It is physical and the expression of the mental, not vice-versa.

We came to the conclusion that our handwriting is poor because the cause was in the mind, in the belief system. It may have been a remark picked up during childhood. Someone may have said, "Your handwriting is poor," and from that point forward, the program is operative. We have to look at the ingenuity of the unconscious mind to really see it. It would be great if one had some experience in watching hypnotic experiments. It has been shown that if a person is told their legs will be itching when they awaken, and then induce amnesia for that suggestion, when the person wakes up, they are asked how they feel. Instantly the mind will start creating the most marvelous and convincing argument of why the person's legs should itch. The person doesn't just say, "Well, my legs itch." The mind always gets creative and starts explaining, "Well, I have wool pants on, and you know I'm allergic to wool, and the heat in this room is steam heat, and that always creates the itching." It is just marvelous to listen to the inventiveness of the mind as it begins to create the reasons for the symptoms, which, as stated above, were placed within the hypnotic subject on purpose. The mind will do the same thing without formal hypnosis, so it is helpful to look at ourselves as though we have been hypnotized for half of our lives and did not even realize it.

What is hypnosis? It is suggestibility, is it not? It means to be in an unguarded, suggestible, relaxed state, so anytime we have been in that state, we have picked up all the programming, and whether we remember it or not, it is still operative. All the times we were half asleep as we sat in front of the television set, hour after hour of programming went into the mind and became unconscious hypnotic programs.

We can discover what we have been programmed with by watching to see what comes up, such as the idea that, "I'm no good. Oh, I'm no good, I'm no good. I never was very good at playing cards." If we have the belief system of not being very good at playing cards, that is what is going to operate in our life and also reinforce that belief system. The belief systems become self-reinforcing and self-fulfilling prophecies. A belief that is held unwittingly can manifest in our life, thus justifying the belief system. By looking at our lives, we can tell what beliefs are being held. If we cannot recall them, then we say they are unconscious or have been unwittingly picked up from the collective consciousness of society.

Health is the automatic expression of higher energy fields. The fields of 540 and over are the levels of gratitude, forgiveness, and healing. The willingness to be forgiving and grateful in itself automatically begins the healing process. Becoming a loving being in the energy field of love is not sentimentality or emotionalism. What the world calls love is more often about dependency, control, sentimentalism, and emotionalism. It is an emotional, sentimental attachment in which control is going back and forth, and there is the satisfaction of desiringness on both sides. This is the Hollywood version of love.

When you hear someone say, "I used to love George, but I don't anymore," it means that they never did love George. What was really meant is that they had a sentimental attachment, sort of a solar-plexus kind of a 'hanging onto', which the person romanticized and glamorized within their life, pouring a lot of emotional energy into it so that when that tie was broken, up came a lot of negative emotion.

Real love is unconditional love. Unconditional love is a decision we make within ourselves. The process is one of intention and the decision to be a loving person. If I decide to love you, that is my inner decision. There is nothing the other person can do about it. Therefore, one is not the victim of what goes on in the world because the decision to love creates a stable energy field of unconditionality. The other person's behavior may not be pleasing or contribute to what is desired, but it does not change the lovingness. For example, the mother who visits her son who is a murderer in prison for twenty years still loves the beingness, the 'is-ness' of who he really is. Of course, his behavior does not make her happy, but the love is unconditional, no matter what he does. We see examples in the world of the unconditional lovingness of the mother, and the lovingness of twelve-step groups, such as Alcoholics Anonymous. Unconditional love is not concerned with what you have or with the past.

The people at the lower levels of consciousness are very concerned with havingness and rate others based on what they have. In the middle of the Map, people are preoccupied with doingness, and their status rating depends on what they do and all the titles that go with that doingness. As they move towards the top of the Map, people are concerned with what they are, with what they have become—their 'is-ness', their beingness, that which they truly are. At that level, there is concern with a person's stature, their value, and the kind of person they have become.

The willingness to become a forgiving person who nurtures all of life nonjudgmentally automatically brings that about within oneself because of the very healing nature of that energy field. It is a condition of good health and the beginning of seeing the perfection of all things and how all things work out for the good. Illness cannot stem from that context.

For the person who is oriented in the direction of health, illness merely becomes something that is coming up in order to be healed; it is bringing up a lesson.

The illness is saying, "Look at me. Please heal what I stand for and symbolize. Please heal the guiltiness, self-hatred, and limiting thought forms. Please move up to loving me so I can be healed." The illness is a demand to grow spiritually. It is an incessant gadfly that tells us that something is 'out' and needs to be looked at. Something needs to be held in a different way.

It is not the events of life but how we hold them in mind that creates our reaction. Events in and of themselves have no power to affect how we feel, one way or another. What does affect us is our position and judgment about them, and how we decide to be with them. Our attitude, our point of view, the context, and the overall meaning give the event the emotional power over us. We can see that we are the creator of the meaning and impact it has on us.

Stress comes from our giving externals power over our life, which comes from the position of victim, of putting the source of happiness outside our life and denying the power of our own mind. The healing comes about through re-owning that power and realizing that we and we alone create the meaning of any circumstance, event, place, position, thing, or any person in our life. We create the meaning, our position, and the way we hold it. That either becomes a source of healing or a source of illness. We are the ones who determine the outcome.

Eventually we begin to see that the body is like a pet or a little marionette. It happily goes along its way as a consequence of the energy fields of joyfulness and gladness. It just sort of does what it does automatically, without thinking much about it. 'Healthy' means that we pay less and less attention to the body and enjoy it out of appreciation. It is an expression of how we are with that body.

Being healthy means we have re-owned our power as source and are not giving away the source of the body's health to the world. The exercising we do is out of the joyfulness of experiencing the body. We do not say that swimming causes the body to be healthy, but we instead come from the position that because we enjoy the body, we enjoy activities such as swimming. Those activities that the world considers healthy are the expression of our inner sense of aliveness. There is joy in allowing the body's expression in ways that the world considers healthy, not because they are causal, but because they are the effect.

The healthy enjoyment of the body is the effect of the mental attitude, of looking at it as something pleasurable, and therefore, we come to a lovingness of the body. It is not a narcissistic self-glorification, or a muscle man's picture in the photo magazine. It is not out of desiringness, pridefulness, or narcissism, but out of lovingness and gratitude. We say, "Ah, little body, you serve me well. I love you, I appreciate you, and I value you." To know that we are not the body and merely realize that if we lose our right arm, we will still say, "I am me." If we lose our left arm, we will still say, "I am me." If we lose both legs, we will still be saying, "I am me." If we remove the ears, etc., the body progressively diminishes to almost nothing, and yet, the sense of self is ever with us.

The healthy person begins to develop a sense of self that is independent of external events and of being the body itself. The person is aware that the body is the body and events are events, but "I am 'me', and that which I am is really untouched by these events." The self that wakes up every morning before it even begins to remember its name and address, where it is, and what it is supposed to do today remains unimpaired. There is the 'hardware' innocence of consciousness that in itself is unaffected by the programs of the 'software' and the events that occur throughout life. A healthy attitude is one that does not base its reality or survival on that which is transitory.

At the lower levels of consciousness, it can be seen that the person has placed their survival on something outside themselves, and that it is always transitory in nature. One thing we know about the world for certain is that all things change. Consequently, if we put the source of our happiness or our survival on that which is outside of ourselves, such as our job, our possessions, or a particular relationship, then we are merely setting ourselves up for the loss of our health because what comes up first is the fear of loss. Even though that is not conscious, we know if the source of our happiness is in our title, position, address, the kind of car we have, or even in the beauty of the physical body, we feel vulnerable. That vulnerability is in the unconscious and stores up a great deal of fear. As a result, our lives become endlessly focused on reinforcing and protecting ourselves from the loss of those things upon which we have based their survival.

Healthy persons realize the true nature of who they really are, and that they are something far beyond that. They realize they are the ones who give those things value and temporary enjoyment, but their survival does not depend on them. Previously it was said that when people move up into the energy field of acceptance, they have stopped giving their power away to the world. They have begun to accept that they are the source of their happiness. If we were to put that person on a desert island and return a year later, we know they would have a coconut business going, would have found a new relationship, would have built a tree house, and would be teaching native children. In other words, they have the capacity to re-create for themselves because they know the source of happiness comes from the realization that "I myself am the source of that happiness. I myself am the source of health. It doesn't depend on epidemics, or what is out there in the world, or what I eat." When they finally realize that, they begin to transcend and are no longer at the effect of all the false belief systems.

What kind of life is possible then? What kind of life evolves from canceling these belief systems? The mind says, "Uh-oh, if I cancel these belief systems, then I am really going to be in trouble." There is a state of mind that places its security on the worship of fear. It says that paying attention to these fearful thoughts and complying with them is why they are alive.

When motivated by the willingness to own and accept the power of the mind, the willingness to undo its mistakes and be forgiving and compassionate, there is the realization that we make ourselves victims when we place the source of happiness outside ourselves. As we begin to recontextualize our life, we ask, "What is it that gives my life meaning? What do I really value? What is it that if you were to remove it from my life, my life would still have meaning? If my job and position were taken away, what meaning would my life have then? What would it be worth? What am I willing to die for?"

Introspection and spiritual movement are necessary to achieve a state of well-being, a feeling that one's life is significant, and that we make a difference in the world. We do not need the attention that illness brings to us because our sense of importance comes through the realization of the greatness of our real Self. General growth in the field of spiritual development brings about a condition of health and can do so quite rapidly if we change our position to let go of certain limited beliefs. It does not take very long at all. First is the realization that we have the power to do it. Second is the willingness to try it out, to verify it through our own experience, and to accept the recovery of other people as an inspiration. We have enough faith in them to say, "Well, if it works for them, then I'm willing to give it a try."

In my personal as well as clinical experience, I have seen illnesses leave in a matter of minutes, days, weeks, or months. The most chronic illness that had existed for twenty-five years took perhaps two years to leave and finally did so by my constantly doing the processes that have already been described.

Some illnesses are persistent despite all one's efforts to clear away contributing factors, and the reasons are often multifactorial. One that is commonly overlooked by citizens of the culture of the Western world is the factor of karma, both individual and collective. In its broadest sense, karma merely refers to the totality of one's inheritance by virtue of human existence itself as represented by evolution, both physical and spiritual. Each human being already has a calibratable level of consciousness at birth, which is also aligned with genetic patterning.

Spiritual evolution itself may well bring up karmic patterns from the individual as well as the collective unconscious; therefore, spiritual work may paradoxically bring repressed patterns into manifestation. This is characteristic of the life histories of mystics who frequently went through periods of illness. Sometimes the basis of a persistent illness can be discerned by simple past-life recall techniques, such as hypnosis or induced altered states of consciousness. The basis for a persistent illness is often quite specific, and processing it through forgiveness of self and others for a forgotten event turns out to be curative.

Another technique is to forgive in oneself that unconscious aspect (from the collective unconscious) that was responsible for occasioning it in others and thereby bring up the inner healer from within. For example, if an illness is characterized by lameness, then forgive the one in oneself that was responsible for the lameness of others, for example. While at first such a process may seem speculative, positive results can be amazing.

Healing ensues from the willingness to accept the power of mind, and the willingness to never allow the mind to say something negative without challenging it and replacing it with a positive thought. The willingness to let go of being judgmental towards oneself and others is the result of letting go of the negative. Why is this so? It is because the energy field of that which we truly are is ever present and gives us an intense sense of aliveness when we let go of the obstacles. It is the energy field of the vibration of life itself that is constantly present.

Like the sun, the inner Self is always shining, but because of negative clouds, we do not experience it. It is not necessary to program oneself with the truth; it is only necessary to remove that which is false. The removal of the clouds from the sky to illuminate the negative allows one to experience the energy fields of that which is positive. It is only the removal of the negative that is necessary—the willingness to let go of the habits of negative thinking. The removal of the obstacles to the experiencing of this will result in an increasing sense of aliveness and a joy of one's own existence. As this joy comes in, first subtly and then more and more strongly, there is a diminished awareness of even the presence of the body, of one's physicality.

As one evolves into higher levels of happiness, there is joyfulness. The body is looked at as a source of pleasure and is held as a pleasurable and enjoyable experience. As we move towards the highest levels of consciousness, the experiencing of the body begins to diminish altogether. There is a pervasive experiencing of diffuse joy, along with an inner, progressive state of serenity, accompanied by a peaceful blissfulness. At this point, the experience of the body may disappear altogether into a kind of sublime state in which one is joyful aliveness. One becomes loving bliss, and the awareness of the body may be almost nonexistent. It is as though it is present in the room, but it is no more important than anything else in the room. There is the loss of identification with the body, and we watch it from that viewpoint as it happily goes about its business. We are no more concerned about it than we are about anything else in the room. It is a loss of identification with the separate, limited self and the limited physical. With this, the body is expressing the absolute truth, the infinite truth that one is included with the infinite Beingness of the universe. Therefore, there is the value of replacing the space that contained the negative thought which was canceled with the statement, "I am an infinite being and I am not subject to that." Because our essence is aligned with the Reality of Truth, we consequently have the power to negate falsity.

We replace everything we cancel with the truth. In place of the negative thought, we put in something that is positive because we choose to love ourselves instead. We can say, "I cancel that; I no longer buy that; I'm not subject to that. Instead, I choose to love myself." We can see that lovingness is the great healer. We have within our capacity, within our power, all the abilities of self-healing. All we have to do is remove the obstacles.

Perfect health is an expression of spiritual awareness. It is the willingness to let go of the negative and allow it to be replaced by that which is loving. The physical expression of sickness is of the lower energy field that is given form by what is held in mind. Physical health is merely an expression of a positive energy field that is reinforced by our willingness to commit to compassion and forgiveness. That which I am includes the body but is not limited to it. That which I am chooses to love it, to value it, to be appreciative of it, to be grateful for it, and to enjoy the sense of aliveness.

We eventually get to the level of the 'experiencing of experience'. We become the awareness of the joy and the thankfulness for our existence and the existence of our consciousness. The body is then included within the field of consciousness itself. We come again to the surprising thought that the body is within the mind. Most people with a limited belief system think that the mind is somewhere 'up here' in their head. Actually, when it is being experienced, it is found to be everywhere. When a thought is being experienced, it is being experienced everywhere. The thought that seems to be occurring somewhere 'in here' is itself a belief system as it is actually being experienced everywhere. It is a thought about a thought. Inner experience will tell us that the experience of the thought and the experience of the body are occurring nonlocally everywhere. Thoughts are occurring in consciousness itself. We understand that the body is sitting in the chair, but that understanding is being experienced in no specific place. It is happening within consciousness itself. Addressing ourselves to health is really addressing the nature of consciousness and appreciation for our own existence as the aliveness of life itself.

In this chapter, certain things have been repeated several times because of the mind's resistance to accepting the truth of it. Right-brain learning is really about becoming familiar with and constantly re-exposing ourselves to the same viewpoint until it becomes natural. It is difficult when we are dealing with healing and health because we are really reversing the mind's belief in causality. We are saying that the physical is the expression of the mental, and not vice-versa. The world would like to say that it is the other way around and that 'cause' is within the world, within the virus, or within the bacteria. Even medications work because of our tremendous belief that they will. It is the belief in the power of the medicine. This is certainly obvious with scientific research into the nature of placebos. Placebos alone will generally cure thirty-five percent of the people with any given illness. Just the suggestion that this pill will heal it thirty-five percent of the time is all that is necessary for it to occur. Realizing that we are making a major move in consciousness allows us to value all our knowledge about illness and health and to use it as a springboard to our own spiritual growth and development.

As in all spiritual work, it is discovered that the mind resists letting go of negative programs despite the suffering that it occasions. The source of this resistance is the secret payoff that the ego gets from negativity. The ego derives pleasure from 'justified' resentments, blame, self-pity, and all the rest. Thus, what has to be surrendered is the gratification the mind gets from the negativity. To undo the addiction to the payoff, it is only necessary to ask oneself if the suffering of the illness is worth clinging to the pleasure of the negative attitude. Secretly, people just 'love' to hate, blame, and get even as well as being 'right' or 'superior', and more. Nursing grievances extracts a cost in being prone to illness as well as resistance to recovery. Self-honesty is therefore the key to making progress and increasing well-being.

Despite all the above, it is also important to realize

that just being a human being means that one has inherited the limitations and vulnerabilities of protoplasm itself, and thus, one's days are numbered. "From dust one has arisen" and "to dust will return" signifies the value of humility and acceptance of the limitations of humanness itself. As the Buddha said, "To be born a human is a great gift for the human has the option of earning karmic merit and undoing negative karma.

CHAPTER 5

Spiritual First Aid

Next, we're going to discuss the need for spiritual first aid and the various principles we have discovered through research, including things not so generally known but of great importance to those involved in spiritual work and the spiritual aspects of life.

Previously, we have discussed the relationship between body, mind, and spirit, how the body reflects what the mind believes, and how the mind then reflects what is held in consciousness. We have also talked about handling problems directly within the area in which they are experienced, which is within consciousness itself.

As explained earlier, the body is experienced via the senses in mind. Mind does not experience itself but is experienced in a greater energy field called consciousness. This 'nonlinear' energy field is directly related to spiritual first aid.

It is valuable to create a safe context from which to approach one's spiritual work, something that is usually not taken into consideration. For the last thirty-five years, we have been researching the nature of consciousness itself. Spiritual research is not common. As a result, we have learned a great deal because not much has ever been written about it.

There are many questions the ordinary person has, for example, what can one bring to the entire field? How can one approach it? How can one create a safe context for personal investigation of these matters that are of great importance?

As we discuss all of this, we will be referring again to the Map of Consciousness. It comprises the research of many individuals and groups over the years. It is a mathematical model that represents stratified levels of consciousness which man commonly experiences. The levels have been calibrated as to the progressive power of their energy fields showing, for example, that Apathy carries much less energy than Fear. Fear has less energy than the level of Courage, and so on. These calibrations start at zero, continue upward to the level of Enlightenment at the energy field that calibrates at 600, and then on to the highest fields of Enlightenment at calibration level 1,000, which is the maximum level for the human domain.

The exact way in which the energy fields were originally calibrated is a whole field of inquiry in itself. It is possible to confirm the calibrations by using the muscle-testing method. As you may already know, it is a simple method of testing the resistance of one's arm. The subject holds out an arm and the tester presses down on the wrist. If anything that is being held in mind, such as an angry, fearful, or hateful thought, is below 200 on the Map of Consciousness (the level of Courage and Truth), the arm goes weak. It indicates nonintegrity of the energy field, and the downward direction of the energy field indicates a negative answer.

If that which is loving and true is held in mind and the arm is tested, it will be strong. You can have someone test you and say, "Anger is over 75; it is over 100; it is over 125; it is over 150; it is over 155," and you will go weak at 155, indicating that anger is around 150.

One can then ask what level Grief is and come up with 75, illustrating that grief therefore has much less energy than anger.

These are very useful calibrations and tell us a great deal of importance as to the direction of energy and whether it has a destructive, or negative, effect on our life, our consciousness, and our capacity to comprehend and reflect truth. The calibrations have a very positive effect, which we will see as we move up towards Enlightenment and Christ Consciousness. As one gets closer to the Truth, one is closer to God. As one moves toward the bottom of the scale, one gets farther away from Truth and God.

If you have someone test you when you purposely tell a lie, the arm will be weak. When you have the person test you again when you tell the truth, the arm will instantly be strong. This is a very useful indicator because it provides an orientation towards any field of knowledge or endeavor. It can also be useful in working our way through the maze of what the world calls 'spiritual'.

In the beginning of the research, we were naïve. We assumed that anything labeled as 'spiritual' must be of the highest truth, valid, and something that could be corroborated through one's inner experience. We found that this is not necessarily the case, and what is labeled a spiritual teaching might range anywhere over the Map of Consciousness, all the way from the bottom of the Map, where the teaching was written by those who teach hate as the way to truth, up to those who are most infinitely loving. We found that many of the books were of a negative energy field, meaning that one would end up in a worse condition from getting involved in that particular field of learning and would move farther away from the truth than before reading about it. Almost half the books in a typical spiritual bookstore are actually fiction.

As a result, we had to look at the value of the research itself. In looking at the field of spiritual research, we found there were no real guidelines for the person approaching spiritual work for the first time or going back into it later in life with a renewed interest. Each approach claimed that it represented the truth, so the self-claims were no indication of validity. We also found that the number of followers and the glamour and riches of the teacher of a certain pathway had no correlation with its validity—the number of followers meant nothing, and best sellers were frequently purely fictional.

A purported teacher could have a great many followers, and yet we discovered that the energy field was in a negative direction, with calibrations being very low. As we got closer to the truth of the great enlightened beings that were acknowledged by all of mankind, the energies always moved upward in a positive direction. The calibrations were always over 600 and on up into the 700s. Therefore, we see how the great teachers—those called avatars—who were on the planet for only a very short period of earthly time, changed the face of the world and the belief systems of mankind, breaking new ground and creating a whole new context and set of values because the power and energy of their words were of such a high caliber.

We will be talking about crisis, conflict, the nature of an upset, and ways of handling, transcending, and breaking through, along with practical measures for spiritual seekers. We will find that all upsets are spiritual in origin and have common sources. We will learn how to survive these inner trials and how to avoid disillusionment, despair, and self-hatred. We will discover how to detect false teachers. (See page 188, *Reality, Spirituality, and Modern Man*, or page 379, *Truth vs. Falsehood.*) We will see that all spiritual pain and suffering is really due to ignorance and will learn how to find the answer. The vulnerabilities that come from spiritual naïveté, along with crises, can be overcome by utilizing the laws of consciousness. We will see what we are hanging onto and how to let it go. We will learn how to recognize the culprit called the spiritual ego, which is behind so much spiritual crises and suffering. The spiritual world is frankly one of great confusion, with its conflicting statements and positions. We need to approach it from a position outside the field.

Referring again to the Map of Consciousness, the energy fields are calibrated as to their relative energies, starting with Death at zero, Shame at 20, Guilt at 30, Apathy at 50, Grief at 75, Fear at 100, Desire at 125, Anger at 150, Pride at 175, and the crucial point of Courage at 200. At this level, the direction of the arrows changes from negative to neutral. Above neutral, the arrows point upward, in a positive direction; this occurs when the truth is told about something. The attitudes or positions now indicate Neutrality at 250, Willingness at 310, Acceptance at 350, Reason at 400,

Love at 500, (which is a very significant level), Joy at 540; and Ecstasy at 560. Level 600 is Bliss and beyond the world of duality. It is a level of Enlightenment that reveals the true nature of God (Sat-chit-ananda).

Awareness of the true nature of God really begins at level 200 as one becomes progressively aligned with truth and then progresses upward through Willingness, Abundance, Acceptance, and an increasing Lovingness that expands in an infinite, upward direction.

Each of these levels of consciousness is characterized by correlated emotions that begin as the most negative and destructive at the bottom of the Map and lead to suicide, self-hatred, etc. Also at the bottom are guilt, the process of destruction, and seeing the world as a place of sin, suffering, temptation, and disaster. The God of that world is seen, therefore, as the ultimate destroyer who is really the ultimate enemy of mankind because he hates man and will throw him into hell forever, which is the ultimate act of hatred.

Above that is the level of Apathy, which calibrates at 50. The emotion is that of a hopeless world of despair, and the process is the loss of the energy of life. The world looks hopeless, and the God of a hopeless world is unloving, does not care for people, ignores them, and views them as sinful worms. There is an abject hopelessness, and God is thought to be truly nonexistent. There is now the existentialist who talks about the hopelessness of mankind and the death of God as coming out of this level of consciousness.

The level of Grief is one of loss, regret, despondence, and loss of spirit. It sees a world of sadness and, again, a God who is uncaring and unloving, having created a sad, hopeless world.

The level above Grief is Fear and is an energy field moving in a destructive direction. This level is characterized by worry, anxiety, panic, and terror. There is deflation, and the world looks like a frightening place. The creator and God of this frightening world is therefore a punitive god who terrifies by his unending threats.

Above Fear is the level called Desire, with which most of us are very familiar. People are entrapped by the emotions of wanting and craving. They are trapped by what they desire, and this creates the worldview of frustration and a God from whom they are separated because this god is always withholding from them what they need to feel complete and whole.

The next energy field upward is Anger and is of great importance. The energy of Anger at 150 is much greater than that of Grief at 75. A person in grief has very little energy, but it is obvious that an angry person has an enormous amount of energy. The emotions arising from this level are of resentment, hatred, and grievance, which occurred in the process in consciousness as one of expansion. From the place of anger one sees a competitive world of war, conflict, and enemies. Therefore, God becomes polarized and a retaliatory and angry god—the great punisher.

Above Anger is the level of Pride, and in its application to spiritual work, the level of Spiritual Pride at 175. It can be seen that as one moves up the scale of consciousness, there is more power. The fields begin to feel better, but Pride is still a destructive emotion, as agreed to by all the spiritual literature. It is characterized by an arrogance and contempt headed by denial. The process going on in consciousness at this level is one of inflation. Because of arrogance and contempt, a person with this attitude about their spiritual work is not going to be willing to talk things over.

The person at the level of Pride perceives everything in terms of vanity, self-importance, and status, which leads to a view of God that can be in one of two directions. It can be the atheistic position that comes out of intellectual arrogance and says that the left-brain intellect is the highest faculty of man, and, therefore, reason will decide whether God exists or not. It can also be from the position of the zealot or bigot who claims that they have all knowledge of the subject, and who is in a prideful state, arrogant and contemptuous of any other position (e.g., "death to infidels"). This obviously comes from an inflated ego. All the positions up through this level are below the line of integrity at level 200.

What happens when we cross the line of 200, the level of Courage and Truth, the level where the muscle-strength test no longer goes weak? Now a person is able to begin looking openly at questions because they are in the power to do so. The level of Courage is one of opportunity, open-mindedness, and the opening strata for anyone who is serious about spiritual work.

The next energy field is called Neutral at 250. Just below it at 200, we had an open mind, but at this level, we become unattached as the energy field now goes upward in a positive direction. We are now released and free to research, investigate, and find out for ourselves. At this energy level, the world looks okay, and the God of that 'okay' world is a God of freedom, and a God who loves one's innate capacity to want to find out the truth for oneself.

The next level is Willingness, where one has let go of resistance and attachment and has begun to say "yes" and join, agree, and align with the search for and the truth of one's inner experience of it. The person has introduced one's own positive intention; therefore, the world in which this is occurring appears friendly, and the future looks hopeful and promising. The view of the God of this kind of world is promising, hopeful, and very positive. It is the God of freedom.

At the bottom of the scale was a very negative-looking God who was more demonic, threatening, and punitive. At the level of Willingness is a God who becomes a friend, one who can be trusted. This is the beginning of a loving God and the opening where one can begin to be willing to perhaps see God as a positive aspect.

From there is the movement up to Acceptance at 350 where a person now starts to feel a certain confidence and transformation of consciousness. One realizes that the power to discover the Truth resides within the self.

The lower levels of consciousness hold that Truth is outside of self. If Truth is outside of self, it will have to be revealed by someone because the energy is so low at these levels. All the energy fields are in a negative direction, preventing one to be able to discover the truth on their own.

At the level of Acceptance, the power is re-owned within oneself. Therefore, the road begins to be a positive experience. The search now starts to become harmonious, and the God of that energy field is a merciful God who is accepting. In the re-owning of one's own power, God is pleased. This God is viewed as having a positive attitude towards one's spiritual search.

From that point, one moves up in a very positive direction to the field of lovingness at 500, which is nurturing, supportive, and forgiving. As one moves into the desire to be a loving person, the inner healings begin to take place, and one gets to experience life as loving despite its emotional ups and downs. The process of life itself and the innate nature of what is happening are loving and come from a God of Unconditional Love and lovingness. This discovery leads to an inner state of Joy. As one begins to periodically experience the joyful states, one's orientation becomes compassionate. It is the beginning of a progressive shift in process, in consciousness, and in seeing God as perfection and incredible beauty. There is movement into the capacity to see God from the viewpoint of Oneness and Unity.

Movement up toward 600 takes one into the levels that the world calls Enlightenment. There is a progressive loss of identification with the small self, which the world calls 'ego' and is commonly referred to as 'I' or 'me' because it is identifying with the various energy fields and the kinds of behaviors that ensue. As that identification and points of view are surrendered, expansion takes place as one's context of experience enlarges, and one moves upward towards the top of the scale and identification with the true Self.

The states that emerge at level 600 are termed 'Bliss'. These are states of infinite joyfulness, of experiencing an infinite Presence, and are the consequence of letting go of identification with the small self. In moving toward Enlightenment, one experiences states of illumination and sees God and the world as Oneness. One also experiences God as the Source of Existence. Within the enlightened states over 600 are the avatars, the great saints, the great teachers of mankind, the sages, and the enlightened beings.

At least now there is an idea of the way to God. God is at the top of the Map; that which is not God is in the other direction, at the bottom. This is rather clear and may seem simple when viewed; however, it is common sense and something we all intuitively know. We will refer to this in the future now that we have an orientation to the field.

That which is truthful carries greater power and calibrates at a higher number. It is a higher frequency, and in physics, the higher the frequency, the greater the power. Electrical power, for example, is not transmitted across the countryside at 120 volts; it is transmitted at 30,000 volts or even higher. The higher the frequency, the greater the power. This is why the words of the great teachers have transformed mankind for thousands of years. Their words are still active and powerful and continue to transform the consciousness of mankind thousands of years later, even though their bodies have left the planet. When we calibrate the energy fields of their work, we see that they are of enormous power, so it is not just what is said, it is the power of the being who says it.

It has been discovered that, historically, there has really been no safe context or orientation available to people approaching this field, so the way to avoid spiritual crises and the need for spiritual first aid in the future is to back up a bit and do some individual research. The first question to ask about any teaching is, "What is the level of the teaching?" This is helpful because the child within continues to be naïve and innocent. The innocence, on the other hand, is what leads to error because the innocent mind of the child has no means of discernment. It needs some way to determine what is going to be beneficial. (See list of Spiritual Teachers in Chapter 17, *Truth versus Falsehood.*)

It is obvious that if one is involved in a teaching that has an energy field below 200, one will have negative experiences. In contrast, a teaching that has a positive energy field and calibrates at a high level is going to lead into a lovingness, which is the best insurance against spiritual catastrophe. One can ask if the teaching, teacher of that teaching, or the books of the teaching are reflecting a high level. This is not to say it is right or wrong; it is just beneficial to determine its level.

If a teaching is below 200, at Hatred, for example, it will say that God hates you, your behavior, your impulses, and your humanness. Thus, this is a God of hatred, and the energy field is negative, calibrating even as low as 20, 30, or 40. At that level is hatred, the killing of others, and suicide. There is a God of death rather than of life. Self-hatred and an inner feeling of being destroyed come from this teaching. If one wishes to follow such a pathway, at least one is going in with their eyes open (e.g., terrorism).

There are the teachings of existentialism that focus on man's hopelessness. They are based upon worshipping the past in which there is a great deal of grief and self-pity toward what has befallen this group of people. There are teachings and teachers who express and exploit the energy field called Fear, in which case the person experiences a fear of God as a punitive God. The energy field is in a negative direction and continues to engender fear.

All these negative fields have proponents who sound convincing. They are like politicians in the religious or spiritual world and very adept at their convincingness. Yet, when we check their energy and direction, we find that their teaching of fear is negative and destructive. When seeing them on television, we can turn off the sound and look at their faces and fist-shaking gestures to see what they reveal when disconnected from the words. When tested, these people make us go weak, indicating that what is being taught is not Truth. Research shows that God is not at the bottom of the scale; all the teachings of hate and fear that come from the bottom of the scale indicate the reverse.

As we move up into Anger, we see those positions that promote anger, conflict, hatred, and religious wars because they are competitive and usually champion a politicized god of retaliation. Because it is a polarized position, it is always viewed that God will punish the nonbelievers, which is usually one of the traditional teachings. It is important to know where this calibrates on the scale so we can see how it correlates with those things that are truthful.

The purpose of all this is to create a safe context, a safe orientation, and a safe space in which to do our spiritual work because in spiritual work, we commit ourselves to certain goals and purposes as a result of our intention, and certain things will come up during that process. Frequently, one cause of spiritual crises is that the person forgets they initiated a process through their own intention, and their experience is a result of having asked the question, made the commitment, and aligned themselves with a search for the truth.

Defining oneself in a certain way has great power. When we look at the power of the mind, we can see how crucial its beliefs are. It has the ability to bring up within one's life the very thing one has asked for. Frequently in the middle of a crisis, the person has forgotten they really asked to bring up that which needs to be healed. Therefore, what is occurring in their life is not a mistake or an error. It is exactly what needs to be brought up, looked at, understood, surrendered, recontextualized, healed, and forgiven. As a result, one needs to maintain a compassionate view.

How can we heal what comes up in our lives unless we hold a healing position? It is obvious how critically important it is to know the energy field of a given teaching. (See Chapters 16 and 17 in *Truth versus Falsehood*. If it requires forgiveness, the teaching of the Christ is based on forgiveness. It if requires compassion and understanding, then the teaching will have to be at calibration level 500 and over because healing begins at 540. That which the world calls sin is obviously something that requires healing, does it not? Then a healing that is at least at the level of 540 is needed.

To ask people to bring up something from within into a negative energy field is to bring about upset; therefore it is unsafe to go into any spiritual teaching whatsoever that suggests introspection, soul search-ing, and purification unless the energy field of that teaching or pathway is positive and at 540 or higher. It is evident how dangerous a lower-level teaching could be—it would be like putting oneself on the operating table and letting one's abdomen be opened up by a surgeon who does not have the skill to handle what he is going to discover when he does so. We don't allow a second-year medical student to open abdomens on the operating table. Instead, it is done by someone who has the power. These energy fields have power. It requires a great deal of power and knowledge to open up someone's insides and investigate them.

We don't advise introspection in the beginning of the inner process of purification until it is determined that the teacher, teaching, and those around a person are in the energy field of at least 540, a field that is nur-turing, supportive, and forgiving and has the purpose of healing through understanding and true compas-sion. The God of that kind of energy field would there-fore be a God who loves us because healing only occurs through loving, and His love would be uncon-ditional.

It we understand the nature of God at all, we realize that that which is godly is unconditional. That which is conditional and therefore limited by definition could not be called godly. That which is God is beyond all condition and is infinite, so the love is infinite lovingness and therefore infinitely capable of healing. To create a safe context and space for ourselves, it is necessary to know that we are in a safe space, that the teacher and the teaching are positive in direction, that the energy field is at least 540, and that it holds compassion and forgiveness in a very high place within the teaching; otherwise, it will be unable to heal that which is brought forth.

In calibrating literally thousands of factors in various teachings and pathways, it consistently appeared that those who calibrated the highest and in a positive direction were characterized by the absence of teachings of hatred or condemnation in any way. It was found that great compassion and a calibration over 600 characterized the great teachers and teachings. They spoke from an infinite, compassionate forgiveness towards one's humanness and viewed it as something that needed to be healed. In the higher teachings, there is a lack of concern with a person's money or status, and there is no desire to control a person's personal life. There is no 'make wrong' or invalidation of life in any of its aspects. How is this so? For example, it is not money itself but the way it is held in mind. It is not the events of life but one's position about them.

The great teachings, which are in a positive direction, present basic principles through which one can experience the truth of oneself through one's inner spiritual work. The creation of a safe space then requires teachers who have no desire to exploit or invalidate anyone and are therefore examples of their own principles. They are devoid of exploitation of followers for 'the sake of the movement' or 'the cause'. There is avoidance of that common polarization of 'us' versus 'them'. There is a necessity to remain clear about the difference between the logical phenomenal world and that which is spiritual. There is no preoccupation with form in the spiritual world but instead with non-linear basic principles that then express through all the levels of reality.

The creation of a safe place characterizes teachers who have no wish to exploit or invalidate, so the great teachers have no interest in influencing one's money, life decisions, or personal life. Many of them actually refuse to answer questions on that level. Instead, they exemplify and speak of the teaching of a principle. It is then left up to the student or the follower to discern how to apply that principle in a given situation. As a result, there are no 'make wrongs'; there is only the teaching of a greater context from which to hold that life experience.

Referring to the Map of Consciousness, we can see how various things can be held. We can single out a world event that, in itself, is of no particular significance. It is how we hold it, the meaning we project onto it, and the significance we give it that makes the difference. In and of itself, it really has no meaning; the meaning depends on our own level of consciousness, or the level of consciousness of the teaching. We will use money as an example because it is often a source of conflict among spiritual seekers, at least in the beginning.

How would one look at money? It would depend on the energy field of the teaching or the teacher. It could be something one feels guilty about or is sinful to have. God will destroy us if we have money, and we can hate ourself for having it. The whole process is a destructive one because it is in a negative energy field with a very low calibration relating to Truth.

Money could be viewed from a higher energy field, such as Fear, in which having money would then be a frightening thing, with accompanying worry, anxiety, and panic. It would be viewed as 'unspiritual', with resulting punishment from God; or it might be the source of hatred, resentment, and grievance, with the money then being used by the spiritual group in a competitive, retaliatory way towards others, leading to anger and religious war.

Money might be held from the level of Pride, in which it is a status symbol that God has given us. The more God loves us, the more money he gives us; this thought comes from an inflated process.

When people move up to a higher energy field, they now become unattached to the money. They are released, and the money does not 'run' them any more. It is now okay to have money because the God of that energy field is a God of freedom. God is not concerned about whether one has money.

As we move up the scale into Acceptance, we might be willing to view this differently. As we move on up into the energy fields of Love and Gratitude at level

540, money might be viewed as a gift from God for which we are grateful. The money would then be a tool, a way of expressing compassion and unconditional lovingness towards the suffering of the world because the energy field of Love nurtures and supports love, life, and all its reflections. It is the beginning of a revelation because there is the release of endorphins in the brain that leads to seeing money as a loving thing and a way to support others. The intention behind it and the way it is held in mind at this level would have one viewing the money as a blessing, a responsibility, a stewardship, and a way of helping and supporting others. The money would then be used for the benefit of mankind and not as an egotistical gesture that would get one's name on a brass plate from the receiving organization. The money would be used as a gift while acknowledging the source as the love of God and seeing it as a positive expression. Everything in Creation belongs to God, including money, of which we have only temporary custody.

As one moves towards the top of the field into Oneness and perfection, one sees that all things are aspects of God, and God is All that Is. One begins to see Divinity within all things, and that this applies to everything in life. Now, instead of seeing money as sinful, it is seen as a tool God has given us so that lovingness can be expressed in a greater field and can help large segments of mankind. Money can then be held in joy from which one can feel an inner gladness that one has been given the power, with money being an expression of God's power on earth, to bring about the healing of the inner pain and suffering of mankind.

The expression and nurturing of love is the desire coming out of compassion for the relief of suffering. Money then becomes a tool to enable one to help relieve the suffering of the world. Assets are held as gifts from God, and the gifts are then used to bring about the increasing knowledge of man and the relief of suffering that occurs through the progressive increase of man's knowledge of Truth.

After the problem relating to money, the next one is always sex, is it not? We will look at sex and see how the conflicts arising around it depend on the energy field. Sex, an event in human life and part of humanness, could be viewed from the bottom of the scale (lust, addiction, craving). The teaching coming out of this energy field would perceive it as negative and associated with sin and suffering for which the God of that level is the great destroyer, with the process being one of destruction, self-hatred, self-pity, and self-blame.

The next view would be that man's sexuality is a hopeless condition—one of despair, loss of energy, and the lack of the capacity to experience aliveness. It might be viewed as sad and regretful that man is an animal. At the bottom of the scale, man is viewed as a body. As we cross the line at Truth (200), man is viewed less and less as a body, and progressively there is the realization that he is spirit. However, that which views man as a body then condemns it and is sad that man is such an animal. Those who are dominated by fear would view sexuality with worry, anxiety, and panic. They would treat the whole subject as frightening and think it best to deny and just ignore it altogether because the God of that level is punitive and would punish one for any sexuality.

Looking at the scale, one can see the various ways, including anger, with which people can hold sex. There are people who hate themselves for their own sexuality as well as those who exploit seduction. There are the perversions of religion, the satanic societies, and others in which sexuality and seduction are now reversed, and their expressions inflate its importance out of proportion.

How would sexuality be held at the level of truth? At this level, one begins to face and handle what sexuality is from a spiritual viewpoint. One begins to become empowered, to take the opportunity, because the God at this level is one of an open mind and freedom, the freedom that it is okay to explore this because at this level, one is not attached to any position about sex. At this level, one comes from humility. This means that one says, "I really don't know the answer to this subject; however, I am willing to begin to look at it." Because the willingness is a positive energy field, it says that this is a friendly, promising, and hopeful subject that one can investigate. When one's intention has been added to clear up the subject, there is a certain confidence that there is the capacity in a harmonious world with a merciful God to now explore it without being thrown into hellfire.

When sex is viewed from an energy field of 500 and over, it is now from a place of lovingness and gratitude. It is seen as an expression of nurturance, support, and healing, and that making love is a healing, forgiving act. People who have argued and fought before now melt in the embrace, forgiving, nurturing, and healing each other. They reaffirm each other's worth and value. Now sexuality becomes a gift and an expression of love. It eventually becomes an expression of unconditional love, joy, and the celebration of one's own aliveness and existence. There is a gratitude to God for the joy of existence, the beginning of transfiguration and revelation, and then the moving on to Bliss. Those who move on to higher states of consciousness see it as an expression of oneness and a way of being. It is a way of being and a way of joining the masculine and feminine energies in the world.

Sexuality, money, or anything else is held primarily as a point of view. In none of these instances can we say what a thing is, in and of itself. It cannot be taken out of the field of understanding that is concordant with its level of consciousness. When a person or a teaching expresses attitudes, beliefs, or opinions, it will be found they are all merely opinions. The essence itself is not being talked about; it is just how the person views it (perception). How they hold it in mind is an expression of their level of consciousness, their degree of awareness of truth. The lower their view, the more negative they will look at any human behavior.

All things can be viewed from a 'make wrong' position because the bottom of the scale is an endless 'make wrong', an invalidation of life in all its expressions. All man's intentions, impulses, biology, psychology, even his spiritual ambitions and the desire to be a spiritual seeker, can be invalidated because there is sure to be a skeptic who will deride it.

We can move out of this by seeing clearly that there

is the event in the world, there is life itself, human nature is what it is, and there is a way of being with that and viewing it, which is expressing a level of consciousness. We are still not saying anything about that 'out there'; instead, we are talking about one's level of consciousness. Nothing is really being said about the world itself (e.g., perception rather than essence).

All the enlightened beings at the very top of the scale say that all is God and that a 'thing' is merely what it is (essence). They place no constriction or valuation of right or wrong on it. They see the sacredness of all of existence; therefore, there is no invalidation. If all is God, then to invalidate any part of it would be to invalidate God. Man, along with his expressions, being God's creation, would least of all be invalidated by God. Instead, the great beings teach a principle that leads to understanding. The highest teachers say that if you follow a certain course, certain things will happen; they then leave the rest up to you.

A very good example of such pure teaching in our society is that of Alcoholics Anonymous (AA). AA takes no position about whether you drink or not. It does not try to close up the liquor industry or try to convince you to stop drinking. However, it does say that for those who have a problem, this is what we do, and these are the results. If you continue to drink, these will be the results. There is no 'making wrong' or invalidation. No one is looking for any power nor do they wish to exploit anyone. AA has no possessions, no royalty, no government, no buildings, and no glamour. It is just pure spiritual principle that allows an individual to have the freedom to see the truth in it for oneself and to apply it in one's own life if desired.

This is an example of a high teaching; AA calibrates at 540, which one would expect. An energy field that heals would have to be a teaching that is in a positive direction and calibrates at least at 540. AA stands, of course, as an example of healing that is based on the physical, mental, and spiritual aspects of man. It is said that no healing from addiction can occur without spiritual growth and development.

What happened in the lives of saints is that they descended to the bottom of the scale, which played a major part in their inner experience prior to their achieving a higher state of awareness. This was a consequence of their research into their inner selves. They finally brought up the very bottom of the scale and faced the formerly unconscious and then conscious conception of self as that which is ultimately separated from God. The bottom of the scale represents the ultimate separation from God.

The agony and self-hatred of the exquisite sense of sinfulness did not bring about the discovery of God within sin but instead brought about surrender. In each and every case, there was the agonizing experience of being so far from God that the person let go. There was the willingness to let go and accept God as Divinity. They then moved up to a situation called surrender, an energy field that calibrates at 575. They removed themselves from the energy field of 30 by finally giving up and surrendering to God, which opened the way to the experience of Truth.

Those who became enlightened often went through agonizing periods of facing the utmost of

negative experiencing that was buried in their unconscious, of owning their own shadow, of looking at what
they had held as most hateful and owning it, and then
letting go of it (the 'dark night of the soul'). The letting
go of what was the farthest removed from the truth in
those positions at the bottom of the scale, the letting
go of those positions that came out of self-honesty, led
to the realization of the Truth.

The progressive letting go of positions and moving
into an ever-enlarging context brings us to the overall
general nature of spiritual work itself. All that is within
the Scale of Consciousness is the ego, from high ego
states to low ego states. The letting go progressively is
beneficial because the levels represent points of
view—the letting go of judgment and vanity that come
out of prideful "I know." Surrender through humility
allows the process of revelation by which the truth is
revealed. There is the progressive process of letting go
of these restrictive positions, all of which block the
inner consciousness and awareness of the truth. This
awareness automatically emerges out of an energy field
and gets progressively higher until it finally reaches a
point where one is open to the Grace of God.

Another difficulty now arises in spiritual work and
brings about crises and conflicts, which is the use of
the term 'ego' in a pejorative, 'make wrong' kind of way.
People will say, "Well, that is only the ego."

In looking at this from the viewpoint of Truth, we
can see there is no such thing as 'just ego'. It would
mean that there is some place where God is not. All
positions represent ego, and the ego is then superimposed on that which is not ego. There has to be some-

thing larger, which is consciousness itself. To safely do spiritual work and avoid crises, it is necessary to reaffirm, look within, and discover one's own innocence. It really is not safe to do spiritual work unless one has a glimpse of that innate naïve innocence and keeps one eye on it at all times, because that innocence is the gateway back to the Truth so one does not get lost in the swamp.

How do we see that innocence and know its presence? We know that enlightened beings say that all are one with God, and consequently, that which is intrinsically innocent is within us at all times. The knowingness can occur as a matter of revelation or understanding.

If we look at the consciousness of the child, we see the child's innocence. Everyone agrees on the innocence of the child whose consciousness is not devious. It hasn't learned to lie; it hasn't learned the values of judgment and criticism. The child is openly trusting and innocent, and out of this innocence and trustingness, paradoxically, it begins to learn that which is not the truth. He or she hears the parents say, "We don't play with certain children because they are the wrong race, creed, or color; they belong to the wrong religion," and so hatred is taught to the child. In order for the child to be loyal to the family, to honor and love its mother and father, the child has to adopt that teaching.

As a result, the innocence of the child is exploited by that which is not the truth, and that which is not the truth innocently comes through, generation after generation, via the parents, grandparents, other family members, friends, teachers, television, storybooks, and novels. So that which is intrinsically innocent now begins to take unto itself programs and beliefs that are not the truth.

We can compare the consciousness of the child to the hardware of a computer, and the programming coming in from the social consciousness of the world itself is the software. We see that in the computer, the hardware, which is intrinsically innocent, is uncontaminated by the software. You can run any kind of ignorance of negativity or falsehood through a computer, and the computer itself is uncontaminated. You put in the next CD, and the computer's capacity is unimpaired. Likewise, that intrinsic innocence within consciousness itself is unimpaired, and that intrinsic innocence is reading these words right now. It is the intrinsic innocence of one's consciousness that is listening, reading, trying to find the truth, trying to tune itself in to what is real. That childlike innocence is unchanged throughout one's entire life; it never leaves.

When looking at what the world calls ego, or what spiritual work calls ego, instead of condemning it, we can see, out of innocence, that is what we believed at the time. What we did was appropriate if that software program had been correct. Therefore, we do not ever really make a 'mistake' in our spiritual work. Everything is on purpose once we set our intention to achieve an understanding of the truth and be open to Grace so that the truth may be revealed in whatever way we wish to hold in mind, in whatever expression is most appropriate. It is important to remember that we have asked for all that is in error (i.e., ignorance) to be brought up for recognition. It is all right to do that if we realize our innate innocence at the same time.

We again ask, The innocence of what? It is the innocence not of us as a person but the innocence of consciousness itself because, as a person, we are merely reflecting that which is universal as consciousness itself. What has gone on has happened as a result of the nature of consciousness; therefore, there is no point in going into personal self-condemnation about it nor, on the opposite side of the coin, going into personal pride about it.

Discovering the nature of consciousness itself and looking into the nature of that consciousness in our own introspection reveals that everything we have believed in during our whole life has happened out of innocence. Compassion and understanding develop, and because of that compassion, we can now see that, through our own innocence, we have come to believe what we believe. The willingness to forgive then allows us to see into the hearts of others. Out of our own compassion, we can see the innocence of the child over and over. No matter what the age of the body, the consciousness has remained unchanged. We can still hear the heart of the child within the adult saying "won't," "don't," and so forth; it is the innocence of the child still speaking. We need to keep an eye on that to prevent spiritual crises. It heals conflicts as they arise.

The reaffirmation of our innocence consists of never buying that anything is 'just' ego; there is no such thing as 'just' ego. Ego, the software, social consciousness, and the programming have been superimposed on that which is not ego but on truth itself and consciousness itself. All spiritual crises come from context, meaning, and the way in which a thing is held. If we think our diet is an unspiritual diet, or our lifestyle or what we do for a living are unspiritual, they are merely reflecting a certain level of consciousness.

Those who have reached very high levels of consciousness condemn nothing. They will affirm, however, that certain levels of consciousness will have consequences, and that a certain lifestyle, one of selling out the truth about oneself, will bring inner pain and grievance. It is left up to the individual to continue the process, and there is no attempt to control anyone. Certain behaviors or self-condemnation will activate energy fields that will be experienced as painful. Again, it is left to the individual to continue or not. However, it is then not seen as a threat but as merely a fact of human consciousness that inner agony can become greater than what it already is if one violates certain principles. The teaching still holds up that it can be a very high teaching even though it may warn us that very agonizing, painful states of consciousness can come about as a result of certain behaviors.

All the experience within human consciousness, including all spiritual work, represents a position, a way of being with, and a way of holding what we are always talking about. Even though we think we are talking about the external world, it is really an inner position as a consequence of a certain level of consciousness, of how we choose to be with something, and the pains and agonies that come about as a result of our clinging onto putting our survival on something that is not the truth. Pain tells us that we have put our survival onto something that is a violation of some principle of consciousness. That is really what spiritual work is about.

The progressive pain of these positions tells us that they are far from the truth, not that they are 'wrong'. As we get closer to the experience of the Presence of God, the inner experience is one of increasing joy and happiness. As we get farther from it, it tells us that we are far removed from the truth. Therefore, it is not a 'make wrong'. It is not right or wrong, it is just that it is painful and does not work.

The Buddha said that all pain and suffering are based on attachment and desire. A greater elaboration is that desire arises out of fear, which is a consequence of a sense of lack and the belief that one is separated from God. Desire itself leads to progressive frustration and a feeling of being separated from the truth. Constant wanting and craving lead to entrapment and bondage. There is no 'right' or 'wrong' about it. The consequences of this endless frustration lead to anger. Acquisition or desire leads to pridefulness and fear of loss. Failure of ambition may lead to apathy or guilt. The consequences of ego positions do not support moving toward the truth.

Noticeable is that negative energy fields tend to bring forth all the ego positions so that desire does not remain pure. It tends to bring with it anger, pride, fear, grief, and apathy. Grief tends to be accompanied by fearful, angry desire, and each of these tends to attract the other.

The critical point in all spiritual work is the capacity to be willing to tell the truth. Very often that truth is "I don't know," and out of the "I don't know" comes the willingness to surrender to God. The truth comes about through the act of surrender. The truth is not 'causing' the pain, and it is a mistake to worship the pain and think that suffering is therefore the royal road to Enlightenment. It is by realizing that the suffering within oneself is not due to the truth but to the unwillingness to let falsehood go. It is by surrender to God that the truth is revealed.

By remembering our inner innocence when we begin spiritual work, we ask to have that which is not the truth brought to our awareness. The process is therefore the evidence of success. As a result, there may be a somewhat chaotic appearance to the lives of people who are labeled spiritual seekers. The inner person is pleased because it says, "I have been asked to see what stands between me and the truth, and that has been brought up from my awareness to be recognized, re-owned, recontextualized, and healed." We provide a safe space and context about our spiritual work by being centered in the Heart—not the physical heart, but from the ultimate compassion, the owning of ourself from this level, the joy of the spiritual work, and the saying "thank you" to all the things that come up out of gratitude. The crisis is the very event of the spiritual healing. It is out of the crises that the healing occurs.

CHAPTER 6

Sexuality

Applying the knowledge derived from the study of the nature of consciousness to common human problems, we will now focus on the area of sexuality, including the difference between sex and making love, between high-energy and low-energy sex, how to transcend feeling guilty, and the effect of social programming about sexuality. We will learn how to experience it from the heart instead of from just the body; how to make it an uplifting and grand experience rather than one of manipulation and control; and how to get out of the energy interactions that result in impotence, frigidity, and sexual dysfunction.

We will explore questions like "Does God approve of sex?" "Is sex all over with advancing age?" "Does 'middle age' mean that we're 'over the hill'?" The answers will be addressed from the viewpoint of consciousness itself and from the position of 'body, mind, and spirit' about which one hears so much in the field of holistic health.

What does 'body, mind, and spirit' mean? Is it a slogan or just a catch phrase? What is 'spirit,' anyway? Is it something we can experience? Is there an energy to it that we can discover through our own research into our inner experiences? The focus will be on inner experiences, on subtle states of inner awareness and the part they play in this important area of human behavior.

Initially, we will again review the nature of the relationship between body, mind, and spirit. We will review where that human experience is experienced, and discuss and demystify consciousness itself, making it understandable. Reference will be made to the Map of Consciousness, which will be very helpful in understanding the nature of the relationship between body, mind, and spirit.

What is that relationship? First, as noted previously, is the fact that the body cannot experience itself. When talking about sexuality, everyone automatically thinks of the body and its allure, physicality, and form. Astonishingly enough, when one looks at it, there is the realization that the body is insentient in that it cannot experience itself. The arm cannot experience its armness, and the leg cannot experience its legness. Something greater than that has to take place before experience happens. The body is experienced through sensations. One experiences not the body but the sensations of the body—where it is in space and motion. The sensations themselves cannot, of their own, really experience themselves. They, too, have to be experienced in something larger, which is in mind.

When looked at carefully, one realizes they are not experiencing the body or the sensations of the body but instead are experiencing what is going on in mind about the body. Even mind itself, curiously enough, cannot experience itself. A thought does not experience its thoughtness; a feeling does not experience its feelingness. Something larger than mind has to be present, something that is unchanging in itself. The reason we become aware of what is going on in mind is because of consciousness, which is a much larger energy field than that of mind. Mind tells us what is going on in emotions, thoughts, and sensations. Sensations tell us what is going on in the body. Therefore, what we experience is always going on in the field of consciousness itself, which is like an invisible screen that is really located everywhere.

Consciousness itself is unaware of what is happening within itself. This is due to something infinitely larger than even consciousness, which is the nature of awareness—that which has no dimension or locality. We experience experience within the field of consciousness itself in handling human and behavioral problems and in understanding human behavior. We can address it directly by going to its experience within consciousness because consciousness itself is more powerful and dominant. We can handle problems that seem to be arising in the body by handling them on the level of consciousness and also on the level of mind.

When looking at human experiences and events, we see that events are one thing, but how we choose to be with them is something else. We may not be able to determine, control, or choose the events that occur in our lives, but we can determine how we wish to be with them. Therefore, the experience of how to be with them is perhaps more important than the events themselves. We all know that when we are in a certain mood, a minor irritation may be trivial. However, when in another mood, that same event can be aggravating or even send us into a rage. Therefore, how we contextualize events brings up the whole concept of energy fields.

The energy field or the position from which we perceive a situation, the way we are holding our own existence, and the importance of all events are arising out of the context created by our position. We will refer again to the Map of Consciousness, which shows the levels of consciousness, their calibrations relative to their energy fields, and the power of each energy field calibrated mathematically. This gives us an understanding in our left-brain way of comprehending things. Each level has a direction of an energy field, either positive or negative. The emotions arise from these energy fields, along with a way of viewing the world and of relating to that which is greater than our individual selves. The entire process is going on in consciousness.

All of this will come together in addressing the question of high-energy sex, that which arises out of the heart, and our way of being in the world as compared to low-energy sex, which is localized in a physical experience about which society has had so much to say over the ages. It can be seen that man's conflict about sexuality is consequent to the energy field of his position about the subject, how it is perceived, and what it means. Problems are best solved not on the level where they appear to occur but on the next level above them.

We are not going to discuss philosophy but instead, clinical experience—that which we can verify through our own experience, through human experience—and look at it from a level that is above the problems. Problems are best solved by transcending them and looking at them from a higher viewpoint. At the higher level, the problems automatically resolve themselves because of that shift in point of view, or one might see there was no problem at all. We are going to look at what appear to be sexual problems that are actually arising from an energy field, and about which we can change our position.

In general, when people talk about sex, they are referring to a type of experience, but they are also talking considerably about an energy field, the one that everybody presumes to be and the media focus on, called Desire. They are talking about a certain perception or way of looking at things; a certain wantingness; the overcoming of frustration or lack; the withholding of this or the manipulation of that; the gratification of it or using it as a trade in relationships; the allure, the price, and the value added to the allure; and, in general, they are talking about the physicality. Morality is related to physicality and the view or holding of sexuality from the physical level, or the lower energy field.

There is the story of what happened in the Garden of Eden. Man and woman were in a state of innocence in a very high nonlinear energy field where they ate of the linear tree of knowledge, the tree of good and evil. They bought into a world of duality. In contrast, in the world of Love, there is no duality. In lovingness, lovingness just is. The heart does not say anything; the heart just 'knows'. The heart is with life. In eating of the tree of right and wrong, of good and evil, what happened? They then saw themselves as mentalized bodies and came down into Guilt, which is at the bottom of the scale. From a high state of joy; a state of lovingness; a state of innocent, infinite being with life; from joy that is beyond right and wrong, they fell into a field in which they were looking at the body as an identity. They then became conscious of its naked bodyness, and out of that arose shame and mankind's sexual problems.

Whether it is an historical event or primarily merely allegorical is immaterial. Psychologically, it is an event that has happened to mankind, so the problems that man has called sexual are really due to a point of view about physicality and seeing sexuality as a physical phenomenon being run by desire. In contrast to desire is aversion, so sexuality is then characterized by desiringness, aversion, avoiding the field, wanting nothing to do with it, and taking the moralistic position that one is superior by seeing it as a physical, animal function. It even degrades that which is termed 'animal,' calling it 'carnal' as though the animal world, which was created by God, is somehow immoral. Therefore, the difficulty is not in sexuality at all, but constantly within consciousness. The view is arising out of how, in consciousness, the mind is seeing sexuality and defining these relationships.

In studying these fields of consciousness, we have learned that the level called Courage is the energy field of 200; the arrow is neutral and no longer negative. Everything below 200 is a position of victim and lack. Guilt, apathy, grief, fear, desire, anger, and pride all come from positions of lack, of not having wholeness, of not being at one with life. Holding sexuality from the physical level of Desire (calibration level 125) and dividing it according to gender into maleness and femaleness create a feeling of separation. Out of that separation comes craving; out of desire comes frustration; out of frustration come anger and resentment; and out of all that come fear, grief, and apathy. As a result, people are prone to guilt about sexuality; some are also limited by apathy, hopelessness, and lack of desire; others associate sexuality with grief; and some are fearful.

Frustration is associated with desiringness, wantingness, and then anger and pridefulness about sexuality. This is demonstrated by strutting one's macho image or sticking out one's feminine attributes in a prideful, tantalizing, seductive kind of controlling, manipulating, and exploiting way, a la Hollywood.

The marketing industry utilizes this—the desiringness, frustration, lack, and feeling of separation—and attempts to control and manipulate people. There is a pretty girl sitting on the hood of a car, but what does a car have to do with a pretty girl? The advertisement is trying to connect the two. If I get this car, or shampoo, or hair-do, or if I wear this perfume, then I will overcome this separation between me and what I desire. That point of view then creates an endless painfulness and source of suffering. The suffering takes various forms, such as impotence, frigidity, sadism, or even violence. They arise from holding sexuality from the view of its physicalness, desiringness, and lustful wantingness. One can see why many people are run by that.

Because of the nature of this energy field of Desire, the accompanying emotions are those of wantingness, greed, and cravingness, leading to an addiction to sex. Sexuality runs the sexually obsessed. Sexual obsession/compulsion results in the endless promiscuity of going to bed with anyone who is available and arises from the need to prove one's desirability.

On the right side of the Map of Consciousness, one can see that the process going on in consciousness at this energy level is that of entrapment. Within consciousness at this level, once a person wants something, that wanting begins to dominate. The desiringness and wantingness run the person. Temporary gratification fails to suffice because of the negativity of the field, and leads to endless frustration, wanting, and craving. There is no completion, no feeling of finality, and no feeling of happiness; there are only enslavement and sexual addiction.

True happiness does not prevail until one reaches the higher energy fields; therefore, trying to find happiness through the endless creation of satisfaction and the cycling of desire creates frustration. Frustration feels good when it is temporarily satisfied. It feels good when one stops banging one's head against the wall, but that is not the same thing as happiness. The desiringness and cravingness continue. It is because of this physicality and the energy field that all the moral questions arise.

Why do religion and morality address this kind of energy field, and why is it called 'carnal'? Lower-energy sexuality is held in mind in a lower viewpoint, and therefore the whole question of morality then addresses itself to that which is carnal. Carnality arises from looking down on one's animal nature instead of accepting it, being happy with it, being grateful for it, and saying it is intrinsically beautiful when it is not judged or held in a degrading manner.

How does one get out of this cycle to experience sexuality from a much different energy field and get relief from it? How does one let go of being 'at the effect of' or controlled or dominated by this instinct and run by the repetitive recycling of it? How can one view sexuality from a different energy field so that it is experienced as a totally positive experience? When it is held and viewed from a different level of consciousness, all the questions and problems begin to disappear. Then there are no such things as manipulation, withholding, frustration, or being run by desire, danger, and resentment. There is no feeling of lack if the desire is not fulfilled. Desire creates the fear that it will not be fulfilled, or grief that is has not been, or apathy, anger, frustration, or self-blame.

The bottom of the Map shows that guilt is accompanied by self-hatred. Holding sexuality from this level links to a view of the world of sin and suffering, of hopelessness and sadness. From a lower viewpoint, the whole subject of sexuality becomes frightening.

Sex becomes competitive when it is used in a seductive manner, or in a manipulative energy field of competition. Used as a symbol of status, sexual attraction becomes an illusory 'power' symbol, and the adornment of the human also becomes a symbol of status and another way of controlling, manipulating, and trying to influence one's sense of self-worth. Worry, anxiety, shame, wantingness, and resentment arise from this energy field, which often leads to hatred. Thus, there are stabbings, violent murders, and suicides based on the infatuation, seduction, and manipulation of one by another, along with the triangulations of the situations and the unconscious exploitations that occur based on this desiringness and attractiveness. The denial about this is visible, along with the contempt (e.g., 'trollop', 'whore', 'bitch', etc., or carnal rap music).

There is also pridefulness about sexual morality, which is seen as contempt, denial, or religious conflict. Prideful people often hold all sexuality from a contemptuous 'looking down their nose' viewpoint and see anyone who indulges in that kind of activity as being debased by a low animal nature. They presume that everyone else is run by it in the same way they are. People who hold contempt for sexuality are projecting their own way of being with it onto others and saying, "Aren't they carnal? Aren't they animal?"

In contrast with such views, high-energy sex, with a different energy field and a different way of being with it, then transcends all these problems—competition, frustration, fright, guilt, regret, worry, and anxiety. How can we imagine enjoying ourselves in a human endeavor that is taking place in this whole energy field while secretly feeling that God is probably going to punish us for it because the view of God that emerges out of this field is punitive? We are certainly separated from Him, and if we get any enjoyment or happiness, very likely there is expectation or retaliation in the end.

Some people cannot stand the intensity of this conflict between a driving biological urge, a psychological need, and religion, so they just avoid it altogether via atheism, which just eliminates the guilt. They have to either let go of their view of God and religion, or let go of their sexuality. For some people, this is an impossible conflict to resolve, and many of them end up as atheists because there is no way for them to handle their humanness and their views of God.

How does one move out of being run by that conflict in order to experience these experiences from a different energy field? We will contrast it with an energy field of lovingness, with sexuality as an expression of lovingness, as a sense of aliveness, and of being with the truth of that which one is. In order to have that kind of experience, one has to let go of the lower energy field in which sex is really experienced as a local physical phenomenon. Then there are all kinds of preoccupation with anatomy, such as men's preoccupation with their fitness as a sexual partner, and women's focus on the physical attributes of the body.

Along with the physicality, there are emotionality and sentimentality. Emotionality plus physicality is the expression of love—the 'mad, passionate' embrace and the expression of the emotionality of wantingness and desiringness. "Oh, how I want you!" "Oh, how I crave you!" "Oh, how I must have you," and the thrill of all that is what the movies and the media often portray. If one lets go of those perceptions, what kind of experience is possible? What kind of experience would happen if sex were no longer just local or a negativity? How would it be perceived if it happened out of the heart, out of an energy field of 500, out of the space of being with the reality and the truth of that which one is?

First, it is necessary to talk about how to let go of this driven energy field, how to avoid being run by it, how to experience sex without conflict, and how to transcend the cravingness of this energy field that causes all the problems. How can we experience it from a much higher level?

There is a technique that has worked with weight problems, with pain, and with a great variety of illnesses.

The basic principle works the same no matter what the situation is. When the energy, feeling, expression, or desire comes up, first, let go of labeling it or calling it anything. Let go of the fantasies, images, and pictures, and instead, allow the experience of what it is and the sensations of it to occur. By letting go of resisting them, they progressively diminish. The solar plexus energy fields of desiringness, cravingness, and wantingness eventually run out.

When looking at wantingness, it is apparent that it is not really a pleasurable experience. It is not pleasant to stand in front of the store window, looking at what is inside with a feeling of wanting, desire, and frustrated craving. If we look at it and cancel the content of the 'what', whether it is diamonds, a fur coat, or someone else's body, we realize that the experience itself is unpleasant. To want and not have, especially at this moment, is unpleasant. To want a steak and smell it cooking but not be able to eat it is really frustrating. If a steak is held in front of a dog's nose and he is not allowed to eat it, what is he experiencing? Is he experiencing happiness? Is he glad to be alive? If this continues long enough, the dog will end up with anger and rage at the frustration of his desiringness. It is not a pleasant feeling.

The illusion is that it is the desire itself that brings sex into our life. Actually, the opposite is true. The wantingness and desiringness are blocking sex from coming into our life, as well as the full enjoyment of it when it is present. With the letting go of resisting this craving, all the desiringess that has been repressed and suppressed comes up. If it is allowed to just be released and flow without doing anything about it, without opposing or resisting the experience of it, it begins to decompress. Eventually, because there is a limited quantity of it, it finally stops altogether. When the cravingness, desiringness, obsession, compulsion, and addiction to the wantingness and cravingness of this physicality dissipate, we are at peace. What a shocking thought! Where there were desiringness, cravingness, wantingness, and frustration; where there was a feeling of lack, of 'not havingness,' and of low self-esteem because this was not being gratified, there is now instead a state of peace.

The same thing happens when we let go of resisting food cravings and the desire and appetite for food all the time. That greediness finally lets go. These are merely varieties of greed. There can be greed for any external thing. What the world calls sexuality is often really a greediness, a wantingness, a forever desiringness that runs and dominates people and their lives.

Instead of that, there is an inner state of peace and serenity. It is as though the whole question has been handled and is no longer a problem. What is the problem now? There is no problem. It no longer drives us crazy or insults our integrity or us. We no longer have to sell ourself out or feel that we have to barter or trade our body or our sexual expression in the endless bargaining that goes on between men and women. There is no longer the tantalizing with it, the withholding, the gift of it, the "Now you owe me," or the "Now you have paid me," or the "I have paid for your dinner, now give me your body." The endless trade-offs and bargaining come to an end. We are now free of manipulation by that. Remember that when we manipulate others, we are equally manipulated in return.

When we let go of manipulating through this variety of sexuality, it means that we cannot be manipulated by it either. We become freer once we are unattached and move into the field of facing and coping with this problem. When we face and cope with it, we become unattached and released instead of entrapped.

What is the released state? It means to be so free that if something happens in our life, it is terrific, and if it does not happen, it is okay also. To be free means to be at the level of choice. Then we are not run by the world or manipulation. Every billboard does not send us to the store to buy chewing gum or whatever the pretty girl is selling. Willingness to transcend limitation moves us up to acceptance and allows us to feel adequate and confident. Feeling adequate arises from an inner knowing that somehow a question has finally been answered by life.

Where there was frustration, there is now freedom, and with it the feeling of being adequate as a human being and having far more confidence. There is the willingness to begin to move into a lovingness. The world begins to seem friendlier. If sex is desired and frustrated, it hardly looks like a friendly world. Upon surrendering desire and its associated mental images and fantasies, the world begins to look more friendly and harmonious, allowing the freedom to enjoy the opportunities for sexual expression.

As we move out of desire to acceptance, we move into an energy field where we begin to approach happiness. There is the beginning of happiness and a sense of mellowness and feeling really good about our behavior and ourself. This lovingness is the beginning of nurturance to support the willingness to forgive. There is the capacity to experience our being with this field of behavior from a different point of view. The energy field then resolves all the problems that arise in the lower energy fields.

As said previously, everything is experienced in consciousness. For example, if our consciousness were colored blue, then everything would be experienced as blueness. If our consciousness were colored pink, then all of our experiences would be experienced as pinkness. Likewise, negativity also colors the entire experience of our sexual life. Coming from lack is characteristic of lower energy fields; therefore, everything is experienced as giving and getting. Wanting means the exchange of giving and getting, so we hear expressions about sexual life by adolescent boys when they get together in the locker room, such as, "Did you get any last night?"

As we move up out of the lower energy fields of giving and getting, there appears the middle energy field of 'doing.' In this case people are preoccupied with the doingness of sex. "Let's 'do' it" is the expression. Therefore, the style of 'doing it' becomes the preoccupation. As a result, there are the endless sex manuals that talk about doingness. Some of the more modern ones even throw in some love. That is often considered to be just romanticism and something that women require to have happy sex.

The energy field of doingness has to do with how well one 'does' it. As a result, people become anxious about their performance. If sex is something we 'do', then we should do it well in our society. Therefore, there is the whole idea of competitiveness and performance. Out of performance anxiety come frigidity, lack of desire, and various forms of impotence in which there is the anxiety about 'doing it'. "Will he like the way I do it?" "Will she like the way I do it?" "Have I satisfied the other person?" It becomes somewhat redefined as a form of athletics.

Eventually, sexuality becomes a way of how to be with someone. It is a way of sharing our being with that person. It is not what we give and get; it is not how we perform as though it were a rating scale. Instead, it becomes a way of being with the person in which the whole barter system falls away. When no longer viewed from a lower position, the whole question of guilt falls and disappears, and the moralistic questions are answered. Lovingness means a connection within the heart, the opening up of a space and a way of being with that person.

The fear arises that if we let go of our desiringness and wantingness, it will mean that it will disappear from our life. Research, experience, and clinical experience show that the opposite is true. Desiringness and wantingness set up a resistance. That which we want and desire also sets up a resistance in the other person. When a salesman addresses people in his salesman style, the people know he is going to want to sell something. When we get that he wants to sell us something, resistance comes up that counterbalances what is going on in the lower energy fields.

Surrender of wantingness creates the space for the

energy field of life itself to enter the body and open up the heart. The letting go of the lower energy field opens the way for the higher energy field to express itself through the opening up of joy, joyfulness, and lovingness. There is then the desire in the relationship to bring happiness and pleasure and to support the other person's experience. There is compassion in lovemaking. There is no longer worry about performance or morality. From the energy field of lovingness, the loving of sex replaces the desiring and wanting it.

Love is nonjudgmental. It is aware of intrinsic innocence and naturalness. It now watches even the animals from a different viewpoint, seeing the expression of the grace of the animalness. When relieved of the negative, condemning, moralistic energy field, it is possible to experience the incredible beauty, perfection, and, indeed, the sacredness of the expression of our aliveness—the thrill, joy, and experience of the energy field of our aliveness. It is experienced as the sexuality of love and the love of sexuality as an expression of love.

In contrast, desiringness seems to bring with it a whole energy field that includes guilt, apathy, or grief, and then frustration, fear, anger, pridefulness, and anxiety about performance. When we are free of the cravingness of desire, we are then released from guilt and remorse, from anticipating that maybe it will not happen, and from all these energies that arise almost en masse, almost as a unit. With maturity, the integrity of the relationship becomes progressively more important, with increasing appreciation for the other person's happiness.

At lower levels of consciousness, people do not

experience the other person's energy; they experience their own energy. Sexual attractiveness, as amazing as it may seem, does not originate in the outer world. It is something that one projects onto the world. In one society, being extremely slim is attractive. In another society, being plump is attractive, or being brunette or blond, or having a bone through one's nose, or many rings around one's neck, or ear lobes that are pulled long, or symbols painted on one's head, or hair piled up. All these kinds of decorations of the human body are only projections of one's own images that are being held within. People are the source of their own sexuality.

Out of lovingness emerges the desire to experience the other person's energy. In that clear space, masculinity and femininity are mutually attractive. It is as though universal man is with universal woman, transcending the personality. Instead of a localized physical experience, now there are quite different feelings of expansiveness and oneness that arise out of being with the energy of that other person. Perhaps a second before, there was no thought of sex in the mind of either one. The couple is waiting for the toast to pop up out of the toaster. Then there is an embrace that is done in a field that is clear. In other words, the partners have let go of any withholds, resentments, or things that were obstructing their being with each other. Out of the embrace itself arises the desire that is now of a totally different nature. It is the desire to be with and experience that person and their energy. The spontaneity of it arises not out of desiringness but out of the space of the essential aliveness and energy of being with the other person. It is a diffuse, overall experience, and there is joy and gratefulness for the opportunity to be with that energy. The high joy and pleasure of that brings a sense of allness of completeness.

At the very moment that this desiringness arises in this type of energy field, it is already simultaneously complete. For example, if the phone rings and the whole setting is interrupted, it can be dropped instantly with no feeling of loss. There is no feeling of loss because the sense of completion within the heart—the oneness, the unification—has already occurred. Wonderful phenomena happen in life when we let go of being run by any particular appetite. When that happens, it is as though the experience is complete at any moment, at all times.

With weight reduction, if we let go of and disappear the hungriness, the wanting of food, and being run by hunger, the sense of wanting and desiring to eat now arises out of the eating itself. When we sit down to eat, there is still no feeling of hunger or appetite, but as we begin to eat, the enjoyment is enormous. If, however, the doorbell rings right in the middle of eating a steak, we can leave the meal and go to be with a friend without a feeling of loss or lack. It is as though the completion accompanies the enjoyment. Instead of coming from a wantingness, it is almost as though we are just this side of the experience and trying to push to the next second. We know how that is in sex, how that is in eating—we are always anticipating the next bite, the next sensation. We are always anticipating. It is like we are reaching, so there is always an internal stream between what is happening right this second and what we desire, want, and crave to happen in the next second.

When wanting, craving, and desiring are released, there emerges the feeling of being with the exact moment so that each moment is complete and total in itself. Because of its completeness, it can be stopped at any second with no feeling of loss. In a very high-energy state of joyfulness and blissfulness, there is no feeling of loss. Someone can turn off the television program we are watching without a feeling of loss. That is because we are experiencing, without control of anticipation. The nature of experiencing arises from completeness in every moment. To be with that person now, to feel at one with their energy, to feel acceptance, to feel the aliveness of that oneness, is already complete at the very moment of its experience. There is no 'have to' to continue the experience as a consequence of projecting completion in the anticipated future. The pleasure of eating is perfect without the anticipation of the next bite. In the energy fields of lower consciousness, life is experienced as going from incomplete to complete. In the higher levels of consciousness, life moves from complete to complete.

The letting go of desiringness allows the experience to be completely a state of oneness and contentment. Each moment seems to be arising spontaneously of its own. Within the embrace, the experience is happening spontaneously. It is like we are a participant in the unfolding of a movie. This happens because one has owned oneself back as source. Instead of putting the experience outside of ourself as something to get, we have owned it as something that we are. It is our way of being with that way about ourself. The experience comes from within; therefore, there is no gap between what we are and the experience.

From a lower energy field, we experience ourselves as separately 'here', and that which is desired is over 'there'. The desire is then pictured as somehow coming across, reducing the distance and the space, but there is always that feeling of space between what we think we are and what we want. Our desiringness and what we want are dualistically separated as the subject and the object. As we let go and become free of that, we then begin to experience life as spontaneously unfolding of its own. We begin to have reverence for the nature of this experience. It becomes like the state described by the mystics.

What is a mystic? It is a person who has really let go of that desiringness and is experiencing completeness and totality from second to second, and within it, the exquisite beauty, reverence, and sacredness. Now the relationship becomes an expression of that which is sacred, and there is the enjoyment of the exquisite sense of aliveness. It is as though we have transcended the world. How has it done that? It could be said that the world is that which is constantly changing, that which begins and ends, that which is limited, and that which limits us. If we identify with it, it then limits our experience to that local wanting and craving. If we let go of that, then the energy field that begins to come through the heart and unite us with that other person in this spontaneous joyfulness means that we have really transcended the world because now the energy that we are experiencing is infinite.

Experientially, the sexual experience now expands.

Instead of a local genital phenomenon, the experience expands throughout the entire body. From the entire body, it now begins to expand into a space around the body. It seems like the whole room is having an orgasm. It seems as though some kind of an infinite space is the source, and the body is merely what is happening in that space. The body becomes like the marionette that is acting out what is going on in an invisible realm that is infinite. The energy being experienced is unlimited because love is unlimited.

If we look around, we see the expression of lovingness everywhere. It has no beginning and no end. It has no limitation. The only thing that limits it is our willingness to experience it and be open to it. It is like an infinite ocean, so when we become open to it by letting go of that which opposes it, we become an expression of that lovingness. It is then experienced as an infinite space that transcends the personality as well as time and space.

The greatest aphrodisiac is that inner sense of aliveness, and as that aliveness intensifies, it is as though it awakens the totality of all of us. That feeling of lovingness and goodness is the greatest aphrodisiac of all. We are talking about the eroticism of the heart instead of the sexuality of the body. The heart is all encompassing, diffuse, and all inclusive, and it generates an intense sense of aliveness. There is that exquisite pleasure in the experience of our own existence expressed now within the energy field of being with someone whose energy matches, yet is its polar opposite. This allows the man to experience his own feminine side. He then owns it in the experience of the embrace. The woman experiences his energy field within herself, coming back to her through the man, and there is that sense of oneness and completeness in the magic of that embrace. The magic is the joining of these two energy fields, the masculine and the feminine, as an expression of their oneness out of that intense feeling of aliveness and joy.

Recontextualization settles the problems that man has talked about having to do with sexuality because, in the subtlety of that inner experience is the reconnection with the joy of our innocence. The whole question of whether God approves of sex disappears.

In the experience of that aliveness, oneness, and joy, as one moves up to an infinite state of inner peace and completion (because completion is peace), it is found that peace is that sense of absolute oneness and the rejoining with oneness. Within the sexuality that arises out of the heart is the return to the experience of being complete. It is the mystical quality of transcendence, a sense of unlimited everywhereness.

When that sense of oneness occurs, it is as though we transcend all of time, as if we have been all of men forever and all of women forever. We own the source; we are that out of which the experience arises. We are no longer at the effect of it but the expression of it, with its incredible sacredness and beauty. There is the subtlety of that inner experience as we look within.

How can this be made practical? Does it sound like fantasy, like the mystical or the unreal? Does it sound mythical, perhaps, and not really of men and women? There are certain practical ways in which one can move into it. A way to unfocus from the localized physicality of the body arises out of the ancient traditional meditative technique of focusing your attention on the point one inch below your navel and keeping it there throughout the entire experience. Just try it. That is a point the Japanese call the 'hara'. It is used in martial arts where one's focus or centeredness is. Instead of paying attention to the movements of the body, the manipulations, and the endless anxieties, concentrate and fix the attention on that spot one inch below the navel. Hold your attention there no matter what is happening, and you will find that you are somewhat removed now. In this state, one becomes the autonomous participant/observer. The entire experience now takes on a whole different dimension. It is now spontaneously happening within you, but instead of being focused on the local, you are now experiencing from a more generalized energy field. Try this as a way to move from that local experience on up to the heart. Just move into that point called 'hara' and notice the change in the quality of the experience.

When we move out of the localization, we move into a different energy field. The entire experience is then one of expansion, an expanded experience much greater in intensity, much more fulfilling and gratifying, subsequent to which we feel joyful and grateful instead of satisfied. The difference is gratitude, which is akin to joy. Instead of the satisfaction of desire, which often leaves people with a sense of loss, there is sadness. Why does it leave one with a sense of sadness, loss, incompletion, and lack? It is the result of putting the source of our sexuality out there someplace in the world instead of re-owning it as part of that which we are. The sense of innocence that arises then puts us back in the Garden of Eden as though we have not eaten the apple from the tree of good and evil. It is as though it takes us out of the field of carnality and puts us back into the field of innocence and the awareness of the truth of that which we truly are. It is, therefore, one of the greatest of human experiences.

This demonstrates the principle that it is not the events of life or what is happening but how we contextualize them that determines the nature of the experience, whether it is a guilt-inducing, frustrating, anxiety-provoking, neurotic type of dysfunction, or it is one of the greatest human experiences.

CHAPTER 7

The Aging Process

How does the relationship between body, mind, and spirit correlate with the aging process? We will learn how to identify with the aspect of ourselves that is real and to let go of those identifications with that which is unreal.

Where is it that a human experiences experience? When our research addressed that area, it was found that we are not subject to many things that the world holds to be inevitable.

Aging is a series of identifications as well as programs, stereotypes, behavioral patterns, and scripts. That which experiences life has no age and is not subject to aging. We have to ask ourselves if we are that which we are experiencing or if we are the experiencers. There are the middle-age myths, health patterns, sexual patterns, and weight problems that supposedly occur in middle age to consider, as well as the statement that the body does what the mind believes, along with the physics relating to that. Several facts and ideas will be considered, such as the fact that the body is really the effect and not the cause and is subject to what one holds in mind. There is freedom of choice to elect these various patterns. There is the adopting of family and social patterns and the influence they have on one's thoughts and beliefs about longevity.

Feeling that one's life is a contribution or a sharing makes a difference and is of value. There are some hypnosis experiments to review, along with some odd things that have occurred in science, including a clinical example called 'progeria', and what that means to us. Aging will be considered as a class phenomenon. We will also look at sex and age. The whole field of aging preoccupies everyone as they grow older, and the facts and fantasies can be examined and redefined utilizing the knowledge of the nature of consciousness itself.

The Map of Consciousness again provides an orientation to the subject of human behavior and 'who I am'. To review, the chart is a numerical model showing the relative strengths, directions of the energy fields of the levels of consciousness, and their relative power, starting with death at zero and Bliss at 600, for example. Apathy at 50 is weaker than fear at 100. Fear has much less energy than that of Courage at 200.

At Neutral, everything is okay yet has less energy than Love at 500. Below the level of Courage, or the capacity to tell the truth, all the energy fields are in a negative direction, and above this critical level, all the energy fields go upward. In other words, positive energy fields are those that nurture, support, and value life, and hold it as sacred.

The energy fields below 200 are opposed to life, do not support life, and in fact, at the bottom of the chart, they become very destructive. Loss of energy, loss of spirit, deflation, entrapment, inflation, and expansion are all negative processes and lead to viewing the world in a negative way. They also lead to seeing God in a very negative way or even denying Divinity.

It is necessary to restate the relationship between body, mind, and spirit to see what this really means because it is very important in looking at the aging process. It is necessary to know and realize through one's inner reflection and contemplation that the body is unable to experience itself. This cannot be repeated too often. The body has no capacity to experience itself. Knowledge about the body and what is going on with it arises from its sensations, but sensations in and of themselves have no capacity to experience themselves. That experience has to occur in something that is greater than the body and its sensations, its sensory mechanism, and that is mind itself. It is because of mind that one is aware of what is going on within the sensations. The sensations reveal what is happening within the body.

Mind alone, as curious as it may seem, has no capacity to experience itself. A thought cannot experience its own thoughtness; a feeling cannot experience its own feelingness; a memory cannot experience its own memoryness. In order for mind to be experienced, it has to be experienced by something that is greater than itself, and that is the energy field of Consciousness, which is greater than mind and more inclusive.

Consciousness itself, and how we know what we are conscious of, comes from an infinite field with no limitations, which is called awareness. It is because of awareness that we know what is going on in consciousness. It is because of consciousness that we know what is going on in mind. Because of mind, we are aware of what is going on with sensations. Because of sensations, we are aware of what is going on with the body. Consequently, that which we are—that which is aware, that which we really mean by the ultimate 'I'

and the infinite Self, and that which is consciousness—
is operationally many levels removed from the body.
The interesting thing is that the body expresses and
does what the minds holds. One is subject to what the
mind believes. In other words, the body, being like a
puppet, is controlled by mind, both consciously and
unconsciously. Few people realize the power of mind
over body.

When looking at the Map of Consciousness, we can
see that the physical body has a relative energy of 200
(the same as the earth). The levels of mind are energies
up to and including the 400s.

The energy field of the body is neutral—it is neither
positive nor negative. In looking at the physics of it, a
thought held in mind from an energy field of 400 then
dominates the body, which has an energy field of only
200. Consequently, the beliefs, ideas, thoughts, configu-
rations, patterns, and scripts that are held in mind are
adopted by the body and begin to reflect in the body's
physical appearance. This has been covered in our
discussions on health, illness, and giving up the various
diseases. This principle is important to consider further.

Later in this chapter are physical examples and
ways to verify the principle for oneself, for example,
how to undo the middle-age myth, the whole of idea of
decrepit old age, the idea of failing health, and the
belief system that all these things are inevitable and
must be part and parcel of the body process itself, little
realizing that they are actually coming from mind. This
can be demonstrated with very simple clinical examples, such as hypnosis.

In hypnosis, for instance, an old person who is quite

feeble walks into the office and says, "Would you like me to sit here? Can I sit in this chair here?" And he sits down as though he barely has the strength and power to sit in the chair. Then he is put under hypnosis and told that he is thirty-five years old. Then amnesia is induced so he will not remember what the suggestion was. When awakened from the hypnotic state, he is asked, "Would you like a glass of water?" and he answers, "Yes, I would like a glass of water." He then walks over to the fountain, takes a glass, fills it, sits down, and the feeble old man is gone. Where are all the shaking and the trembling? Where are the weakness and decrepitude? What has happened to the feeble old man? He seems to have disappeared!

Through this clinical example, it can be seen that through the hypnotic state, the body is reflecting exactly what the mind believes—the way it stands, the way it holds itself, and its attitude toward the body. The old man is looking at the body as though it is frail. He is preoccupied with the thought that he might fall and break his hip. As a result, holding that in mind might bring it into his life experience.

Another example is in the case of the multiple personality where one of the personalities has totally different views about health, life, and aging than the other one has. The body reflects the beliefs of the personality that is dominant at the time. If one personality believes in asthma while in the body, the body literally has asthma. But when that personality is replaced by a more pleasant personality that does not have a belief in psychosomatic illnesses, then the asthma is not present and the person has no allergies. Consequently, the physical body reflects one's unconscious belief systems as well.

In looking at how these belief systems arise, the mind first erroneously concludes that it does not have any options and thus thinks it is at the effect of the body and the ongoingness of time. In this case, the mind is giving away its power to the calendar. It pictures that the body must of necessity get older as the years go by.

A very interesting clinical example is 'progeria', a genetic condition in which the person progressively ages and becomes an extremely old, old person by the age of five, six, seven, eight, and nine years, and is often dead by the age of ten from literally decrepit old age. Death can actually occur from old age in a span of only ten calendar years.

If calendar years were the cause and the physical body was at the effect of the calendar, no such thing could occur. This information is provided to begin to open the mind to see that there are options and that what we believe, buy into, and allow ourselves to be programmed by now becomes the source, the program, and the script, and that this script begins to express itself on the physical level. When seeing it occurring on the physical level, the mind, due to its naïveté, concludes that the cause is happening on the physical level. The naïve mind sees causality on the physical level as 'A causes B causes C' within the physical realm, the turning of the calendar, and the seasons. Thus, it is causing the aging process of the body on the physical level.

In truth, something from a higher level is sequentially causing both A, B, and C. If we hold the concept in mind that goes A → B → C, then within the physical world, we first see A, then B, then C. Therefore, the left brain, because it thinks linearly and projects its concept onto the phenomena of the world, holds that A must cause B must cause C. It never suspects that the causality of ABC is simultaneously arising from a different level altogether.

The level of cause, where the power is, is the level of mind. The world of the physical is the world of effect. It creates ABC. If we hold a pattern in mind of what aging looks like and think that is what must be and happen, we create on the physical level ABC—the decrepit people—because that is what old people looked like in our childhood. We were convinced that is what someone looks like when they are eighty; thus we will look like that when we are eighty years old. If we were to look back into that person's mind and see their pictures of what an old man looks like, we would see that he looks exactly like the person standing in front of us because that was his picture of what it looks like to get old.

An experiment demonstrating what the mind believed was done with the menstrual periods in women in which they were given an injection and told that it would result in their skipping their next menstrual period. They were given an injection of a placebo, and about eighty-five percent skipped the next period and about fifteen percent experienced a lengthy delay in its onset.

These examples are not exceptions. Our interest is in the basic principle, which is that this is going on all

the time. The mind continuously reflects the patterns
and beliefs of what is being held in mind. These clinical
examples from hypnosis and research experiments are
merely isolated ones to demonstrate it clearly. We can
see that under hypnosis, the body will do exactly what
the mind believes. For instance, a patient can be hypnotized and told he is allergic to roses, and when he
wakes up, his nose will become stuffy. He will develop
hay fever and have an asthma attack right there in the
office. This experiment has historically been done
many times and recorded in the annals of psychoanalysis. This is always going on; now you can become aware
of the constant programming affecting us. The expectations of middle and old age and what they are supposed to mean are brought on by the mind out of its
naïveté.

As mentioned previously, one of the basic principles of consciousness itself is its intrinsic innocence.
Because the mind is innocent, we have to begin to carefully watch and guard it. We have to become like its
mother. The mind is like an innocent child who goes
out in the world and believes everything it hears. It
believes every billboard, every commercial, and every
remark that people make. It believes what it sees. It has
no way to evaluate it and has no sense of discrimina-
tion. We have to begin to take responsibility and say, "I
can see that my mind is intrinsically innocent, and
because the innocence of the mind of the child is still
with me throughout life, I should start looking into
what it has been buying."

In looking at the lives of many who are very
creative, one can see that they characteristically live

well into their nineties, frequently getting married at eighty-five, and even having children at ninety. Dr. John Diamond wrote an entire chapter about that and the energy of life in one of his books, *Behavioral Kinesiology*. He studied the life patterns of those people who were devoted to classical music as conductors, composers, and performers, and found that they all characteristically lived and remained productive to a very old age. It is accepted that an eighty-six-year-old conductor can lead a whole symphony orchestra and have a thirty-four-year-old wife and a young baby at home. It is a somewhat accepted occurrence with that lifestyle. Many humorists and writers live to very advanced ages, as do many people who do research and study physics. Performers such as George Burns and Fred Astaire also lived long lives.

In other words, the numerical, chronological age has no power within itself. It is our beliefs about it, how we hold it in mind, and how we genuflect to all the belief systems that go with it and that we have bought into throughout the years that have power. How is it that some people are dancing and performing at age eighty, and other people at age fifty-nine are ready for the grave?

I have a friend who, at age fifty-nine, looks like he is seventy-five. It is as if life is all over for him. He has already had two coronary bypass operations. The way he holds himself—the weakness and his whole body stance—shows what he believes old age must entail.

The first thing to realize is that we have options. We can choose to be different and to let go of the belief systems in our family. We can look back and begin to find where the belief systems about middle age and the aging process came from. What constitutes them? We can look at our own childhood and see what the relationship was with our parents, and also look at the time when their parents were middle-aged. When looking at our middle-aged parents, we can remember the pattern, which can be seen like a photograph.

To some people, middle age means having a beer belly, sitting at home feeling tired and discouraged, watching television, and complaining about life with remarks such as, "I don't have the energy for that anymore." Or getting the thought, "Well, you are over the hill," and the men start to wink at each other. "Hey, George, what? Are you a little over the hill there?" meaning middle age and forgetting about a sex life. All these programs go into the impressionable mind of the naïve child who is creating a picture of what mother looks like—tired and bedraggled. She no longer cares for her appearance and does not bother going to the beautician anymore because middle age to her now means sort of retiring from life.

Then we see people looking forward to retirement and their views of that, including retiring from life. The whole attitude is, "We'll go to Sunset Hills now and slowly wait for the sun to set. We'll join the old people's fadeout club, get progressively weaker, and watch each other go." That is an option. However, George Burns did not buy that option, nor did Alan Greenspan, or Fred Astaire. Think of all the great composers and writers, the politicians, and the powers that run this world who are well into their sixties, seventies, and even eighties. As they got older, their power, wisdom, and ability in the world grew ever stronger, not weaker. Look at all the thought systems and beliefs about what is supposed to happen to the body, all the thoughts about what we think aging must entail.

We can look at our pictures and the relationship with our parents. Did we love our parents? Interestingly, that love can be the very reason for that identification. It is because we love them that we pattern ourselves after them. If we admire our father who then develops this middle-aged pattern, we identify with and pick up the pattern, not for negative reasons, but out of admiration, innocence, and love for him, along with family loyalty. The same is true of the relationship with grandparents. We get an idea of what old age looks like.

Interestingly, I had a relatively negative view of middle age, but I also had a relatively positive view of old age; therefore, I looked forward to that time. At age seventy-six, my grandfather was up on the roof putting on a new one, and my other grandfather was dignified and elegant, so I looked forward to old age. That is the time when we can put on our spats and best hat, dress up in our best clothes, and live a really aristocratic, enjoyable life. For once, we can just be who we really are. It is going to be over before long, and therefore we do not have to cater to anybody any longer. We can really be an elegant and very loving, wonderful person, so to me, old age was not something of a faltering decrepitude. It has been that way for other people, however, so we can see that there is an option. It is about whom we love and identify with. It is all the programming that we got from television and the movies, along with the image of what aging means. The television commercials are designed to appeal to those fears of aging.

Of course, what we fear we hold in mind, and what we hold in mind tends to manifest, so the fears of old age, the very things we begin to fear, are the very things that begin to manifest. It is helpful to return to the realization that there is an option to not buy any of these pictures. Whatever picture is bought is what is going to manifest in our life; therefore, we have to be careful about what we buy into. We become the guardian of our mind. We look at it and see what it does believe, and then we forgive it for what it picked up over the years. It did not know of its own innocence and therefore picked up all of the programs, stories, and scripts, and unwittingly, we find that we are beginning to act them out.

If we want to know what life scripts we bought into, all we have to do is look at our own life and our physical self. The physical self is a reflection of what we have bought, and we may not even remember having done so due to amnesia about remarks overhead throughout childhood. People look into their memory and say, "I don't remember ever believing such a thing." Actually, we are unconscious most of our lives and have amnesia about most of it because of the millions of things we do remember. What we do not realize is how many seconds there are in one day. Do you remember what happened each second of each day? We are lucky if we can remember what we had for breakfast yesterday. Therefore, a great deal of what went on in our life is operationally forgotten in that it is not available for immediate recall. In looking at the body, we can see what programs were picked up; what its belief systems were; what was thought to be valuable or loved, or its reverse; and what it feared and brought about into manifestation because the fear was being held in mind.

The patterns of aging also follow a certain class phenomenon, and in the picture of age and aging, there is increasing longevity. It is now very normal for people to live longer, and even though they live longer, they are energetic and functional into a very advanced age. They see old age as a time of increased stature and value. This can be contrasted with a different social view where power and value come out of physical strength, and the aging patterns are more rapid. For example, in the area of sports, a participant at age thirty-two is already considered old, and at forty is considered to be an old man in the field. When certain classes of laboring people reach age sixty-five and retire, it is pretty much over, and from sixty-five onward, there is the pattern of moving into Sunset Hills, along with indolence and the loss of energy, interest and aliveness. There is the giving up of life as though retiring from a job means retiring from life. It is as if the job was the only thing that gave meaning and value to life, and now that the person is no longer classified as a 'worker', they no longer have value in the world.

There is the failure to look at oneself in a more holistic, total way and see value as something other than productivity in the workforce and the capacity to bring home a paycheck every Friday. There is the failure to see oneself as something other than just a provider, or just the mother of the children.

In women, the pattern of the aging process does

not really start until the children grow up and leave home. Suddenly, the mother joins her husband in the pattern of retiring from life. The father retires from the job, and the mother retires from raising the children. Both of them are now unemployed, with lessened value in their own eyes. Although they make a few sporadic attempts at being of some use in society, they do not really believe it. Therefore, the aging process can become progressively rapid and many people often die within a few years of retirement.

It is important to look earlier in life and constantly challenge these belief systems in order to discover something about our life that is of such value that, whether we work, bring home a paycheck, raise children, or follow a traditional, solid middle-class-America way of life or not, life still has value, and we see that we are making a difference in the world and that our life is significant. There is the willingness to share our life with others, to be a source of enthusiasm, and to contribute to the lives of those around us. We have to reevaluate the worth of our life and recontextualize it, adopt a different way of being with it, and view it differently in order to give it a different value in our own eyes, thereby raising our own energy pattern consequent to a more positive way of looking at life.

Previously we indicated that one is subject to what is held in mind. We can identify these belief systems and patterns and know that we have the option to change them. The choice is up to each one of us. We can be very active and vigorous into old age, we can have a very significant and valuable life that is highly enjoyable, and our physical health can continue right to the very end.

Everybody has life-script fantasies and looks at the advantages of different programs. That is one of the reasons we choose them. It is necessary to look at whether we are willing to let go of those that are not beneficial for the gain and benefit that we would receive from doing so.

Our life, our body, and what goes on in our life are projections of what we have been holding in our own mind. Over-experiencing is the projection of our own belief systems into the physical world. What we hold in mind manifests, and we have a choice when we see this pattern. We begin to realize that if what we experience is the result of what we hold in mind, then we can change what we experience by changing what we hold in mind.

We have to exchange the belief system we are holding for the truth that we are infinite beings and subject only to what we hold in mind. Every time negative beliefs come up, it is necessary to cancel them and insist on the truth. The collective consciousness, the energy field of the world, has to be constantly countered because the world reprograms us with it again. It may even return due to hearing a chance remark. It requires vigilance to undo all the belief systems within the mind.

The same thing happened with vision and glasses. I wore bifocal glasses for fifty years. Of course, there is the belief system in our society that middle age brings about changes in vision. Many people start using reading glasses during middle age, so when we think of a middle-aged person, we see them wearing reading glasses. The people in magazines for retired people almost always wear glasses. It is just presumed that by middle age, a person is going to need them.

Well, I already had glasses because I had the image in my mind of the intellectual bookworm, which I was, as wearing glasses. Part of the image of what I was as an adolescent included wearing glasses. Of course, if we already wear glasses, it is presumed that our vision is going to get worse by middle age, and that we are going to need bifocals. By late middle age, we are certainly going to need trifocals.

It was during this trifocal stage that I was involved in this kind of research and study. One day I was sharing with my class about all the physical illnesses that I had let go of using these consciousness techniques. There was probably a list of fifteen or twenty different diseases, and then somebody said, "Well, then, how come you are still wearing glasses?" I said, "You know, I never thought of that." I never thought of the fact that the eyeball itself and its capacity to see—the whole mechanism of vision—would be another manifestation of my belief systems about it.

I looked at the belief systems and began to cancel them, saying that I am an infinite being who is not really subject to any limitations such as the belief that I need glasses. The process took six weeks, and I could hardly see anything during that time because I was not wearing my glasses. However, I never put the glasses on again, and during that six weeks, my mobility was somewhat limited by the inability to see anything more than a couple of feet in front of me. I was myopic as well as farsighted, and I also had astigmatism. I could not read anything, nor could I see anything distant.

After about six weeks of constantly and consistently letting this go, I finally just surrendered to it and realized that part of the technique is to let go of resisting what the belief system was. Then I said, "Well, God, if I'm never going to see again, I guess I am just never going to see again." And then I just totally let it go, totally surrendering it to a higher power. And then I said, "Whatever your will is to be, I will agree to that."

What is the will of God for us? The will of God for us is complete and total happiness, wholeness, and oneness. After surrendering to God's will, suddenly, in one instant, the vision returned and was absolutely perfect after a lifetime of wearing glasses.

It does not matter how long we have had a belief system. The belief system that was present throughout my entire life and literally limited my vision was surrendered many years ago. This example is just a demonstration of the principle involved, which we experience in the level of consciousness itself. The body is a reflection of that which we believe, so if we address ourselves directly to those belief systems, to the mind itself, and to where it is being experienced, we can undo belief systems. We have that freedom and option.

Returning to the commonly held belief systems about middle age, aging, and old age, two things are occurring. There are the belief systems about what aging entails, and there is our position or the way we feel about it. In truth, it is not the events in life that have any importance, but their meaning to us. The importance of a fact or an event comes from how we feel about it, which creates a context. It creates a way of being and decides in advance how we are going to feel about that event, decision, or fact.

In referring to the Map of Consciousness, we can see there are various energy fields and levels of consciousness. The bottom of the chart represents the most unconscious level, which is farthest from the truth and closest to death itself. At the top, because of increasing truth, there is an alignment with life, with truth, and with a sense of aliveness; in other words, we might say that at the top is God.

Emotions reflect the energy field of a positionality, and out of that comes a certain view of the world as well as the view of a certain kind of God in that world. At the bottom of the Map are the levels of the lowest energy, which lead to almost passive suicide. Many deaths from old age are not due to old age at all but are forms of passive suicide, the result of having given up out of hopelessness. There is a sense of guilt, as though old age, its decrepitude, and illness are almost the punishment for one's sins or failures in life. It is as though one deserves all this, and out of self-hatred, the person chooses destruction. They see their life and the world as the experience of sin and suffering. They really fear dying because, out of their guilt, they picture God as being very punitive. There is a fear of old age as well, along with the view that it is a process of destruction, which comes from this belief system in their life that allows them to fall into the domain of this destructive viewpoint.

An energy field somewhat above but still very close to passive suicide is that of just allowing oneself to die by not caring enough about oneself. This is in the field

of Apathy, with a calibrated level of 50. It is again a negative attitude, one of hopelessness and despair in
which there is a loss of energy. In this view of old age,
the whole situation is considered hopeless. It is as
though the grim reaper—the skeleton riding on horse-
back and carrying a scythe—has the power over us,
and it seems that old age and all its conditions and
physical elements are hopeless. There is a loss of energy
with this view of the world. The loss of energy means
that, out of hopelessness and despair, we do not have
the energy to handle this life. Therefore, we see the
personal life and life in the world as hopeless and see
God as uncaring.

The next higher energy level from which to look at
middle or old age is that of Grief. This is a very common
view. There is sadness over middle age and seeing the
absence of youth as a great and terrible loss—the loss
of vigor; the loss of one's sex life; the loss of one's physical attractiveness and seductive sexual abilities; and
the loss of mental acuity, position, and power in the
world. The endless grief over these perceived losses
results in the emotion of regret, where one looks at
middle and advancing age as decline. People become
dispirited about their own lives and life in general.
There is sadness at middle age. They look at life, the
future, and progressive aging as sad. It seems as though
God is ignoring them and does not really care about
the aging process.

The next higher energy level is that of Fear, and that
energy can be utilized in a positive way. What people
need to fear are the consequences of these negative
belief systems, not old age. The danger is not in age

itself but in the negative belief systems that they have
been holding in consciousness. However, the ordinary
person fears old age itself and is full of worry and anxiety. Grief has to do with the past, and Fear has to do
with the future. The mind looks at old age out of fear
and holds worry and anxiety about the future; therefore, the world and the whole aging process look
frightening. There does not seem to be any God they
can rely on.

Next comes Desire, and out of that, the intense
craving and wanting to change all this. One aspect of
that is becoming addicted to being young and seeing
that life is where youth is. There is the resulting youth
cult expressing its fear of old age in a frantic desire to
hang on to that youth. Some people are unable to age
gracefully, as expressed through inappropriate behavior, because of their inability to let go of the desire for
youth along with misidentifying youth as life. Life is
present throughout. The same energy of life is in the
child as well as in the 'old' person.

The next energy level is that of Anger. There is anger
at the thought that one is subject to, at the effect of,
and victim of the whole progressive aging process, and
that the calendar has power over one's life. These are
all negative energy fields, and in practice, they are usually mixed with other levels. Rarely is there just one
level. Anger is also mixed with some sadness, some
hopelessness, and some guilt, and all of them tend to
occur together. There is the anger of old age and the
frustration and resentment about it. People hate and
resent the aging process and the loss of youth. There
are many young people who have not had good expe-

riences with their grandparents and hate older people; they don't want to be around them. Out of anger is a world of conflict and competition, and the projected anger of God leads to an unconscious guilt and the fear that God will retaliate.

Denial is another way to be about aging, refusing to see the options mentioned above, and holding a certain arrogance and inflated position about the process. This would be a totally negative positionality.

All these things have more to do with the truth, and to begin looking at them would then allow people to move out of these negative positions. They would be able to let go of resisting them, of being attached to them, of giving value to them. They could be released from these positions, thus allowing middle age and protoplasmic aging to start to look okay. The God of that kind of experience would be a God of freedom. There would be the freedom and willingness to see that perhaps they are the source of what happens in their life. They might say they will agree with that because their intention now is to find out the truth about the aging process. Now, middle age, aging, and the world begin to look friendly. The God of such a world is promising and hopeful.

In moving up to the level of Acceptance, people begin to re-own their power. The willingness to accept the truth now shifts the energy field from negative to positive. The truth is that we are the source of what happens to us in our life. We are the source by virtue of buying into and owning these belief systems; we bring them into our life. The truth is that we have a choice. The minute we see that there is a choice and begin to accept that, it all begins to look harmonious. The God of such a universe begins to look merciful.

We can now move into a condition of lovingness and begin to take responsibility for really loving ourself. We can begin to nurture, support, and forgive ourself for falling into these thought patterns. Why do people fall into these thought patterns? It is done out of innocence and naïveté. We think that that is the way it is; there is no thought to question it. People have not been so conscious or aware. It is only by giving examples that one can say, "Wow, it looks like I have a choice here." We stop saying, "Well, it must be that person's genetics." Or, "If I were like that, I would be glad to be alive at ninety, too." We stop excusing it and begin to really accept that it is because of the patterns we have held in life. This comes as almost a revelation to us, a sudden opening of the mind.

The way to avoid limitation is to begin to have an open mind and the willingness to look at the options and see that we do indeed have choices. Then the world starts to look loving. We now begin to love the prospects because we begin to see the advantages of middle age and old age. There are many people who look back and say, "Frankly, I wouldn't want to be young again. I mean I would hate the thought of going through the teens, the anxiety, the acne, the unknow-ingness, the stumbling around, the awkwardness, and the endless social anxiety and self-consciousness. I don't think I would care for the twenties, either, won-dering what I am going to be in this world and having terrible anxieties, such as, Will I make it through col-lege? Then there is the struggle of the thirties, when one is trying to establish a family and all those kinds of things."

Instead of now saying that the past was better than the present, one begins to say, "Hey, right here, right now, in the present, I have some beautiful options." It is like the whole world suddenly opens up anew. "I can become reborn at age sixty, so why not?"

As we move from a negative energy field into a positive one, we get closer and closer to the truth and become progressively aware that we are the experiencer, and that the phenomena which have been going on through life have not really affected the experiencer. It is like we are the hardware of the computer and the experiences are the software. The hardware is not affected by the software; that which experiences is unaffected by the experiencing, so that which we are has remained unaged. It is not subject to aging.

The inner experiencer has been unaware that a change has been going on in the body, which sometimes comes as a surprise. People look at us differently, and we wonder why. It is because that within, we have not experienced the passage of time. The real self, the true self, has not experienced anything such as aging. No such thing goes on within the truth of that which we are. This progressive awareness increases our freedom of choice and the way we wish to be with ourself.

We realize, for instance, that sexuality in old age does not decline at all but remains active, very often until the very end of life. A personal friend of mine, a world-famous person who was seventy-six, said that his sex life was better than it had ever been at any time in his life, and that it had improved to a quality he had

never even thought of as a younger man. As a young
man, he was interested in the calisthenics, the acrobat-
ics, and the performance, but as an older person with
more maturity and greater wisdom, he was interested
in the greater dimensions. He confided that, at age
seventy-six, he had just discovered what sex was really
all about, that it was incredible, and that he was just
boggled by the quality of it and what he had discovered about it.

That brings us to some of the belief systems that are
so common in our society having to do with what happens in one's sexual being at the time of male and
female menopause. There was a clinical experiment in
which a group of thirty women was given a placebo
injection and told it was a hormone that would bring
their periods two weeks earlier. The result was that the
whole premenstrual syndrome, with the bloating,
weight gain, belching, abdominal pains and colic—all
the things the various women complained of—
occurred two weeks early because they all held in
mind that it would happen. This demonstrates the
intense suggestibility, the whole belief in the premenstrual syndrome, and the symptoms that are supposed
to go with middle age in both women and men. The
belief of women in hot flashes and all the phenomena
that are supposed to occur can be induced by hypnosis, which has been demonstrated repeatedly. A young
woman is put into a hypnotic trance and told she is
going through menopause. She is asked to report her
symptoms, which are identical to the ones reported by
women experiencing menopause. The menopausal syndrome varies from culture to culture, and from class to

class within each culture, and what occurs is what is held as the inevitable. It can be seen that the mind holds the woman as a victim. It is as though the mind says, "And this is how it is." The situation is hopeless. She can only give in to it, buy into it, and be at the effect of it, thereby giving away her power.

There was the example of the middle-aged man and what is supposed to happen to him—the cold hands and feet, feeling tired and discouraged, loss of energy and libido, and the occurrence of the middle-age diseases, including diverticulitis, gout, and all the other things associated with that age group.

All these things are the consequences of the belief systems of a naïve mind. It is out of innocence that we buy into all these belief systems. By accepting our humanness, there arise compassion and a willingness to forgive ourselves for what we bought into. It is just that we did not know any differently.

The purpose of all this is to share what has been discovered—that we have an option, a choice, and that we are not victims. The way to move out of that is to choose to move up out of the bottom of the Map of Consciousness and realize that it is not hopeless. Just by education, by hearing and knowing about it, we begin to realize that life is not hopeless, yet the mind would also like to excuse its own responsibility.

If we look at the Map of Consciousness now from a slightly different view, people at the lower levels of consciousness value life and rate themselves and others based on what they have. Because that is aligned with survival, 'havingness' is important. A person's value of himself and others is based on what they 'have.' As certain people get progressively older, they cling more and more to what they have in order to give themselves a sense of value. There are certain subgroups in our culture in which havingness is predominant. It is what one has and whether they have more millions than another person that really counts, and if they lose all their money, now they are out of that society.

Moving up into the middle range, closer to the Truth and Courage, there is the energy field that sees life as opportunity. It is the part that settled America and created all the big industries. There is a powerful energy center coming out of this level where it is what we do that counts. Doingness is very important, and what we do is seen as cause. Since we are important because of what we do, there is therefore a great emphasis on doingness. We want to hold doingness as the effect rather than the cause. What we do comes from what we hold in mind, or the belief pattern, so doingness is a result and not a cause.

It is not because of playing tennis that we are happy and healthy; it is because we are happy and healthy that we express that joy of our aliveness in the form of tennis. Therefore, the doingness that is so important begins to fade out as we move and progresses in our level of consciousness.

As we get closer to the awareness of what we are, then it is who and what we are that become important. As we progress in life, it is what we have become. This is true in other cultural groups where it is what one is, what one has become, what one stands for in this, one's beingness. It is the beingness that counts, so spiritually sophisticated groups are not interested in or care about what someone has. Everyone knows that 'having' is a result of doing, and if one wants to work harder and more effectively, it will bring about havingness. They know that doingness is just a matter of exercising options. Someone can join the Board of everything and run themselves ragged; therefore, doingness no longer has status or value.

True value results from what we have become and the principles by which we live. These include committing ourself to the principle of becoming increasingly conscious and aware, committing to spiritual principles and those things that are universal and transcend the temporary, and, finally, identifying with the progressive awareness of that which we truly are. With this progressive increase in consciousness, we are no longer at the effect of the world. We no longer need to 'have' in order to realize the significance of our beingness. It is the awareness of that which we are.

This provides a different position from which to view the body. We can now look at what our relationship is with the body and see that it is something we have, not something we are. It is something that belongs to us, and now we can begin to enjoy the body and see that we have an option. We can look at it as a fun thing that belongs to us and is there for our enjoyment. If we let go of our identification with the body and realize we are not the body, we see that we are experiencing the body. That gives us options and choices. We can decide to enjoy it and see that it sort of bounces around happily, doing what it does with little effort.

By letting go of all our negative belief systems

about sickness, we can be willing to let go of all those things, and as we get older, we can enjoy a progressively healthier body. The body that I enjoy now is considerably healthier that it was thirty years ago. With progressive age, or what the world calls 'aging', the body has gotten increasingly better. I enjoyed the body much more at age sixty than I did at age forty. The body at forty was very tired because it had migraine headaches, ulcers, diverticulitis, colitis, hemorrhoids, swollen ankles, elevated cholesterol, and gout. I had to carry a cane around in the trunk of the car. So at age forty, the body was old. Now, at a much older age, I enjoy it greatly as all those illnesses are gone. With the letting go of those belief systems and limitations have come the progressive enjoyment of the body and being able to see it now as something with which to express one's happiness.

If we hold in mind that the passage of time automatically means the progressive deterioration of the body, then we are subject to that. If, on the other hand, we view time as this space that gives us the freedom to grow, to become more conscious, and to become aware, then time becomes our friend. It is over the passage of time that these illnesses of the body of middle and old age disappear. We have the time in which to explore and to become aware that there are options for how we limit ourselves by belief systems.

Recovery from many illnesses and personal human conditions can occur when these basic premises are consistently applied, but possibilities are limited by the general circumstances inherent to the human condition itself. Thus, the human body is protoplasmic and inherits the human genome. There are also karmic influences and propensities as well as programs that are inherent to the collective consciousness of mankind.

CHAPTER 8

Handling Major Crises

All of us are beset by the major crises of life at one time or another, but how many of us know how to handle death, divorce, separation, disfigurement, injury, accident, catastrophe, and those other serious events that result in emotional overwhelm? What techniques can be utilized to handle these experiences?

We will refer again to the Map of Consciousness as a point of reference for greater understanding of the question. This map is a mathematical model that represents the human ego, the self (with a small 's'). Included are the various levels of consciousness and their names according to the common human experiences of shame, guilt, apathy, grief, fear, desire, anger, pride, courage, willingness, acceptance, reason, love, and joy. As we move towards the top, we get closer to the truth. As we move toward the bottom, we get farther and farther away from the truth.

The Map shows that the numbers indicate the relative energy or power of the various levels. For example, Apathy is far less powerful than Fear. Fear has much less energy than Courage, and Neutral has less energy than Love. The relative power of these different positions reflects different points of view.

As mentioned previously, the arrows below Courage go downward, indicating that the effect is destructive, does not support life, and is in violation of truth. At the level of Truth, which is denoted as Courage, the arrows are at neutral. They then go upwards as they move into areas of lovingness, indicating that these energy fields nurture and support life and are aligned with truth.

In the time of acute catastrophic experiences, life abruptly becomes a nightmare, and one is suddenly overwhelmed by an emotional storm. However, techniques are available to handle these acute events, to shorten their duration, to relieve the pain and suffering, and to diminish the stress to the minimum.

All these major life experiences have something in common in that they all represent an acute catastrophic loss to the mind and a threat to survival. They indicate a major change and have in common the feeling of powerlessness due to their finality and permanency. The mind perceives that it is stopped and cannot do anything about them. It is this phenomenon of the permanence of being stopped and that one is powerless and cannot change the event that contributes to the intensity of the acute upset. How to handle it will depend on one's orientation to the subject and one's knowledge of the whole field of consciousness.

All these experiences unleash a storm of negative feelings, such as shock, disbelief, denial, anger, guilt, tenseness, self-blame, resentment, being undone or abandoned, rage at God and oneself, self-pity, rage at the world, and rage at the family. All these negative emotions surface and come on at once, sometimes in sequence and sometimes in combination, but in general, there is the massive overwhelm of the negative emotions of separation, loss, and intensity that all the experiences share in common.

First, there is the sequencing of shock and then resentment, disbelief, and anger. The sequencing of these emotions varies from experience to experience and from person to person; the exact sequencing is immaterial. The significance is that they unleash everything at the bottom of the Map of Consciousness.

The energy fields at the bottom of the Map are in a negative direction, and when one of these energy fields becomes strong, it tends to pull the rest below level 200 down with it. The grief over loss then seems to bring guilt with it, along with a sense of hopelessness, a fear of the future, a desire to change the whole event, and anger. The whole negative energy field is unleashed in one giant emergency. The problem is really that of being disorganized by the massive unleashing of energies.

The mind tries to use reason to handle these energies. It tries to think its way out of the dilemma and looks for explanations and reasons. The mind cannot succeed in this because the energy-field overwhelm is so massive that the thoughts really become a reflection of the negativity of the field; therefore, the thoughts themselves become negative.

Another characteristic common to all these experiences is that they are all at the top of life-stress rating scales, which numerically rate the degree of stress of certain life events from zero to 100. The ones mentioned earlier are at the top of the list. The death of a spouse, a child, or family member, along with divorce, are at the top of that scale, so they are all the maximal catastrophes that we can face in our overall experience of life. The problem to explore is how to convert them into acute gains, how to maximize them, and how to use them as springboards for major leaps in consciousness.

It is necessary to again review consciousness itself
and the relationship between body, mind, and spirit.
What is the exact nature of that relationship and how
can it help us to learn how to handle major crises? As
mentioned previously, the body is unable to experience itself. The body just is, and it is actually insentient.
We know where the body is because of sensations. We
don't experience the body; instead, we experience the
sensations of the body. Sensations themselves have no
way of being experienced but are experienced in
something greater than themselves, which is in the
mind. Our awareness of what is going on in the body
occurs because it is being reported and experienced
within mind.

Mind has no capacity to experience itself. That
seems like a shocking thought, but a memory cannot
experience its own memoryness, a thought cannot
experience its own thoughtness, and feelings cannot
experience their own feelingness. This is because they
are experienced in something greater than mind,
which is consciousness itself. Because of consciousness, one is aware of what is going on in the mind.
Mind then reports what is going on with sensations,
and sensations report what is going on with the body.
Therefore, the experiencing is several levels removed
from the body itself. In line with this, consciousness
itself is unable to actually experience itself. It is
because of the energy field of awareness that we are
able to know what is going on within consciousness. It
reports what is going on in sensations and then reports
what is going on with the body. Therefore, where we
experience experiences is considerably removed from

the physical body itself.

Because experiencing is going on within consciousness, we can address the solution for human problems directly within the field of consciousness, thereby effectively shortening and relieving the amount of pain and suffering and bringing about a far more effective result. The results of this technique and approach were demonstrated in the handling of physical pain, sickness, suffering, depression, anxiety, and fear. The same technique will work in meeting these acute emotional catastrophic emergencies since where one actually lives is in the experiencing of one's own experiencing.

A person thinks, "Well, I live in the world. I'm experiencing the world," but what is really being registered is one's experience of that experience (e.g., the 'experiencer'). We can handle anything if we address this exact focus. If we focus on where we are experiencing experience, we can handle things with precision. In moments and minutes, we can handle things that would take weeks, months, years, and, in fact, even lifetimes. We can handle within an hour something that others have been unable to handle over an entire lifetime. We know people who have experienced these catastrophic events in early life, and when we see them at an older age, it is still not over for them. The resentment, bitterness, anger, disillusionment, rage, and the major decisions that come out of those negative feelings are still with the person fifty years later. It is as though the event happened yesterday; it is still unhealed and undone, and the knowledge of how to handle the overwhelm has not been available to them.

We will relate how to handle the overwhelm at the level where it is being experienced. We look at the field of experiencing to be aware of where experiencing is happening. It is not happening out in the world, in one's foot, or in one's stomach. It is happening within consciousness. As one examines where one experiences experience, one will find that it is everywhere. One does not experience things in a focal point; that is a belief system of the mind. For example, I ask someone who is not aware of this, "Where do you experience your thoughts?" Out of habit the person points to their head and says, "Here." That is a belief system—one's thoughts about thoughts. One thinks their thoughts are in their head, but that is only a thought. Where does one actually think the thought that one believes is thought in the head? As one really considers this with a little contemplation and reflection, one will see that the actual experiencing is diffuse and going on everywhere. One could not put their finger on any particular place where experience is happening. It is simultaneously everywhere and nowhere.

Working with that point will reveal something surprising which makes this kind of work precise. I know this because I have worked with it clinically for over fifty years, and because I have been through most of the major life crises. In fact, a few years ago, I went through a half dozen and will share my experience of the truth of these things because one can experience all of them within oneself.

It is surprising that the only thing to be handled in these acute catastrophic events is the energy of the emotions themselves. If we look at the experience, we see it is not the event that happened or we think happened in the world that is the problem but the way we feel about it. Who cares about facts? They do not mean anything in and of themselves. It is one's emotional reaction to the fact. The fact is only a fact, a 'nothing'. How we *feel* about the fact is therefore the only thing we really ever have to handle about the events in life.

Our feelings come from our attitudes, beliefs, our way of being with them, and the way we view ourself in the world, thus giving variety to the emotions. However, in a state of overwhelm, the problem is the handling of just the emotional energy itself. We do not really even have to handle the emotions, just the *energy* of the emotions. "Yes," one says, "but what about the events out there? What am I going to do now with no money? What am I going to do with no husband?" and so on. Surprisingly, the events are very easy to handle. There is no acute catastrophe. The events themselves are really just handled in a mechanical way once the feelings are set aside.

There may be some reluctance, resentment, or regret, but these are minor things. The handling of the actual issues within the phenomenal world, within one's daily life, is, in contrast, much easier. They are not the real problems. The thought that they are is just coming out of the energy field of negative emotions where they seem catastrophic, hopeless, unbearable, and insurmountable. Once a person comes out on the other side of it, life adjusts itself. Something else comes in to fill the vacuum, and life goes right on. Those issues were simple to solve once the emotions were out of the way.

Life presents the solutions to all problems. Necessity is the mother of invention, so whatever dilemma appears in one's life will resolve itself, and the energy of life resumes. Life goes right on no matter how major the catastrophe seems at the moment. Therefore, the problem is not handling the event 'out there' or the circumstances of life because they will handle themselves. Usually relatives or close friends will handle a situation for the person who is impaired by the overwhelm. The problem is handling the energies that arise.

When one of these major negative energy fields starts to unleash itself, it tends to drag the rest with it. Rarely does one experience just grief alone. Guilt is almost always associated with it in blaming oneself. It may take the form of questions, such as, Why didn't I look as I went around the turn? Why didn't I put chains on? Why didn't I take her to the doctor sooner? Maybe we could have cured her cancer. Why did I bet on that horse? There is a sort of retrospective self-recrimination. There are also apathy and hopelessness—life is hopeless; life seems hopeless. It looks like we will never be happy again. It is like the source of happiness has left one's life. Of course, the grief is natural to the loss, and then there are the fears that arise—how will I live without whatever it is that I have lost?

The constant, incessant desire drives us crazy to try to change it. What can we do? There is the bargaining, the trying to manipulate, the arguing with God, and the making bargains with God: "Oh God, if you will only let so-and-so live, I'll do this and that." Then there are the anger, the rage at life and the nature of life, and the anger that is displaced onto the people of life—it is somebody's fault. All these negative energies usually unleash all at once, and from moment to moment, one or another may be dominant. At the same time, the mind is thrashing around wildly, trying to come up with explanations, trying to figure it out, and it is swamped by the overflow of energy. The problem is that the energy is just too much for the mind to process. It goes into disorganization, into adrenaline and stress-hormone biologic overwhelm, and that acute stress throws a person into a state of acute emergency within consciousness itself.

The problems are not handled on the level at which they seem to be occurring but on the next higher energy level. Higher energy means greater power. When dealt with there, they are handled automatically, which is not possible on the lower levels. All we have to handle are the energies of the emotional overwhelm. Does that seem surprising for a psychiatrist to say? Most people would expect a psychiatrist to begin talking about the psychology of the intricate relationship between the person and the events and what they mean symbolically, that is, the psychological components.

In this instance, we are going to bypass all that and instead address the energy that the emotions release; whatever the psychology may be makes no difference. There is a massive release of the negative emotions, and it is appropriate to deal with the energy of those emotions. A very effective technique to use is to ignore the thoughts because the mind will never figure them out for it does not have the capacity to do so. It is in a state of massive overwhelm. The issues are extraordinarily complex, and it would take a lifetime to unravel them if a person really wanted to know the full significance of each and every contribution from every level of one's psychological self to the total meaning of the experiences. It is not necessary to do that, and it is a very good thing to not do it. A person only has to go into the feeling itself.

Notice first that the feeling is being felt in a general way, and that there is an energy below it. It is as though consciousness works this way, as though there is a diffuse body of energy that really has no name. One might call it the energy of emotionalism, the energy behind feelingness. Given a moment of time, this diffuse, unnamed energy begins to take the form of, for example, grief, anger, rage, indignation, self-pity, or jealousy. This emotional field at first was diffuse and formless but now resembles the form of grief, but there is also some fear and anger in it. It is the energy of emotionality in general.

When given a split second longer, it will take a greater form of a specific fear, for example. "How will I live now without money or something?" The fear begins to take form, and then thoughts begin to arise out of the specific emotion of fear. It is like a sequence of events and an ocean of suppressed energy.

We are going to learn how to decompress that. If one can disconnect the fuse and pull the plug, then one is disconnected from the whole experience and left with an inner state of peace.

It will be helpful if one can accept the fact that one does not have to do anything about external events or even figure them out. A person cannot make any

progress by looking at the thoughts because they are
endless. One is not going to make much headway in
handling the problem by looking at the specific emotion, but there will be a very profound effect if one
allows oneself to focus on the energy below the upset.
As one catches the experience earlier and earlier, one
will notice that the energy is diffuse and almost nameless. It is like a container of pressurized gas that is
seeking release. Its energy has been accumulating for
a lifetime, and now it has a way out. The event that
has happened in life has opened the sluices, the
gates, the doorway, and now this container of compressed, suppressed emotional energy is using this
opportunity to escape. Once the barn door is open, all
the animals run out.

How can one get out of the way of the running
animals? One cannot; however, the experience can be
cut through quickly by accepting the fact that one
cannot escape it. To try to escape will only prolong it.
The mind will try to figure out ways to escape the
emotional energy as though that will reduce the pain;
however, the pain actually comes from resisting the
experience. To handle this, one just sits down and lets
go of resisting it, choosing instead to be with it. The
faster one opens it up, the faster the energy is let out,
and the quicker the experience will be over. The
whole thing can be released instead of allowing it to
drag out endlessly, agonizingly, through hours, days,
weeks, months, years, or even a whole lifetime.

Remember we said that when someone has an
acute injury, such as a burn on their hand, if they will
stop everything and use this same method of letting go

of resisting by just opening the door and welcoming it and saying, "In fact, I want more of it," more of the energy of that experience, and if they will ignore what goes on in mind—ignore the thoughts but allow the experience of the energy field—the mind will say, "Well, I'm experiencing grief." That is a label, so we will say that all thoughts are labels and have no reality—in reality, none of these things exist. If a loved one dies, the mind automatically says "grief," which is a label. Because the mind has power over emotions and the capacity to give them form, the belief that to lose someone causes grief gives form to the emotion. The energy field of the emotions is actually formless, but when one insists that it is grief, it then takes the form of grief. If somebody holds a gun to our head, we are naturally convinced in mind that this calls for fear; therefore, the same energy now assumes a somewhat different form labeled "fear."

It is preferable to decrease the form of the energy field and stop labeling it anything. We don't tell people, "You know, I'm going through grief; I'm going through fear; I'm going through an upset." An 'upset' is closer to the truth. It is a general term because it is very hard to say what the emotion is in an acute upset. Initially, one usually experiences a sense of shock, numbness, and disbelief that this could have happened. That is the moment to begin this practice. A person is prepared if they know about the technique in advance.

Several years ago, I went through such an experience and instantly began letting go of resisting the experience. I constantly canceled out the thoughts. For instance, the loss seemed like forever, a lifetime. It is not the loss of a lifetime that is the problem, it is the energy of the emotion that comes up about that. Once the energy of the emotion about the loss dissipates, it becomes sort of a "So what?" The problem is the acute catastrophic emotionality, so one just has to be with it. The technique is to allow oneself to experience it. In fact, to get over it in a hurry, just ask for more! Say to yourself, "I want more of it; I want more of it."

We can eventually see that this is a major opportunity. The cause of all pain and suffering is the accumulation of this compressed energy field, and life events give us an excuse. It opens the gate so we allow ourselves to feel some of it. For example, somebody bumps the fender of our car. All the suppressed anger that we have accumulated over our lifetime now has an excuse to pop out. It gets angry over the dented fender; it gets annoyed and goes into self-pity and blame. The events in life are the excuses for letting go of the compressed energy. Because it becomes unbearable, the mind finds a way to discharge it that is acceptable to us.

A person who is familiar with this will feel the compressed energy and begin to release it without waiting for the mind to create an excuse that justifies its release. The more sophisticated mind does not need an outside event to release its angriness. It just knows that it is building up some suppressed angriness and sits down and says, "I had better look at this." It then starts letting go of the energy of it before the mind gets around and creates something 'out there' to relieve itself. It is as though the events in our lives are almost like safety or release valves, providing a way to decompress this energy tank.

The technique is one of decompression. It is looking at the energy as it is being experienced. We do not have to handle the thoughts or the problems that the mind creates around this particular event. When a person looks at any life experience, they will see that they live within their feelings about it. The life event itself is really a 'nothing'. In the morning, it may look catastrophic, but by noon, it might be amusing. The event has not changed at all. The dented fender, at the moment it happens, may be an outrage of indignation. The minute we think about it, we start to feel guilty. We know very well that we turned a little too sharply ourself. Maybe an hour later we are feeling sorry for the other guy because now he has an insurance problem. We realize it really was not his fault, and we have a desire to make it up to him. Now we are into feeling guilty and blaming ourself again. Then we think about it all again, and now we go back into rage. We see what we are living with. Are we living with a dented fender? The fact is that we never really lived with a dented fender; we only lived our own inner experience of that. How we are with that is what we are experiencing. People never experience the dented fenders in life, only their emotions about them.

When we look at it from this perspective, it is not quite as bad an overwhelm. The only thing we are ever going to have to handle is the same energy, the subtle, inner feelingness, and then let go of resisting it, surrender to it, and welcome it. Saying yes to it releases its energy. After doing this for a few minutes, or maybe even an hour (it depends on how adept one is—some people get it right away and some need a little practice), a person gets where it is and no longer has to even handle or experience the emotions as such. What was fear disappears and is not felt as fear any longer. Anger is not felt as angriness; guilt is not felt as guiltiness per se. The emotion is felt as an overwhelming, upcoming flow of a negative energy that is actually generic and nameless.

When we stop naming, labeling, or calling the energy something, we no longer have to handle it. When we stop putting constructions and interpretations of the mind onto it, when we let go of wanting to make it right or wrong or the event or ourself wrong, when we bypass all that, we then get the feelingness of it and see that we do not have to handle all that. We do not have to handle the thought or even the emotions of it. All we have to do is handle the same upcoming energy.

Can we do that? Yes, we can because we are doing it all the time anyway. It is a more effective technique than wildly racing around in our mind trying to figure it out, or running around inside our feelings and trying to handle the catastrophic emotions because, at the same time, this letting go of the energy field is happening anyway.

It is helpful to become conscious of it, to cut through the confusion and get right to the essential point of what is effective. Dealing with the thoughts and the events with all the reasoning, logic, and figuring it out, and dealing with all the probing into the psychological significances is entertaining but thoroughly ineffective. It is a waste of time and energy and really delays the recovery.

The healing of an acute burn of the hand takes only a matter of seconds. How long should it take the bleeding to stop if we have cut off a thumb? It actually takes a matter of seconds. For example, when I unintentionally cut my thumb off, I instantly used this technique, and the thumb bled exactly eight drops. The instant releasing of it, the releasing of the pain, and the letting go of the resistance of the catastrophic overwhelm allowed the bleeding to stop instantaneously.

Those people who have tried this technique have had the same experience on the physical level, demonstrating the truth of this. It can be done with any emotion. One goes into the emotion, then past the emotion, and stops calling it anything. One gets in touch with the generic energy of what is coming up. It seems to come right up through the solar plexus, or it seems to be everywhere. One goes right to where the experience is being experienced. One has to use a little discipline with the mind and refuse to have the mind fool oneself. The person says, "Well, I'm experiencing the death of that person out there." One is not experiencing it 'out there'; one is experiencing it 'in here'. Where is that? It is the same place where one always experiences experience—within the feeling self.

The only problem is one's own feelingness. The real problem is not actually the death of someone 'out there'. A person is up against the energy of one's own feelingness, the overwhelm of the energy of that. If one directs their attention and focuses it there with precision, it aborts what could be a prolonged and very painful experience; it is brought to an abrupt end.

What happens if we keep on letting go of this energy? What happens if we welcome it? What if we say, "What an opportunity to decompress all this"?

What will be the experience then? It will be relatively brief compared to what it would be with an ordinary state of consciousness. Suddenly, the energy field stops. It is as though, when the pressure gauge on the compression chamber reaches a certain point, the overflow stops, and then we experience a state of peace. Right out of acute catastrophe come profound states of peace. If someone has been through this, they understand what is meant here. ***The core of relief is surrendering the energy at great depth.***

Suddenly, all the agony stops and instead, there is almost a silence, an infinite presence, an infinite state of peace, something that may be greater than any experience a person has had in their life previously. They are not the same when they come out on the other side of it. From then on, they are lighter, freer, and less subject to pain within their own emotional experience.

Clinically, what usually happens is that the person now sighs with relief. They realize that life is going to continue and they can live with it. As bad as it seemed, somehow they can survive. Peace continues for a variable period of time, and then a wave of the emotionality comes back. It tends to return in waves, with periods of relief in between. When the wave comes back, they welcome it again and try to release as much out of the pressure as they can before the valve closes again. They welcome it as a very valuable opportunity, and since it may not happen very many times in life, it is one to be treasured. The value of it comes only when a person is really on the other side of the experience and can look back on it with the wisdom that has been gained and understand that the mind is not going to be of any real help in the experience. This is because the mind looks in the wrong direction and says, "If I could only change the circumstances of the event out there, then I would feel all right." There are some good clinical examples of that.

There was the case of a woman who received a telegram saying her son was killed in Vietnam. As a result, she stopped talking, sat in a rocking chair near a window, and just kept rocking back and forth, staring numbly out the window. She was in the state called apathy, with complete loss of energy. The world looked hopeless, and to her, God was dead. She rocked back and forth in this hopeless state, not responding verbally to her family. She refused to eat, barely slept, with naps perhaps during the night, and just stared blankly out the window in a state of total apathy. We found that certain changes had taken place in her brain chemistry as a result of this, with the neurotransmitters being depleted.

In the meantime, the family did not know what to do and was very disturbed. About ten days later, the family received another telegram from the U. S. Department of Defense saying that it was all a mistake, that the son had not been killed in action, that it was another serviceman with the same name and an ID number that was just one digit different, and there had been a computer error. The family told the woman, "Mother, Mother, he's not dead!" She went right on rocking, staring blankly out the window as though she did not even hear them.

So, changing the circumstances in the outer world is not necessarily going to change the upset because it has started a process. It is the process that has to be handled. It is not the events that have happened out there that have to be accepted, because that is just what we cannot do. We cannot accept the circumstances that have happened in our life. What we can do is accept and surrender to the fact that one has to bite the bullet and be with the situation right now. For example, if our leg is caught in the bear trap and there is no way out, we surrender to the experiencing itself—the necessity to sit through it, face it, handle it, and surrender to the experiencing of the experience, using the techniques already presented.

To be effective, one pays little attention to the mind because the mind really has no solution to the problem. The mind says, "If only we could change those external circumstances." This is where people's experiences with prayer often come in. Not knowing what to pray for, they may come out of it with bitterness because they were praying in the wrong direction. Very often the prayer goes in the direction of "Please undo that, please bring joy back to life. Please bring my thumb back; please change what is happening out there." Prayer in that direction is very likely to be ineffective because the form of the prayer is like, "Dear God, please let me be one foot taller." Is the problem God's, or is the problem the lack of comprehension about how to pray?

At this point, the prayer might be, "Please be with me; show me how to surrender and handle this experience," and ask for conscious awareness of the Presence of God. We would be asking God to take on the experiencing in place of ourself. Curiously, as we keep surrendering the experiencing to the experience, as we let go of resisting and labeling it, we are progressively surrendering it.

We have to refuse the attraction to pay attention to the thought and to 'do something' out there to try to change the situation. Then arises the willingness to surrender the labeling and cause the emotional energy to take form. The total surrendering to the energy itself takes us to an inner state as we keep getting deeper into the surrender that something is experiencing, and something is handling the experiencing of the experience for ourself. It is as though the personal self now withdraws, and all we can say is that the energy is being handled.

Those who pray in that direction become aware of that which is handling the experience because, as one gets deep into the surrender of the experience, one realizes that it is being handled. It is as though some energy field, some infinite mode of existence, some aspect of beingness, is handling it. Then comes the surprising realization that one was never handling it at all to begin with, that it was some kind of illusion that was projecting oneself into it, giving it form, and identifying with what was causing the pain. The pain comes from resistance and the insistence that the personal self and all of its aspects have to handle it, that it must do something about the experience out there—sue somebody, change the house, or move to a different location—as it surrenders that along with its thinkingness. It surrenders wanting to control and change it. It surrenders to the inner experience and eventually sees it as a great gift but only when coming out on the other side of it.

To those who are aligned consciously in their lives with spiritual work, what does spiritual work look like to you? What do you think of spiritual work? What is the nature of what you call spiritual, or consciousness, or dealing with your unconscious or your superconscious? What does it look like to you?

Some people who have spent many years at it have said they see a person kneeling down and praying, or they see a person in church. They see a person at a gathering with everybody holding hands and saying "Om," and they see light in the center of the circle. They picture themselves sitting with a book and studying late until midnight or 1:00 AM. They see themselves listening to audiotapes of well-known spiritual speakers, or see themselves at convocations for 'body, mind, and spirit', or at healing services. This is a whole panorama of what the mind encompasses and calls 'spiritual work'.

When faced with a life crisis, however, it does not seem like 'spiritual' work. Spiritual work is pictured as studying a textbook, looking at a picture of a guru, and singing songs. Then an acute catastrophe occurs, and the spiritual work is bypassed. It then resumes after all the various emergencies and tasks in one's life have been handled.

It is as though we do not really see the essence of spiritual work. We do not see that the spiritual work brings up these acute crises, brings us into them, and that they are an opportunity. This is where the spiritual work is happening. The other was preparation, gathering of information and experience, deciding on direction, and accumulating spiritual knowledge. Then suddenly comes the moment of truth, the time to do it.

There are people who have been in spiritual work and around metaphysical circles for many years, and nothing changes in their lives. They have the same illnesses and problems; their personal life is the same. They have not had any of the experiences of inner truth that they hear about, and why is that? When life brings the golden opportunity to them, that is the time to make the spiritual knowledge real. It is the time for transformation, the time to take that leap in consciousness. These are golden moments.

Acute catastrophes are the times when we make great leaps, when we face them directly and fixedly say, "I will not veer from this spiritual work." Now we are really confronted with truly spiritual work. It is not reading some pleasant-sounding phrases in a book or looking at some happy picture. Instead, we are right in the thick of it, in the teeth of it. The teeth of spiritual work occur when we are confronted with that which we cannot avoid. It is the direct confrontation that requires a leap in consciousness.

These are the golden opportunities that are priceless if we see them that way, if we are willing to be with them and say, "Okay." The willingness to go with them, no matter how painful it may be, enables a giant leap in consciousness, a real advance in wisdom, knowledge, and awareness. That which we read about in the books then becomes our own inner experience.

There is something below the emotionality that is experiencing this energy out for a person. It is literally being handled by something far greater than one's personal self. If only the small personal self were present, one would be totally swamped and obliterated by the energy released during these experiences. One survives the experiences because there is something greater than the personal self that is more than capable of handling them.

The trick of the mind is to not see that. It tries to change what goes on 'out there', tries to figure it out, and then falls back on the intellect and finds that the intellect is not going to resolve this kind of problem. When we have dropped a big oak log on our foot and broken all the bones across the front of the foot, what is needed at that moment is our readiness and willingness to handle what life presents. Having the tools and the willingness brings about very rapid healing.

There is the awareness in acute overwhelm that we really can handle the experiences. Part of the panic comes from the realization that what we think we are—our powerless, limited self—is no match for the power of this experience. That is precisely what is going on—the limited, individual, personal self cannot handle the overwhelm. This is the precise spiritual value of it. What do we really want to change about the experience? We will see that what we want to do is change how we feel about it. What we can know is that the feeling will come and go. The event is not going to bother us after the feeling state. All that we have to experience through is the acute upsurge and energy of the emotion. The events will take care of themselves.

The desire to change what occurred and how we feel about it have to be surrendered. The confrontation is there, and all we can do is say yes to experiencing it through, no matter what the nature is, such as the death of a loved one, divorce, separation, an acute emergency, or a catastrophic injury. All bring about a state of shock that is the same, no matter what is the precipitating event. The shock is the sudden realization of our powerlessness, the fact that the will has met a brick wall, that we are stoppable and have been stopped, and that the personal will cannot have its way. Therefore, the shock and realization of all this is the same in all the experiences, along with the fact that it is unchangeable and permanent. That is the shock. It is as though we come up full speed against a brick wall, and every time in life when we do this, it releases the same energy field.

If you have been through more than one of these experiences in your life, you can look back and realize that this is so, and that each time the state of shock was the same. The experience and sequence were the same. There was the experience with the feeling of sudden numbness, the state of disbelief, and then the unleashing of all the negative feelings.

When we look at the negative feelings precisely and at some of the experiences we have had, we realize that we experienced all of this. We experienced the totality of that negative energy field. In the morning it would be present, and in the afternoon it would still be present. In fact, within a minute's time, we fluctuated back and forth. It is like a scintillating energy field in which the form of the emotionality is flickering from anger to resentment, to self-pity, to jealousy, to getting even, to revenge, to hate, to hating God, to hating oneself, to blaming the family and society, to blaming the government and laws. The mind wildly races around in this negative energy field. We can see the diffuseness and formlessness of it. It is like a basketful of negative energy, and we only have to handle the basket, not all the little things that are flickering around in it. We only have to handle the 'all' of it. When we see that it is decompressing the 'all' of it, it moves us rapidly through it and out the other side. We see that it is an inescapable experience, and we must have the willingness to surrender to the work that has to be done now. How can we tell when that work is finished? When we suddenly come out into that inner state of peace.

We know that years later people continue to have resentment and anger and are still caught in some aspect of that negative energy field because the events were not handled in the first place. The person was unwilling to sit down and handle them until completed. People are unwilling to do this because of the pain involved and because they do not know the techniques to use. Every time they go at it, they again start trying to change the events in the world and handle the thoughts. The intellect and the mind try to figure it out, and the person runs into the same impasse. By not having an effective tool with which to handle the events, the work remains incomplete.

What happens with the incomplete work and the emotions that were not released? That which is left undone begins to express itself in emotional attitudes and in the body in the form of illness. The unconscious guilt that was not let go of over the catastrophe that happened many years ago comes forth through the autonomic nervous system and the acupuncture energy system and connects with something from the mind.

The energy field of the intellect of thinkingness is in the 400s. The energy field of guilt, fear, or anger then couples with some belief system in the mind about a particular illness that results in a physical illness. In psychoanalysis, it would be called psychosomatic, and in this case, the contribution of the psychological element is on the surface and quite visible. The end result of the unresolved emotional handling of a catastrophic experience is often an illness that may occur many years later. The grief that was left undone at the time of the death of some family member twenty years earlier, for example, may now express itself as a heart attack.

A thing has been handled when we feel at peace and complete with it. It no longer recurs or brings up pain when we think about it; we feel satisfied. There may be regret about having to live through it, but somehow we come out on the other side of it as a different kind of person, and with that knowledge, there is a certain sense of peace that lets us know it has been handled now.

Catastrophic experiences are the seeds, the very essence, of the ultimate spiritual experience. Within it and following it to its very center core, totally walking off the cliff in complete abandonment, the full surrender to the experience is the very seed and core of that which the spiritual seeker has been searching for all along.

With many catastrophic situations in ordinary life, there is an incomplete resolution of the experiences, along with a lack of awareness of the jewel-like qualities and opportunities within the events. We are overwhelmed by the 'whatness' of them and look in the wrong direction. The mind also gets a secret payoff from negative emotions (e.g., attention, self-pity, drama) plus indulgence in martyrdom, etc.

Many times when drugs are introduced, altered states of consciousness occur, and the person is taken to the emergency room. What could be a crucial spiritual discovery is covered over with a band-aid, and the family tries to distract the person from the spiritual work.

The essential aspect of the spiritual benefit comes from running directly into the experience. There is a saying in Zen to "Walk straight ahead, no matter what," so when this catastrophic experience comes, it is beneficial to center oneself right into the core of it, say "yes" to it and experience it through.

There have been catastrophic experiences in my life when band-aids were available, and I refused to accept them because by then I had learned the value of experiencing them through. The band-aids really prevent the experiencing through of what might be called 'hitting bottom'. The concept of hitting bottom, which is well known in handling many serious problems, such as alcoholism, means to let go completely.

In an acute catastrophic situation, the mind tries to cling to that which is familiar. It tries escapism, distractions, tranquilizers, drugs and alcohol, and various other ways of trying to ameliorate the situation rather than face it directly and work through it.

The essence of a catastrophic situation is total surrender to the discovery of that which is greater than the personal self. The experiencing through completely of a catastrophe brings us into a connection and a real-

ization that there is something within ourself that has
the power to sustain, no matter how catastrophic the
experience appears to be. As a result, we come out on
the other side of it as a greater person with the awareness that there is something within, that there is a
Presence, a quality, or an aspect of life within that has
the power to sustain us through the most seemingly
impossible situations.

If the catastrophic experience is not worked
through completely, there are certain residuals. It is like
we have only halfway fallen off the cliff. Some people
think they have walked off the cliff, but actually we
find that they were secretly crossing their fingers and
hanging onto some little outcropping or lifeline. The
abandonment to God was not really total, so a doubt
remains, and out of that doubt is the residual of, for
example, grief or fear of the experience. If we do not
experience something greater than the personal self
when going through the experience, we may end up
with a limitation, a certain crippling, the inability to go
beyond a certain point, and the willingness to participate becomes limited. The person says, "I would rather
live a limited life than face that kind of experience
again. I would rather never love again than to love and
lose." The saying is, "'Tis better to have loved and lost,
than never to have loved at all." The experiencing of
lovingness puts us in touch with our Self, that which is
greater than our own limited, small self.

The complete resolution brings us into conscious
contact with something that is greater than the personal
self. Many people who have tried this attest to the fact
that when they surrendered the small self to some-

thing greater than themselves, they came into contact with that which they considered to be 'real'. That personal inner experience of spiritual reality takes one from book learning to a profound inner conviction. Out of this inner conviction comes the willingness to re-enter life again, to participate in it, and to take the risks and chances.

What is the inner experience of hitting bottom? It comes out of the feelings of hopelessness and despair; the person's small self is saying, "I, of my own self, cannot handle this." The person surrenders out of the hopelessness, and from that comes the willingness to let go, to surrender to something greater than oneself. At the very bottom, in the pits, one realizes and accepts the truth that "I, of myself, my own individual personal self, my own ego-self, am unable to handle this. I am unable to resolve it." It is out of this defeat that victory and success arise. The phoenix rises out of the ashes of despair and hopelessness. It is not the despair and hopelessness that are of value but the letting go and the realization of the limitation of the small self. In the middle of the catastrophe, the person says, "I give up. I cannot handle this," and then may consciously or unconsciously ask God for help.

Due to the law of free will and the nature of consciousness being what it is, it is said that the great beings that are willing to help all of us are waiting for us to say "yes." It is the sudden turning from the bottom of the barrel to the willingness to accept that there is something greater than ourselves that we can turn to. When the person says, "If there is a God, I ask him to help me," then the great transformative experiences happen that have been recorded throughout history from the very beginning.

The beginning of the great worldwide organization of Alcoholics Anonymous (AA) came out of such an experience. Bill W., the famous founder of AA, had hit bottom. He was in a state of total despair and hopelessness and gave up the personal self. At the time, he was a nonbeliever, but he said, "If there is a God, I ask him to help me." At that moment came a great transformative experience, the spiritual power of which is evidenced by the millions of lives that have been affected by the energy that flowed out into the world as the result of this man's sharing his spiritual experience.

Obviously, letting go and hitting bottom are crucial. It is out of the awareness that we cannot change things and are limited and powerless that we discover what does have the power in the universe. That power comes in and handles the experience, and we know when that happens because of the profound state of peace. Where there was agony, there is now a state of infinite peace and an ineffable awareness of an Infinite Presence.

Historically, it has been a special occasion when a realization of the truth has arisen, but that is not at all necessary; it is only one type of experience. Actually, this is the nature of spiritual work all the time. The person who is involved in spiritual work is always looking at what is occurring in life, seeing it as the teacher, as the grist for the mill. What is happening represents that which is being worked on, so an acute catastrophe would just be a continuation of the process that is going on anyway. As a result, the person who is intensely involved in spiritual work would then see it as a golden opportunity, painful and regretful perhaps, but one of great benefit.The essential nature of spiritual work is to remain focused on what arises from instant to instant and become aware of 'what' is experiencing and where it is being experienced.

There is a meditative and contemplative technique that can be used to bring about the same result. It is the process of constantly letting go of wanting to control the experiencing as well as experiencing itself. There then occurs the sudden realization that awareness is being handled by some infinite aspect of consciousness (the Self); this may have been suspected previously but not actually realized. After this realization, the awareness of the Presence occurs more frequently.

Out of this experience comes an ever greater willingness to rely on that inner Presence, with less and less reliance on the small self. Less frequently, then, does the person look to the small self to handle life's problems, as there is a progressive willingness to surrender to one's higher Self. The progressive loss of identification with the small self and the increasing identification with the Presence, along with the willingness to surrender life and all of its aspects to the will of God, become the very core of the person's spiritual exercise and experience.

The acute catastrophic experience is a key learning opportunity that teaches us to go to the very core, to the very essence of the experience, to see what it is and handle it at the level of experiencing within the energy field of consciousness itself. There is the willingness to surrender and to let go of wanting to change what happened 'out there'. There is the letting go of wanting to control by thinking about it and trying to handle it with the intellect and the emotions. There is the willingness to surrender to the essence of the experience without calling it anything, or labeling it, or putting names on it. There is the willingness to handle the energy field of it and go directly to the inner experience. The surrender to the inner experience is the open doorway to the experience of something greater than the small personal self.

Each catastrophe, therefore, is a repeat and representation of another opportunity for this great spiritual learning experience; therefore, people who have been through great catastrophic experiences express their gratitude. Often people say, "Although I wouldn't want to live though it again, I am very grateful for that experience."

How could a person be grateful for what the world considers a terrible catastrophe or a dreadful, progressive illness? What they learned out of the catastrophe was of such a great dimension that the price was worth it because, through the realization of truth, they discovered the reconnection with the essential core of their beingness.

As we grow spiritually and become spiritually educated, it takes less and less to bring about the willingness to face this inner experience. It could be said that a person's 'bottom of the barrel' gets progressively raised. The person does not have to go through agonizing pain before they are willing to let go and surrender. More and more there arises a willingness to do it on a daily basis so that it becomes part and parcel of one's life, with the constant looking at how one is trying to control things, or trying to change God's will, or how one is going to try to change and control God. More often there is the willingness to totally surrender at great depth, and then one sees that surrender occurs at different depths.

In ordinary life, we surrender a little bit. Under greater pressure, we are willing to surrender more and realize that we do not have to put ourselves under catastrophic pressure in order to be willing to surrender at great depth. The transformation of personality, the whole shift in one's spiritual position, traditionally comes from surrendering at great depth. What does it mean to surrender at great depth? How can we surrender at great depth without having to put ourselves through a terrible emotional catastrophe in order to accomplish the same spiritual work? By seeing the essential nature of the process, we become educated. Our positions shift and we are different in the way we are. We are willing to be with life in all its expressions. The willingness is then experienced as an inner state of aliveness. Arising from that is the willingness to take the chance because we now know that we are accompanied by something greater than the personal self. It is not the personal self that has to handle what comes up in life. The Infinite Presence that is always with us is more powerful than the human will and ego. The self brings pain and suffering; the Self radiates healing and peace.

CHAPTER 9

Worry, Fear, and Anxiety

As discussed previously, holistic health uses the phrase "body, mind, and spirit" frequently, so it will be helpful to understand more about it. What does it really mean? Is it just a catch phrase or a slogan? Is 'spirit' a meta-physical abstraction or a religious dictum? Is it a fantasy of people who are not very well connected with the real world? Defining this relationship again will help us to speed up our work through greater understanding.

Again, we want to review how human experience comes about and also look within ourselves to see where this phenomenon actually occurs. In looking at the relationship of body, mind, and spirit from the viewpoint of experience, some things may sound somewhat startling, such as the fact that the body cannot experience itself. That may be a surprising thought because all of us tend to think of ourselves as being the body and to think, "I am the body." However, this is not true because the body is unable to experience itself. For example, my left arm cannot experience its own left armness. There are sensations coming from the body, but I am not experiencing the body. Instead, I am experiencing the sensations of the body, but curiously enough, they cannot experience themselves either. The sensations coming from the arm have to be experienced somewhere, however, which is in the mind.

If we have an incision in the brain that deletes part of the operating mind, or at least the way it operates on the physical plane, we fail to experience the opposite side of the body. This is very common after a stroke where the patient is unable to experience in mind even the existence of a portion of their body. Thus, the body cannot be experienced without the sensation, and the sensation can only be experienced in mind. Interestingly, the mind cannot experience itself. A thought cannot experience its own thoughtness, a memory cannot experience its own memoryness, and a fantasy cannot experience its own fantasyness. That which goes on in mind actually has to be experienced in an energy field that is greater than mind itself, which is called 'consciousness'.

Consciousness enables one to be aware of what goes on within mind and is the basic reason for anesthesia. With anesthesia, consciousness is deleted, which results in there being no awareness of what is going on in mind. With no consciousness, there is no awareness of mind or body; with no mind, there is no awareness of sensations or the body. Consequently, we will notice by watching ourself throughout the day that all of our experiences are being experienced in a more general way than realized and in a more general field of experience that is almost diffuse. It is almost as though it is everywhere in space, and this is within consciousness itself.

It is an interesting experiment to find out where we think we really experience a thought. Most people think it is in their heads, but that is the thought about a thought. If we ask them to now let go of any belief about where they think they are experiencing a thought and instead point to exactly where a thought is being experienced—the radical truth of where the phenomenon is occurring—they learn that there is no particular place that thoughtness occurs. All they can say is that thoughtness is occurring, and they have an awareness of the thoughtness, but they cannot put their finger on where it could possibly be—no particular place where it is being experienced in a general, overall way.

It is very necessary for us to know this because some of the techniques we will use cancel a lot of the belief systems that are at the basis of human suffering. Consciousness itself is like a movie screen upon which what is changing is experienced. If we look at it, we will see that all experience is experience of change. The movement we experience is the coming and going, the ebbing and waning, and the flux. The reason we can experience that which changes is because it is being experienced from a background that is unchanging. It is because the movie screen is standing still that we can see the movement of the movie. Therefore, what changes is what is experienced, and it is experienced in consciousness itself, which has no exact location.

The Functional Hypoglycemic

Before explaining fear and anxiety as an emotional level of consciousness (the major source), it is important to identify a frequent source of those emotions, which has a physical basis. A frequent source of anger and other negative emotions is the physiological problem of 'functional hypoglycemia' (low blood sugar), which is associated with an overreaction to dietary sugar input. This is also termed 'hyperinsulinism,' which is an overreaction to glucose and sucrose. The sudden drop in blood sugar can precipitate emotional reactions of anger, rage, fear, shakiness, panic, or even violence.

The diagnosis can be made clinically by simply stopping all sugar intake and noticing the disappearance of the negative symptoms. It can be verified by a five-hour glucose tolerance test. In a normal person, glucose levels first rise rapidly and then slowly subside. The hypoglycemic pattern, however, shows a rapid drop in blood glucose level, and the sudden drop may then precipitate mild to quite severe negative emotions or physical shaking, weakness, or even fainting. It may also result in a craving for alcohol or sedative drugs. The disorder is well known in recovery programs, such as Alcoholics Anonymous. A famous book about the disorder is *Sugar Blues* by William Duffy (1986).

When prospective patients called my office, I told them to stop ingesting all sugar (and alcohol) until I saw them for their appointment. Over the years, twenty-five percent of the patients were 'cured' (asymptomatic) by the time I saw them. Because of the high prevalence of this clinical disorder and its various forms of expression, it is worth investigating as a contributory element in all emotional disorders. It can even be the trigger for psychotic episodes as well as physical violence. Some undiagnosed persons even end up in jail or prison for assault and other crimes of violence. It is a frequent cause of marital or other social disputes, family friction, and behavioral disorders.

In the clinic, we had a diagnostic laboratory and often did the five-hour glucose tolerance tests. By the third or fourth hour, many patients developed negative emotional reactions. One woman suddenly disrobed and ran down the sidewalk stark naked with the laboratory director in his long white coat running after her, yelling "Stop!" She kept on running wildly for several blocks. (Traffic came to a halt at the wild, frantic scene.)

Fear is a level of consciousness to be addressed where it is, not in its expression and extension into the world—fear of this, fear of that—and not trying to handle it on the level of the particular but handling it instead as a level of consciousness. This is done by becoming aware of that which we are, which is greater than the fear, and learning to disidentify with the emotion so we are not that. We are an overall field in which fear is being experienced. It becomes a small thing occurring within the greater context in which we become aware of ourselves as that which we really are.

One of the biggest obstacles to handling and letting go of fear is the fear of fear itself. We will describe a technique that disappears the fear of fear. Once we are no longer afraid of fear, it becomes a very simple matter. Is it not the fear of fear that is the problem? A person is afraid of the fear, just as the person going to the dentist is afraid of the pain; it is that initial fear. When we begin to look at the nature of fear, we can see that the number of fears is endless; therefore, people become victims and convinced that the source of fear is outside themselves.

If people think the origination or source of fear is outside themselves, then there would be very little they could do about it. In fact, there really is nothing

they could do about it. So long as the belief continues
that the source is outside themselves, they will always
be the victims of fear until they begin to realize that it
is a present condition within themselves, and that they
are the source of the fear they project onto the world.
Of course, they are sure to see it 'out there' because
they have just projected it out there.

When we look at fear, we see how all pervasive it
can be. If we realize that fear is a level of consciousness, then we realize that from that level of consciousness, fear can be attached to everything. Trying to
overcome particular fears may have a certain limited
value, but it does not change one as a fearful person,
personality, or human being. The fear of a specific fear
may be clinically valuable, and it may be of practical
use in one's life, but it does not alter who one is. The
conditions of fear can be changed so that one no
longer feels like a small self that is powerless and at
the effect of being the victim of fear itself.

Fear can be like a prefix that gets attached to anything. We can see from the Map of Consciousness that
Fear is at consciousness level 100, indicating that it is
a negative emotion, as shown by the direction of the
arrow. We see its relative power in this mathematical
model that shows the calibrated energies of the different fields. As we go up from the negative emotions of
30, 50, and 75 into the positive emotions beginning at
200, we see that their power, from the viewpoint of
physics, actually increases.

As we address the energy field of Fear, we begin to
realize that being fearful can attach to anything and
everything in our lives. There is nothing in our total

experience as a human being to which fear cannot be attached. We love our mother, and up comes the fear of "What if we lose her?" We love our body and up comes the fear of death or sickness. We love money and up comes the fear of loss or of being accused of being greedy. No matter what we think of, fear can be attached to it. We love our automobile and up comes the fear of an accident. A fearful person attaches fear to everything; therefore, everything that comes into the mind is coming into an energy field of fear and thus gets colored with fear. There is even a fear of life itself, as shown by the song, "'Fraid of living and 'fraid of dying." In other words, this energy field has now contaminated everything.

If we are the source of that energy field, then all our experience comes into the field of fear, and everything in our lives can become fearful. The future is fearful: old age, getting older, what is going to happen to the body, what is going to happen to my finances, what is going to happen to my relationships, what is going to happen to my family, what is going to happen to my bank account, what is going to happen to my country, and what is going to happen to the world?

People who develop global fear will tell you about their fear of nuclear annihilation, or intergalactic wars, or meteors, or cataclysmic 'end times'. The expansion of the fear does not change the fact that it is still just fear. Glamorizing it and making it sound dramatic does not change that it is just fear. The fears of intergalactic war, human demolition, and the expiration of the human race are no different from the child's fear of the dark or his fear that a dog might bite him. Experientially, fear is always just the same emotion.

Characteristic of all of this is the energy field called Fear. Fear of 'what' is really immaterial. We have to learn to look away from the thoughts and look instead at the feeling. We actually have to look below the feeling to the energy field out of which the feeling is originating and then learn how to handle this energy field. When we do this, we lose our fear of fear, and as that happens, we begin to learn how to handle fear directly. It is an extremely simple thing to handle once we are familiar with some rather easy techniques.

The world pretty much runs people with fear because their personal lives are also predominantly run by fear. But once we have learned a way to avoid getting cornered by fear, we begin to transcend the world as well as transcend being a victim because the world can threaten us only by fear. If they cut off our bank account, conduct an audit, run away from us, leave us, or fire us, the gun at our head is always the same gun—the gun of fear. There can be the fear of losing a part of the body—there is no end to the number of fears, but there is an end to fearfulness and of being a victim of fear.

We will learn how to lose our fear of fear, how to enjoy the process, and how to really start feeling good about ourselves when we realize that we are no longer the victim, the worm that is at the effect of this all-pervasive fearfulness. The problem is not fear itself but the energy field of fearfulness. We can begin to

see that we are in control of it because we are the
source of it. We start with admitting the truth that "*I
am the source of my fearfulness.*" We know that in a
different mood, a fearful thing is no longer fearful. We
might say about the thing we fear, "I'm afraid of that,"
but when we are accompanied by someone else, or in
a different mood, such as a humorous one, and we are
having a good time laughing, then the thing no longer
engenders fear, so the source of fear is not out in
the world.

There is no way of overcoming one's fear of the
world because there is no way the world can be controlled to end one's fears, nor can fears be overcome
by changing society, by changing the law, or by
changing the rules. The source of fearfulness is within oneself.

Picture a big event. There are two aspects—one is
the event itself, and the second is how we feel about
it. Having more police at the event might make us
feel better, but, in fact, where are the police going to
be while our apartment is being robbed? At the other
end of town, naturally. Therefore, our handling of
fear is really up to ourself. It comes out of our willingness to own that we are the source of that fear,
which is occurring within our own consciousness.
Therefore, we want to address it where it is actually
being experienced.

Most people experience fear in a somewhat physical way, so the first thing to do about a fearful experience is eliminate paying any attention to thought. A
fearful feeling will engender literally millions of
thoughts. There is no end to fearful thoughts because

they are coming out of the energy field of fear itself, which generates an endless series of thoughts. Clinically speaking, handling the specific thoughts themselves has a limited value, and the fearfulness merely generates more thoughts later on, so we want to use a technique that will handle fear itself.

A person might just picture something fearful in their life, or something fearful that they expect to happen or has happened, or they can just fantasize a fearful experience, such as being tied to the railroad track with a locomotive bearing down on them. As they look at what is being experienced, they will see when they look past the thought, it is being experienced first in the body. They may notice a tenseness in the stomach muscles, a queasy feeling in the stomach, shakiness in the arms and legs, or a dryness in the mouth. Some people have intestinal cramps or difficulty breathing. Whatever it is, they look within themselves to see what is actually being experienced. Radical truth means what is being experienced, not what one is actually thinking about it or the concepts that one is projecting onto the experience; it is not the labeling of it but what one is literally experiencing within oneself.

The technique is to let go of resisting the experiencing of what is literally being experienced. Let go of resisting the dryness of the mouth. Let it be there and welcome it. Let go of resisting the flip-flop feeling in the stomach and the trembling in the arms and legs. When we do this, we are focused away from thought about what is being experienced. We fully let go and surrender being those sensations. The letting go is like being the willow tree in the wind.

The ancient wisdom of Taoism states that the oak tree, which resists the wind, is susceptible to breaking, and the willow tree, which bends with the wind, survives. Like the willow tree, we bend with the incoming experience. We let it be, blend with it, and welcome it. We say, "Let's have more of it." As we do that, we will discover, much to our surprise, that there is a limited amount of that sensation. It is as though the amount of fear we have is limited in quantity. How can this be? It is as though this fear is like a pressure tank that contains all the suppressed fear we have had throughout our lifetime, starting in our childhood. There is all the fear that we could not allow ourselves to experience or express, or were not allowed to express. We were not allowed to have that emotion. For example, a man in military service was not allowed to express the fearfulness because it was thought to be unmanly or showed cowardice, so the fear got suppressed, repressed, and pushed down out of awareness.

Fears we were not aware of have come up by the thousands in our lifetime. The fear comes up and we unwittingly brace our back. The fear is just pushed out of awareness, or we drum our fingers on the desk. The fear is so quickly suppressed that we do not even realize it was there. As the years go by, we have accumulated energy of this fear. The energy behind this fear increases in pressure, and when it reaches a certain point, it is as though a needle has reached a red line on the dial, and the pressure of this fearfulness now begins to express itself. It spills out and over into our experience and begins to color it. If we do not examine it, we think that this fear is coming from the world, and we blame the world for it. We think that it is a fearful experience happening out there. Little do we realize that it is merely our own fearfulness that is being projected out into the world.

Then we own this source of the fear, which is our own accumulated fearfulness. We start to welcome it and look forward to the opportunity to allow this fearfulness to run out. The basic release from fear is by surrender at great depth. The sensations and the inner experience of fear itself remain the same, no matter what we think we fear. If somebody holds a shotgun to our heart and says, "Give me all your money," what are we going to experience? We are going to experience the dry mouth, weakness in the knees, and that old, familiar flip-floppy feeling in the stomach. If an enemy tank rolls up to our house, knocks it over, rotates the gun barrel, and points it right at our forehead, what are we going to experience? The same thing happens if somebody holds a mouse over our head. We are going to experience a dry mouth, queasiness in our stomach, cramps in our intestines, and that shaky feeling in our muscles.

All we ever have to handle is those sensations, and with experiencing this technique, we will learn that all we ever have to handle is what we are experiencing within consciousness itself, whether it is localized within the body or elsewhere. After meditation and working with this technique, we will notice that this experience is actually happening in a general and diffuse everywhereness. The phenomena of the queasy muscles, the flip-flop in the stomach, and the dry mouth are being experienced in a vague, diffuse everywhereness. We just allow the experience to be present without resisting it. Because we are focused on that, the fear begins to diminish because we are no longer paying attention to the thoughts. The thoughts themselves are engendering further fear.

If we are very busy with this technique of just letting go of resisting the fear, we are now focused on the energy field itself. Behind this fearfulness is an energy, and we are letting go of resisting the progressive release and discharge of that energy. By doing this, we lose the fear of fear. It is no longer an awesome terror that awakens us in the middle of the night. It is nothing but an inner emotional experience, the sensations of which can be easily handled. We can ask ourselves, "Truly, can I handle a dry mouth? Of course, I can."

Another technique to eliminate the negative emotions is to let go of their associated mental images that attract and amplify associated emotions. Just refuse the image and cancel the temptation to indulge in it.

While doing research and experimenting with this particular technique, I had an experience that demonstrates one of the principles being described. I had had a lifetime fear of heights which was so severe that when I went to visit the Grand Canyon for the first time, I literally could not walk within one hundred feet of the edge. It created that panicky feeling even when I saw somebody else get near the edge. I was using this technique whenever I could and enjoying the progress I was making with it, but I had never gotten around to working on my fear of heights. I had been working on fear from all its other origins within my experience. The next time I went back to the Grand Canyon about two years later, much to my amazement, I could walk up to within about twenty feet of the edge before the tight feeling occurred in the stomach again. I continued to utilize this technique over the next year or two and again went back to revisit the Canyon. Much to my surprise, I could walk right up to the very edge. Subsequently, I later went up in a hot air balloon without any anxiety. I was so pleased at this demonstration of the principle that what I had been releasing was the accumulated pressure and energy of all that fear from a lifetime. Similar to a pressure tank, as it released itself, there was less and less to spill over into life experiences.

The letting go of resisting is so effective because resistance traps us into a certain state of consciousness; resistance is within. Fear is a negative energy that calibrates at 100, and traps us in the field. We cannot get beyond it so we become the victim of our own fears unless we own that we are the *source* of them. As long as we rationalize and say that the source of fear is 'out there', we cannot overcome it. Once we begin to own that we are the experiencer, that we are the one who sets up the way in which we experience things, then we become the one who is master of the situation. Our self-esteem becomes affected. We are no longer the one who is the victim or subject to fear. We are something other than the fear. Fear is nothing but an experience in consciousness, and we no longer have to give it reality by labeling it as a fear of something, which can be an endless process.

Fearfulness is attached to everything in the world by fearful people. Changing the world will not handle it. A person can be terribly afraid in a very safe situation and not at all afraid in a situation that is hypothetically very dangerous. For example, a person is being mugged, which is one thing, and then there is the fear of being mugged, which is something else. The fear of being mugged is not the same as actually being mugged. It is quite possible to have very unfortunate circumstances occur in one's life and not experience fear at all. In fact, one might even experience that one is merely the witness of the phenomenon.

Such a thing happened to me when I came face to face with a very large rattlesnake on top of a nearby mountain. As I was about to step into a cabin, a giant rattlesnake was coiled up right in front of the doorway, and as I lifted my foot to step over him, his head snapped back, his tongue flickered out, and he was poised to strike me. In that instant, there was a flash of fearful thought, and then the thought that I could get a club and hit it, or I could run, or I could yell for help. I did not have a gun, but somebody might shoot it. All the self-protective thoughts that social consciousness had programmed me with were present.

Happily, and luckily for me or I would not be telling about this, I had learned this technique. I instantly realized that my life frankly depended on my utilization of it, so I automatically went into this exact technique. I automatically let go of wanting to do anything about the fear, of wanting to handle or change anything about it. Instead, I went into my inner Self

and just allowed the inner experience to release itself
without any resistance. I welcomed even more of it
because somehow, when we really get into the experience of our own inner consciousness, we see that
our survival depends on this and has all along. I saw
that my survival really depended on the excellence
with which I let go, surrendered to God, and released
and let go of resisting the experience. As I did, the
fearful thoughts instantly disappeared, and I felt a profound state of peace settle on both the snake and me.

It was as if I had become the witness—not the witness confined to this body, but the witness in consciousness, which seemed to have no dimension. This
formless dimension was then the experiencer of the
presence of a state of peacefulness. This profound
state was of such power that it prevailed over the
consciousness of both the snake and the personality
of this person telling you about this. The snake looked
at me with interest, probably not having seen a
human being in his whole life, much less a foot away,
and I looked at the rattlesnake with great curiosity
and thought of him as a brother. The two of us were
included in the oneness of this space of our own
beingness together in a state of extreme intimacy. Out
of it came a sort of inner joyfulness, and I felt love for
the snake arise out of the field from which fear had
been removed.

In looking at the Map of Consciousness, we can
track what happened. The snake would have instantly
sensed the fear, which has a negative energy field,
along with my anger and desire to strike at it.
However, his responses through his energy system

were so fast that the strike would have happened before I could have moved my shin out of the way. Instead, because of the severe threat of the circumstances, I really, really let go. Did I ever! I moved right through the willingness to let go, right through the acceptance, love, and joy, and right into a state of profound peace. If we calibrate the energy field of that experience, it started out at 100, but almost instantly, it moved up to 600. Then a Presence prevailed—an Infinite, profoundly still Presence whose essential nature is one of peace, whose power is infinite—that controlled the whole experience. Thus, both the snake and I transcended fear, and we moved to a timeless silence. The snake was as though enchanted. We looked at each for minutes, and I was reluctant to break the spell by leaving. The snake then slithered away and never rattled its tail.

This is valuable because it illustrates the falsity of another one of the mind's belief systems that we have to learn to release, which is the idea that fear is the source of our safety. We will notice that the mind seems to worship fear as though it is some kind of a demigod. The mind has a program that says, "The reason I'm alive is due to my fears. I am alive because I allow fear to decide what I am going to do." A little introspection will show that this belief system is going on. A person says, "Well, if I wasn't afraid of being poor in my old age, I wouldn't get insurance. If I wasn't afraid of an automobile accident, I wouldn't drive safely." So the person begins to ascribe the source of their aliveness, the source of their life, to fear, which is the god of their life. They really begin to worship fear.

We can see from the above example that just the opposite is true. What insures our survival is the absence of fear and its replacement by caution and realistic common sense. We have managed to survive in spite of our fears, not because of them. We can make decisions based on rational choice, on our knowledge, and on value coming from the beingness of that which we really are without fear entering the picture at all. All day long we make decisions based just on our awareness of reality, with no fear particularly involved. Fear is not necessary. There is the idea that fear is good for us, that it is beneficial and has all kinds of hidden, mysterious values. People will look back and rationalize how fear got them to do this and do that, and all I can say is, "Too bad." Too bad they did not do it out of love for themselves or for their fellow human beings. Too bad that they did not do it out of love for life itself, love for their own aliveness, and love for their body. Why not do things for our body out of love for it instead of out of fear of the consequences? Why not keep it healthy and happy because we love and value it, not because we are afraid of a heart attack or something else?

There is another technique for letting go of more of this fear, which I call "the worst-case scenario." If we follow fears and ask, "Why am I afraid of that?" we will see that it leads to another fear. Why are we afraid of driving a car? We might have an accident. Why are we afraid of an accident? Because we might get injured. What if we get injured? Then we might suffer pain, and so on. We will find that every fear ultimately leads to the fear of death, the fear of the body's dying.

It will lead to the fear of whether other people like us or agree with us. If we look at fear and keep asking ourselves what fear does that bring up, and what fear is the basis of that, we finally get to the worst-case scenario.

For example, let us say that our financial fears are that we will totally run out of money, have no place to live, no money for food or clothing, and that we will end up semi-naked somewhere on a street corner in the cold with no place to go, and no medical help. What we do is constantly let go of resisting the feeling of this and picture the worst possible thing that can happen to us, such as ending up in the poor farm or sitting on the street corner as a bag lady or a bagman. We then allow ourselves to picture the worst possible scenario—there we are with our bag next to us, sitting on the cold street corner at midnight, friendless.

We imagine whatever the worst possible fear could be and continue the practice. If we will go within ourselves and keep letting go of resisting the inner experience of what is coming up, pretty soon the fear of the worst scenario will run out. If we continue this practice long enough, eventually we will finally sit down and handle 'the biggie', which is picturing ourself in the casket with everybody walking by it. That is the worst scenario that most people can visualize—physical death.

There is the belief that we are the material body, and that is all there is to us. Sooner or later we come to that fear, and when we do, we sit with it in the same way as we sit with any other fear. We let go of death, which is a label, a thought, and a concept. We have no experience of the truth of that, only our fantasies, thoughts, and beliefs; therefore, we have to label it as only a fantasy in our mind. What people actually experience as they picture that and let go of resisting those feelings and sensations is a very surprising thing. When they have gone through the process and become that which is greater than the entire experience, they realize that they have survived the worst possible scenario.

First, I imagined being a bag person. By the time the fear ran out, I enjoyed it. I thought it would actually be fun to just do what I wanted to do—hang out with the people I wanted to talk with, not have to go to work or pay any bills, and have no health or automobile insurance premiums to pay. It would be okay because it would be from choice and not from victimhood. It would just be a different experience that is in great contrast to the rest of my life.

From choice, there is no fear; the fear disappears. The worst thing that can happen is to end up on a street corner and live that kind of life, but the fear about it is gone. I may not choose that kind of life, but if it should happen, it is not filled with fear. I am no longer run by the fear of that, so I do not have to lie in bed at night worrying about what would happen if I run out of money some day. No matter how much money one has, that fear is present. The thought that we can earn more and more money and pile it up in the bank is futile. I know somebody who was worth sixty million dollars, ended up bankrupt, and had to sell off his personal possession to pay his bills.

Could sixty million dollars protect us from that which we fear? Of course not. Money will not protect us at all, nor will barricades, putting six locks on our doors, or hiring more police. The only protection is owning that we are the source of our own experience, that we are the master of it, that we can handle it, and that we are greater than it.

The mind always tries to justify our fear, of course. It says, "Well, there are a lot of muggings; therefore, my fear is justified." Why is there such a thing as justified fear? Who needs it? Why not walk home out of choice in a way that we know is not going to bring on such an attack? Why not out of loving oneself enough? Why not out of just enjoying life and valuing it to the point that we do not want to risk it, out of choice?

Survival does not depend on the fear of being mugged or robbed. It depends on pre-choice, which is made by a mind that is not fearful. Because of the 'not fearfulness', I am alive today. It was not being afraid that held back the rattlesnake from striking me when it was really only inches away. It was due to the loss of the fear and the letting go of it. It is possible to be in very severe, dangerous situations (such as World War II, etc.) and experience only joy, happiness, and trust in those circumstances. I have walked through a crowd of cut-throats who would have readily attacked a person who was holding fear and done it with happy, gleeful smiles on their faces. They 'got off on it' when a guy like me walked right through them while they were holding their intimidating guns, chains, and knives. Had I come from fear, they would have challenged that boldness and attacked me. Safety came from letting go of the fear. Without fear or bravado, there was nothing for them to play off of emotionally.

Letting go of the worst-case scenario is extremely

beneficial. As we do this, we will become aware that something has been setting up the fear within us. Now that we have lost our fear of fear, when it arises, we just walk around with it. One time I walked around with fear for two solid weeks. With that trembling electric feeling running through the body, I went about my business and just kept letting the fear run because I realized it would run out. However, as we do that, we may realize that there is another source underlying the original fear to begin with, which is guilt.

Now we begin to see the value of the work that the world calls spiritual consciousness or something similar. We can see the benefit of techniques such as concentrating on the value of forgiving. In forgiving ourselves and other human beings and turning over any judgment to God, we begin to find that by letting go of condemning ourselves and others, the unconscious guilt begins to alleviate fear since fear was held in mind because we unconsciously expected retaliatory return of our attacks. We expect revenge and counterattack. Every negative or hostile thought that we hold about others engenders our own fearfulness because on the psychic or mental plane, which is invisible to the naked eye, it is as though we are building up for ourselves that which threatens to come back to us. We learn that fearfulness begins to diminish as we let go of our anger, hostility, criticisms, and thoughts that condemn others. We learn the value of letting go of the thoughts that make other people wrong. We begin to value and love them for their beingness, for what they are. We begin to see ourselves as different, and, therefore, we begin to see others as different. We become willing to forgive, forget, and overlook.

As a result, we start to see that all the things we condemned in others are really just expressions of their humanness. What we have been condemning in ourselves and in everybody else is the humanness, the innocence of the little child within that believed everything it heard while growing up. The consciousness of the child is innocent, is it not? It loves and trusts its parents. It loves its mother. Therefore, the innocence of the child gets programmed. It is the innocent child that believes everything it is told by the parents, teachers, and the political/social programming that occurs via television and the belief systems of the country.

Who or what bought all the belief systems in our mind? Who bought what we believe? It was the mind of the innocent within because that innocent child's mind, the nature of consciousness itself, has not changed since we were born. That which is reading this right now is the innocent consciousness of the child saying, "I believe this. I take it within myself." The innocent child never dies; that innocence is still present. We see in today's world the actions of ignorant, susceptible young men who are being programmed to hate (paradoxically by religion). They then believe hate and killing the innocent are 'good' or even 'holy'.

We begin to see that intrinsic innocence and realize that all the things we have ever learned which ended up being wrong were bought out of the intrinsic state of not knowing the truth and also from learning that which was not the truth. Therefore, we are willing to let go of our condemnation of others and ourselves. We are beginning to own our own innocence and that of others. It is misfortunate and perhaps regretful that the misinformation came into the innocent mind.

We might look at the mind as the hardware of the computer and its belief systems as the software. Can the five-year-old child question the political system he hears described in his kindergarten from his fellow students, his parents, or his grandparents? We can see that it is from his 'not knowingness'. It is out of the innocence of his 'not knowingness' that he believes what he believes. As a result, we are willing to forgive others, and instead of condemning them, we understand them.

From this understanding develops a certain compassion. A compassionate person has no fears. What is there to fear in a compassionate world inasmuch as we are the source of our own experience and our compassion when we own it back within ourselves? We see our own innocence and the innocence of other beings and have the experience of a compassionate, loving world. No longer do we walk around fearfully because we are no longer creating it within ourselves. We see that we were the source of our fears. The world was never the source of our fear; we were. Having let go of creating fear and propagating it through endless guilt, which comes about through endless judgments that social conditioning has thrust upon us, the unconscious guilt diminishes. The letting go of unconscious guilt progresses outside of our awareness.

Every time we decide to stop condemning a person and instead try to understand him, our own store of unconscious guilt goes down. In the unconscious, it is an eye for an eye and a tooth for a tooth. If we wish that somebody would drop dead, what do you suppose its equal is in our unconscious mind? That we should drop dead. We do not think that our thought about "If only so-and-so would drop dead" has anything to do with our fears of a heart attack, but, of course, they do. As we let go of wishing for other people to drop dead, we will find, curiously enough, that our fear and obsession that we might or will get a coronary and all the dietary precautions that go with that, will diminish. Instead, we are very peaceful about the whole thing. When we go, we go. If we stay, we stay. Big deal!

What we value is life, and we no longer focus on the potential ending of that life; therefore, we come into a different experience of the experiencing of life and who we are. We are that in which this experiencing is happening. Then, as the classic ox-herding pictures depict, instead of being dragged about with bleeding knees and rumpled clothes against our will by the ox of fear, we can now tie this ox to a tree because we have located the culprit. Having let go of our fear of the ox, we now become the master. We get on top of the ox, and the ox becomes tame; we are the master. We have identified with that which we really are and are no longer the victim.

Victimhood comes out of unconsciousness. It means being unaware of this game setup that has been going on within our minds. Merely becoming aware of this means that we are already out of it. By the time you have finished reading this, you have gotten up from being the victim; you are already tying this ox to the tree. As we practice these techniques that have been described, we will soon be sitting on top of the ox.

When fear comes along, we welcome it and say, "Great! What an opportunity to let go of more of that," because by now, we are feeling the benefit of the decrease in the fears we have had our whole lifetime. Little do people realize the extent of the fears they are holding until they begin to disappear, and then it is mind-boggling. We say, "I never realized I was such a fearful human being." This is perhaps more easily understood by referring to the Map of Consciousness so we can see how the energy fields relate to the way we experience the world.

Mind is so powerful that the way it holds our experience literally determines our experience. Fearfulness creates a certain view of the world and tends to become a self-fulfilling prophecy. Recent university research, as well as our own research, shows that what one holds in mind tends to manifest within one's experience of the world. The world of our own experience then becomes the external representation of what we have been holding in mind, so our life is really a world of mirrors. What we are actually seeing and experiencing is a projection of our own level of consciousness. This is difficult to believe and fully grasp, but to give us a glimpse of it is a whole field of study in itself. The sage Ramana Maharshi taught that the world you see (perception) does not even exist and is illusory (the Buddha's "Maya").

On the Map of Consciousness, let us compare the level of consciousness with its emotion, our view of the world, and how this would give us a view of God. At the bottom of the Map is a negative energy field called Guilt that calibrates at a power of 30. It is the world of self-hatred, self-destruction, and a person who is guilt-ridden. They see the world as one of sin and suffering, which indicates what kind of God in that context would rule over a world of endless suffering and sin. The consequences of sin in the collective consciousness field would be that God is our ultimate destroyer. He punishes with earthquakes, volcanic eruptions, floods, pestilence, and more. God has created the world of sin and suffering in which we are destroyed, and our soul is thrown into hell forever. That is the worst possible scenario.

As one's consciousness rises to the energy field of Apathy at 50, which is the level of hopelessness and loss of energy, the world and life in it are seen as relatively hopeless. As a result, there are some famous philosophers who said that man is nothing, God is dead, and this is a hopeless world. The view of God from that level is that God is dead, or at least cruelly indifferent to suffering.

If we raise our level of consciousness and advance our awareness, we then move up to the level of Grief, which offers a negative view of the world and ourselves. The emotions are regret, loss, feelings of despondency, and being dispirited. A person holding the energy field of Grief sees this as a sad world as they walk down the street. When this person looks at older people, they see how sad it is that they are old. When they look at children, they think how sad is what these poor, innocent children are going to have to experience in life. When they open the newspaper, they see the sadness of all that goes on in the world.

The kind of God that would fit that sadness would be a God who ignores them. Out of this, the person is worthless, so they say, "I am just a worm, and God couldn't possibly have any interest in me. If He exists at all, He would just be a God who ignores me."

What about the fearful person who holds the energy field of Fear? We see that they are the creator of that, the owner, and the source. The emotions of worry, anxiety, panic, and the deflation of self-esteem lead them to see this as a frightening world. As they walk down the street, they see danger everywhere. They open the newspaper with alarm and read about bankruptcy and murder. They walk down the street and see automobile accidents and the potential for starvation. The God of a frightening field of consciousness would be a very punitive one who really sort of hates them and throws them into the world of an endless nightmare. The creator of such a nightmare is a very punitive God of revenge and retaliation and becomes the punisher.

As we move up into Desire at 125, the area of the solar plexus, there are craving, wantingness, and what makes Sammy run, and there is no satisfying it. No matter what the person gets, it is not enough. The millionaire has fifty million dollars and is going for sixty million. He has sixty and is going for seventy. He never gets to the end of the road for there is no end. When he is old, his fingernails are long, he lives on a yacht, he is paranoid and thinks the world is against him, and he does not understand why he cannot find happiness. But happiness is at level 500, not at 125.

The person is trapped by wanting and craving

more and more and therefore sees the world as frustrating. If one is always wanting, then the world is always holding back from that person. As one looks at the jewelry-store display cases, that cravingness comes out—one wants, wants, wants those jewels. They want the wantingness. If they get the jewels, they will feel a satisfaction but not happiness. There is a temporary satisfaction, but what kind of God would hold back from a person what they desire? Then the person feels separated from God, if there is a God at all. There is the person, and then there is God, but the two of them have no relationship.

The exasperation of this frustrating world of desire leads to anger, resentment, hatred, grievance, war, and murder. There is the overexpansion of the angry person, which shows in the protrusion of the blood vessels, and the angry animal within flares up with anger. The angry person sees this as a competitive world. When somebody opens up another used-car lot next to him, he is angry and thinks the person is going to take his business away. He has not moved up to a world of cooperation which knows that the more there are used-car lots nearby, the greater the business because they draw people from everywhere. But he would not even think of cooperating; instead, he thinks of competition and becomes polarized. It is he against them. Therefore, he sees a competitive world and a retaliatory God who, out of angriness, is very punishing, retaliatory, and seeks revenge. "I am a jealous, vengeful God who will get you. I'm out to get you," so God is his enemy, out to get him. How can he relax and reach any kind of awareness in that kind of angry energy field?

From Anger, we move up to pridefulness. Pride at level 175 carries with it the downside of denial, arrogance, and contempt. The process in consciousness is one of being inflated. This person lives in a world of status. When he walks down the same city street, he sees not only your Cadillac, but also the year and model. I did not even realize they came in models. I thought a Caddy was a Caddy. No sir, I have discovered that there are different models of Cadillac—I forget their names, but whatever they are, one has more status than the other—so the interest of that person in other human beings is in their position. "Oh, he's president of so-and-so," or, "He's only a blue-collar worker." It is not the money but the status that money gives them.

What kind of a God can that person see from the level of pridefulness? There are probably two options. Because of denial and intellectual arrogance, one can say that the left brain denies that there is a God, or, one can say that their position is the right one, and therefore everybody else is wrong; thus, they end up with skepticism or bigotry. This is the source of all the religious wars. "My view of religion is right; therefore, yours must be wrong." Pridefulness leads one into a polarized position of "me right, you wrong." The anxiety that accompanies this puts the person on the defensive because he lives in a world of win-lose.

As we move up to Courage at level 200, there is appropriateness for the first time. The person is able to face, cope, and handle, and they become empowered because they have begun to tell the truth about themselves. The person from the level of Courage walks down the same street and sees a challenging, exciting world of opportunity. It is a thrilling world of growing, learning, expanding, and watching others grow. There is an inner joy that comes from expanding one's own space. Courage settled the United Sates of America and the West. It created all the industrial empires and scientific enterprises. It got us to the moon. It is the world of growth and expansion.

What kind of God is the God of that level of consciousness? The person on that level of consciousness has an open mind for the first time. He does not pridefully presume that he has the answer. He is not aligned with vengeful negativity. He says for the first time, "I wonder if there is such a being. I wonder if there is something greater than the personal self. I am open to learning about this." He then treats the God question the same as he does the world question, as an exciting opportunity for exploration, and discovers that spiritual research is exciting, and the things that are discovered are intriguing and beneficial.

The next energy field, Neutral at level 250, results in being unattached. This person says it is okay if they get the job and okay if they do not. They are unattached and not run by the world. Their power greatly increases because they are no longer a victim. The world does not control them anymore. They say, "If this person stays in my life, great; if they don't, I will find somebody else to be with." They no longer live in fear, they have moved up to a certain okayness, and their view of the world is now okay. The God of an okay world would be a God of freedom to expand and explore. "If there is a God, it's okay with me, and if there isn't, that's okay with me." There is an inner fairness about God. "If there is a God, He will be fair, and I will learn about it when the time comes; if there isn't, that is okay with me, too."

At the level of Willingness at calibration level 310, the person now declares an intention and says "yes" to life. "I join; I align myself; I agree with things." The person begins to experience a willingness to be of service, along with a certain happiness, and views the world as friendly. When one is willing, the world is friendly. Now the person walks down the street and sees potentially friendly people. All one has to do is walk up to an old lady and say, "Hi, what a beautiful day." She says, "Hey, nobody has talked to me all morning. Isn't this nice?" The world is a friendly place, and God perhaps becomes a promising and hopeful concept. The God of a friendly world would become a friendly God. Even if one does not believe in Him, one begins to trust Him. If one does not have a belief in God, at least the friendly person says, "Well, if there is one, he will be at least as kindly as my grandmother. He is going to understand human nature and is not going to throw me into the pit fires of hell for being human. He created me as human; I'm his handiwork. What is He going to do? Condemn His own creation?" Therefore, there is a certain trust in a God.

As we move up to Acceptance at calibration level 350, we have begun to own ourself as a source of our own power. We are the creator of the happiness in our own life now, and that transformation in consciousness brings a feeling of adequacy and confidence; the view of the world now is harmonious. When we walk down the street, we see the subtle, beautiful naturalness of how everything interacts, how everything is really where it should be, and that everybody wants to be what they are. The bag lady is there because she wants to be a bag lady; nobody has forced her to be that. She has chosen to be that which she is. We stop blaming things, and we begin to experience that the world is expressing harmony to the degree to which we are willing to own the truth about ourself and express it. The whole movie is harmonious, and God now begins to look like a merciful and forgiving God of a harmonious world.

With the quieting of emotionality that is consequent to acceptance, the way is now clear to facilitate the use of reason, discernment, and the intellect without interference from stressful feelings, such as fear of survival, anger, and the rest. Free of the distortions and distractions, the mind becomes clear enough to utilize logic and the benefits of education and higher learning, including academic study and abstract thought, which is the level of mind that includes the calibration range of the 400s. This is also the realm of science, which is based on the Newtonian paradigm of proof, evidence, and the laws of cause and effect. The 400s include the *Great Books of the Western World*, as well as celebrated geniuses, such as Newton, Einstein, and Freud.

In the 400s, personal power increases markedly by maximal use of the prefrontal cortex of the brain with which fear, worry, and anxiety can be handled with the tools of logic and reason rather than just raw emotion. The world therefore looks less fearful because its risks are comprehended from a higher, more mature level rather than from the raw emotionality of the child. The mind thus discovers safeguards and limits in order to arrive at a balance and the capacity for rational judgment and reality testing.

Via good will and a rational worldview, inner anxiety diminishes, and the shift in brain physiology, plus intention, allows for the emergence of Love as a dominant life principle at consciousness calibration level 500. At this level, the nurturance of relationships and the welfare of others become predominant in contrast to lower levels of consciousness that are the consequence of domination by the narcissistic core of the ego.

With further evolution, the level of Love becomes unconditional at 540, and the way is paved for consciousness to evolve to the higher spiritual levels that calibrate at approximately 600, which is the level of spiritual Bliss and Peace.

As we move up in our willingness to be of service to this world, our lovingness emerges as Unconditional Love to nurture and support life. We are willing to forgive, and beginning revelation occurs. Due to the release of endorphins, we begin to see the lovingness that is everywhere. We see it in nature and in the animal world. We see the natural lovingness of the child within everybody. The loving heart of the child is still alive in everyone. If a person does not experience that, it is because they do not know how to tune in to it, but the innocent, loving heart of the child is in everyone. It can be appealed to, and that is why the merciless killer in the presence of a loving person can become harmless. In contrast, in the presence of a fearful person, it creates the space for him to attack, and he does attack. The loving person then experiences a safe world, and God must, of necessity, be at least at the same level of consciousness as he is and therefore be unconditionally loving.

The experience of the truth of this brings the person into a joyfulness. Joyfulness brings about a transfiguration in consciousness. It brings one into compassion. The inner serenity of the compassionate person begins to see the perfection of creation. The unconditional love of the Creator creates a oneness. The person begins to experience the oneness of all beings. Therefore, all of life in all its expressions is sacred. There is a beginning awareness of the sacredness of life and a merging into an illumined and enlightened state of blissfulness and infinite peace in which the total oneness of Creation brings an awareness of God as the essence of beingness itself.

As I stood on top of the mountain in the presence of the rattlesnake, what was it that entranced and fixed both of us into a state of infinite peace and oneness? I could not really say in that state of aliveness that the life of the snake and my life were two different lives because it seemed as though they were one. The two were being controlled by the nature of the One—that which brought what seemed to be the two of us together as one experience. There was really only one experience occurring. One might say that the one experience was being experienced through the two, or, the two were experiencing their oneness.

Therefore, no thought of attack arose because the energy field of that experience had already arisen. The feeling of infinite peace is often called the Peace of God.

There are certain teachings that say there are really only two emotions—love and fear—and all the negative feelings below Love are nothing but variations of fear. We can see all of these expressions of fear—fear of moral wrong, fear of the inability to survive and exist, fear over the loss of the source of one's happiness, and anger over the intrinsic fear that 'not getting' brings to a person. Therefore, we could say that these are forms of fear.

There are really only two expression of emotion— love, which starts at 500 and becomes infinite in its expression, and fear, which begins at 100 and goes ever downward in its expression. Therefore, the handling of all the negative feelings arises out of the willingness to accept that we have the power within us to handle this inner fearfulness, to recognize that we are the source of it, and to stop projecting it onto the world or God. No one created a fearful world; there is no such thing. The fearful world is within us. We carry it with us and thus we can let it go. We can let the fear of the fear go, as well as fear itself, and move into the presence of Love.

CHAPTER 10

Pain and Suffering

This chapter will cover the subject of the alleviation of pain and suffering. The world thinks that they are the same thing, but we will show how suffering and pain are actually different from each other. We will look at the relationship between the physical, mental, and spiritual aspects of the experience of the body.

It is said that all diseases, illnesses, and human problems are physical, mental, and spiritual, but what does that really mean? As a physician for more than fifty years, I have learned about the physical aspects; as a psychiatrist, I have learned about the mental components; and in consciousness and spiritual research and experience, I have learned about the spiritual dimension.

What is meant by spirit? Is it a fantasy, or is it something real that we can work with? Is it something that is only useful for religious people? What do we need to know about 'spirit' in order to experience the truth of it for ourselves, and how can we utilize this knowledge for the alleviation of our personal problems and those of the people we love?

We will learn how to handle acute and chronic pain, and even more importantly, how to be with that pain. There are two problems to address: The first is how to handle the symptoms specifically and discover what part hypnosis, acupuncture, and other modalities play in the alleviation of pain. The second is to look at the levels of consciousness and how they relate to the experience of pain. Again, we will be referring to the Map of Consciousness, which shows the calibrated levels of energy, their relative power and direction, the emotional component of each level, the process going on in consciousness at each level and how that influences our view of the world and of God, and how the problem is resolved if we do not have a belief in a God.

There will be clinical examples of problems I have personally experienced and worked through using these techniques, along with examples that have worked for others. With these clinical experiences, we can demonstrate certain principles of consciousness that offer a benefit for our lives as a whole. What we learn in studying one specific example then has other applications, so we will be turning lemons into lemonade. We will learn how to transform something that the world considers to be awful, such as pain, and how to derive benefit from it and have our life prosper as a result of the knowledge gained from the one specific experience. In order to do this, we need to know something about the nature of consciousness itself and how that will help us in our lives in general.

What is the nature of human experience? Where is experience experienced? We will again look at the relationship between body, mind, and spirit. Everybody uses that phrase, "body, mind, and spirit," but what does it mean in a practical way? I became a scientist with a skeptical, pragmatic mind. I am very impressed by what works and am very unimpressed by the hypothetical and the theoretical. I am very interested in what brings about results and what one can replicate through one's personal experience.

As said previously, the first thing to realize is that the body has no capacity to experience itself. This is a surprising thought because we think we are experiencing our body—we all think we are our body. How does the body get experienced? For example, the arm has no way of experiencing its armness; the leg cannot experience its being a leg. These parts are experienced through sensations, as is the whole body. We do not experience the body but experience the sensations of the body. And where are these sensations of the body experienced? They are experienced in the mind. Without a mind, we cannot experience what is going on in the body, and we cannot experience the sensations that tell us about the body. The experience of the body is not occurring in the body; it is occurring in the mind. That is the first surprising thought to get used to.

The next surprising thought is that the mind cannot experience itself. A thought cannot experience its thoughtness; a feeling cannot experience its feelingness; and a memory cannot experience its own memoryness. The mind has to be in something greater than itself in order to know what is going on in mind. And what is that? One knows what is going on in mind because of consciousness itself.

The content of mind, and what is going on in mind, is known through consciousness; therefore, all experience is occurring in consciousness. One's awareness of what is happening is occurring within one's consciousness. For example, if a part of the brain is cut, then that part of the mind is no longer operative in the physical domain. If the area cut out is the sensory region, then the opposite side of the body is no longer experienced. Therefore, the body is experienced by the mind via the brain.

We know that if consciousness is eliminated, there is no awareness of what is going on in the mind. That is the purpose of anesthesia. Interestingly, consciousness itself is experienced from an even greater domain. As this progresses, one realizes that the lesser is always experienced from that which is the greater. The greater encompasses and allows the experience of the lesser. Consciousness is then experienced in the greatest domain, which is the one without limit that includes awareness. It is the nature of awareness being itself to know what is going on in consciousness. It is the nature of consciousness to know what is going on in mind. It is the nature of mind to know what is going on with sensations, and it is the nature of sensations to know what is going on with the body.

It is important to know that all ordinary experience is going on in consciousness alone. Where is that consciousness when we experience something? Where do we experience it? Is there a place where consciousness is located? Does it have a specific space or location?

It is important to know that consciousness has no particular space, no physical area, and no limitation. The common fantasy is "I experience things in my head." Actually, we do not experience them in the head. Where do we experience a thought? We experience a thought nowhere; there is no specific location or space in which we experience a thought. The nature of consciousness is that it has no particular form; it is without form. Its content is with form, but the field of consciousness itself is like space, having no particular locality. This will be important later when we discuss one of the techniques for handling pain, which can be handled both locally and generally.

There are several ways to handle pain and the specific sensation and experience of it. Where we are as a being with the experience of pain, and how we evolve in our own consciousness, will determine whether the pain involves suffering or not. The pain is one thing, and the suffering is another.

The first thing to eliminate is the belief system that pain equals suffering because that sets up a whole series of programs that need to be undone. Pain is one thing, and it is quite possible to be with pain yet be totally indifferent to it. It is possible for pain to exist in the body and yet have relatively little or no experience of the pain or suffering with it at all because of an analgesic or altered (e.g., hypnotic) state of mind. It is as though the pain is still present, but one is not connected with the pain. The pain exists on its own but without the person being at the effect of it. In other words, it is not necessary to be the victim of the pain. One can be with the pain in such a way that does not involve suffering or any kind of agony. To realize that this is possible is the first step that leads one out of it. It is the letting go of the belief that pain and suffering are the same thing.

An example is the belief that going to the dentist is necessarily painful. At one time in my life, many years ago, going to the dentist was agonizing. I remember that I always put off going because my pain threshold was so low. I literally had to have analgesia to get my teeth cleaned; I was pain prone.

What is it that sets our pain threshold or our readiness to experience pain? As the years went by, I learned various spiritual and consciousness techniques and began to apply them to pain. The experience of pain began to diminish, and much to my surprise, I could go to the dentist and experience only moderate pain instead of agony. Gradually the pain became mild and then only just a discomfort. When I go to the dentist now, I don't even notice any discomfort. It seems as though I am in the chair for only a minute, and then I am out and say, "Are you done already? I can hardly believe you are done already!"

At the end of this chapter we will discuss some self-hypnosis techniques, a kind of autosuggestion, that will reinforce what we have learned, such as how to utilize a somewhat altered state of consciousness on our behalf, how to come from a suggestible space to learn more quickly, how to relieve pain, and how it is a medium for quickly educating ourself. When you next go to the dentist, you may not have much time to learn these techniques, so we share some ways to speed them up.

The first thing to address is the handling of acute pain. A person is walking along and suddenly sprains an ankle, resulting in agonizing pain; or they break their leg or suddenly have a gallbladder attack, renal colic, or a coronary; or they just have an ordinary accident, such as barking the shin, or hitting the head on something, and there is that stunning moment of pain. How does one handle that acute situation? We will reveal a technique to use in dealing with a variety of illnesses as well as in healing both acute and chronic pain.

There is a shock when we suddenly find ourself facing an accident, such as scalding ourself by pouring hot water on our hand, or burning ourself on the stove. The technique that we will get a lot of mileage from is the whole concept of letting go of resistance. We want to look at the benefit of letting go and compare it with what the mind usually does. The mind normally resists an experience out of the expectation of suffering. It already has a program set up: "Pain means suffering, and I'm going to resist it." The fantasy is that if we resist it, we will eliminate it.

The first thing we have to know is that the relief of pain and suffering comes rapidly by going 180 degrees in the opposite direction—by capitulating and letting go of resisting the pain. How does this work in everyday life? We will provide some clinical examples of rapid healing resulting from techniques that are completely different from those ordinarily used by the mind in an average situation.

To let go of resistance means to completely be with the event and totally surrender to the sensation. It means to ignore the thoughts that we may be having about it. Instead of thinking about it, we go right into the direct experience of the sensation and totally let go of resisting it. For example, if we get burned by accident and let go of resisting the sensation, at first it will be like an overwhelm. We open the doors, the pain rushes in, and we totally surrender to it and let go of resisting it. The way to do this is to say, "More, more, more." The way to hold this in mind so that this is acceptable is to know that there is only so much pain in any experience. We open the door to it and let it run out rapidly. "I let go of resisting this experience. I let go of resisting being with it. I ignore the thoughts because

the thoughts are not going to be useful. Instead I totally surrender and allow myself to experience it totally."
It is as if the doors open, there is a rush, and the pain is
totally experienced out rapidly in a very few minutes.

I remember twisting my ankle in San Francisco. It
was a severe twist that ordinarily would have required
seeing an orthopedist, getting the ankle taped, or
maybe even having a cast put on for six weeks or so.
Instead, I sat down on a park bench, just closed my
eyes, and surrendered to it. It came in waves of excruciating pain. If I had resisted it, I would have ended up
in a cast. In other words, if one resists the pain, it turns
an acute pain into a chronic condition. I just sat down
on the park bench and let it swamp over me. I surrendered to it and waves of pain came over me. Yet, curiously enough, it was devoid of suffering because I was
choosing to experience the experience. In doing that,
I was the master of the experience and no longer the
victim. I was the one saying, "I choose to experience it;
give me more of it." As a result of that, the amount of
suffering involved was really minimal. The alleviation of
pain was very rapid, and within three to four minutes,
I was up and walking again. The pain had decreased to
a very minimal level, and as I continued walking, I kept
letting go of resisting the pain.

At a later date when I broke my left foot, I did the
same thing. When I was chopping wood, a huge oak log
fell on my left foot and crushed all the bones across the
top of it. A short time later, at Christmas, I was back
dancing in the ballroom. My foot was never in a cast; I
did nothing about it except consciously choose to let
go of resisting the experience. After that, I had an injury

that resulted in an amputation. Again, there was the same shock of the experience and then the knowing of how to handle it by letting go of resisting the experience, constantly letting go of resisting the sensations. As I did that, what the world would call miraculous happened right before my eyes. The first thing I did after inadvertently cutting my thumb off with a circular saw was to instantly stop resisting the experience. I just stood still and allowed the experience to sweep in over me, and as I did that, within seconds the bleeding stopped. I have the piece of board that I was cutting, and there are just eight drops of blood on it. By letting go of resisting the experience, the digital artery that had been severed should have pulsated in a grotesque manner, but no such thing happened.

A friend who severely burned himself in the kitchen just stood still and consciously chose not to resist that burn; the pain of the burn was gone in a matter of a minute or two. Later, there was no blister at all. Ordinarily, it would have become a big water blister and taken months to heal, but the only thing that happened was a discoloration.

One time, a cabinetmaker in one of my classes burned both of his hands. He followed the same technique, instantly letting go of the resisting. His hands would normally have been covered with blisters and been in bandages for weeks; instead, he said that in a matter of three or four minutes, the pain was gone and there never was any blister formation. These are just a few examples of instant healing which demonstrate that the body knows how to heal itself the minute we let go of resistance.

Why should this be so? There is no magic involved; anybody can experience the truth of this. This has been a common teaching for thousands of years. Those who have tried Zen meditation know that the first thing taught is the handling of discomfort of the physical body by letting go of resisting the experience, canceling out thoughts about it, and becoming one with it, thereby disappearing it.

In consciousness work, the process is called 'disappearing'. By totally letting go of resisting something, we disappear it out of our experience. One can see that the experience is prolonged by resistance. As long as we resist a thing and hold it, it continues its existence. Resistance gives it the power over us, and we then become the victim of that. We are at the effect of that which we resist. The minute we let go of our resistance and become one with it, it disappears. This also means letting go of all associated images and their accumulated energy.

The reasons for this can be understood from referring to the Map of Consciousness. As stated earlier, each of the levels of consciousness has been calibrated mathematically to show its power relative to the other levels. The arrows indicate whether the energy is in a negative or a positive direction, which is very important in determining the way that we experience things. Those things in a negative direction are experienced as pain and suffering and are detrimental and destructive to our lives.

The various energy fields influence our emotions and are indicators of a process going on in consciousness. They influence how we see and experience the work as well as how we experience our relationship to something that is greater than the personal self, which the world calls a Deity. It is a relationship to a greater field of consciousness and the powerful fields that come about at the higher levels.

The only reason to review this is to understand what happens in the technique of handling acute pain. Resistance to pain is a negative energy field that calibrates at about 150. If one tries to control the pain or use will power against it and resist it, a negative energy field that calibrates at about 150 occurs within the self. This would be about the same level as the emotions of resentment or grief where we resent the pain and are angry about it. If we move up to letting go of resistance, if we have the courage to use the technique and are unreservedly willing to try it, then we move up to the field of 250 called Neutral. Moving into Neutral means being in a positive, detached energy field where "It's okay with me, and I'm willing to experience this thing out." Willingness moves us up to an energy field of 310 where we say yes to life and its experiences, where we agree and align with it, and where life expresses itself as a positive intention.

Instead of resisting life, we go with life and surrender it to God. This is the wisdom of the Tao, which teaches that the willow tree bends with the wind, but the oak tree, which resists it, breaks. Instead of resisting what has occurred when barking our shin, we just become like the willow tree and go with it; we let go of resisting it. We allow that experience to flow through the self. By doing that, we move out of a negative, painful energy field full of resentment, anger, and fear. Fear is at the negative level of 100, a low energy field and far away from joy. The higher the number, the greater the feeling of happiness. We can then actually choose, be willing, and even accept that it is what is necessary to handle this, which moves us all the way up to 380, a very high energy field.

When we choose to go with life, whether it is running across a rattlesnake or some other challenging event, and surrender to that experience, we invite and bring forth from within ourselves a greater power, a higher energy. Those people who have utilized this technique end up calling it a higher power, and we will hear them say, "I called upon my Higher Power." Those who have not heard that expression may say, "It is not real to us, so how can we make the experiences real?"

We can make them real by doing them. It is actually through the doingness of it that these things become real. By doing this exercise, we then begin to experience that something other than the personal self is handling the experience, and within moments, what was agonizing is now very bearable. We are out of the resistance and fear of the suffering. We want to avoid or bypass the negative energy field of a lower energy power and instead move up to a higher one, because, as we move up to higher energies such as love, we are then in the energy field of 500.

When we move into unconditional lovingness at level 540, the field has the capacity to heal; it is the level of healers. The field that healers generate calibrates at 540 and up. It is an immensely loving field, and the emotion is experienced as lovingness—that desire to be with life, to say yes to it, and to let go of resistance.

The healing from acute pain that results automatically from using this technique can be experienced by anyone. I have used it over and over again as have the people who have tried it. Many people have had the opportunity. I remember describing the technique to a Sunday night class, and during the week, several members had acute injuries where this information was life-saving for them. It literally enabled them to carry on through the terrible experiences. Not long after, a big, burly friend visited me and gave me a hug, which broke three ribs. I felt them snap but did not say anything about it because he would have felt guilty. The ribs healed, but later that winter, another friend gave me a hug and broke three ribs on the other side of the body. Needless to say, I did not mention that either (so much for my 'rib karma').

How can this technique be utilized in handling chronic pain, which is different from acute pain? We handle it in the same way as used for acute pain; however, it is done in a somewhat different manner. As we said before, all experiences are being experienced in consciousness. We look to see where the pain is being experienced, such as in the thumb that got cut off. First, we could say the pain is in the thumb. Actually, where is the pain being experienced? It moves our attention away from the thumb. If one says, "I move the focus of attention to the top of my head," then, from the locus of the top of the head, we look at the area of the thumb and experience the painfulness of it, but where is the painfulness of the thumb occurring? When we do that, we begin to notice that the painfulness is being experienced everywhere—all around the body and the energy fields of the body—it is really sort of occurring everywhere.

Most everyone has experienced the pain that makes one sick to their stomach and feel flip-floppy and weak in the knees. We experience it everywhere. If we go into the top of the head, just as an exercise that we do, from that point we begin to experience the pain. We notice the pain as being everywhere and then use the same technique that was used in handling the acute pain. We let go of resisting what is being experienced everywhere; it is not going on in any specific place.

It is desirous to clearly differentiate the feeling, sensation, or experience from the thoughts. We are going to be going on with all of life's problems, especially with physical illnesses, with an absolute sensation coming in of what is really being experienced. The mind then elaborates about the experience, labels it, and puts concepts on it. For instance, one cannot experience an ulcer or a sprain. Those are labels, concepts, or diagnoses. 'Pain' is a concept as is the word 'sensation'. The experiential phenomenon is beyond words, concepts, or labels.

What is a person actually experiencing? Experiencing what the world calls an 'ulcer' is a sensation in the abdominal area, 'right here'. Then the mind says, "Well, if I can't call it an ulcer, I'm going to say it is burning." That again is a concept. We have learned what that means and that it is a thought form. We are not actually experiencing a burning; instead, we are going inside to an experiencing of the experience, which has no words. We go beyond the words to the experiencing of the experience.

When the animal experiences it, it has no words about it; it is just what is going on. Why do we not call up our animal nature and just be with what is being experienced without saying anything about it? It is because all these thoughts bring in complicated programs and belief systems, and we then become subject to the effect of these thoughts. If I say to myself, "I have an ulcer," then a group of programs arises that go with 'ulcer'. Because of the nature of the mind, we begin to experience all the programs because of the power of the mind. The most difficult concept for people to grasp when they enter research work in the field of consciousness itself is the realization of the power of the mind and how influential it really is. We just cannot be careless about our thoughts.

Once we understand the power of the mind and the nature of thought, we begin to realize that one of the principles of consciousness is that we are subject only to what we hold in mind. This one sentence is the key to the healing of all illnesses, pain, and suffering. *We are subject only to what we hold in mind.* The mind is extraordinarily powerful. The great difficulty that people have is in comprehending how powerful the mind is. Therefore, in dealing with pain or suffering of any kind, it is first necessary to discontinue, let go, and cancel all our belief systems about that. Research has shown that it is the belief system itself which literally creates the experience. The incident is an expression of that belief system. It is as if the mind justifies what it believes to be true.

We can know if this is true by beginning to cancel

the belief that pain and suffering are the same thing. In handling pain, either acute or chronic, we have to cancel all thoughts since they are really belief systems. Instead, we have to go for radical truth, radical in that we release everything except the wordless experiencing of what is literally being experienced and let go of the resistance to it. When we do that, we will experience relief from the suffering, and curiously enough, we will reach a point where we do not care whether the 'pain' is present or not.

That may be a difficult thing to accept in the beginning because the mind wants to be rid of the pain. This therapeutic approach is to accept it instead, to let the sensations be present but move away from them. In other words, it is like the pain is circumscribed, and now we begin to disengage from that localized pain. It is the same as when we experience morphine with the pain of a broken ankle. The pain is present, and then we begin to feel ourselves move away from that pain. It is no longer us or ours. In that example, the narcotic does what we are explaining can be done by consciousness. The narcotic does not actually do it, but it enables our consciousness to make this very move. However, we can learn to make this very move without being triggered by a narcotic.

In the past, I have had to do that. I have been severely allergic to any kind of analgesic, narcotic, or anesthetic for many years, and over those years, I have had all kinds of severe illnesses and accidents, plus surgery without anesthesia. Out of necessity, instead of resorting to those usual methods of treating pain, I have had to investigate and discover the capacity and power of consciousness itself. I found that all the analgesics did was allow consciousness to exercise its own power. Therefore, we can own that we have the power within our own consciousness to achieve the same results without the analgesic.

We begin to move away from the pain by letting go of resisting it and not wanting to change it. We just let the sensations be present and then shift our way of being with them to the point where we do not care if they exist. It may sound amazing that we do not even care if they are present. It is very simple. We have been upset over many things in our lives. We have felt that we have to do something about them, but suddenly at one point, we let them go and are indifferent to them. For example, there might have been a problem in the back yard that was driving us crazy, and one day we said, "Oh, the heck with it." Suddenly, we moved from trying to do something about it, to control it, to change it, and exert our will, to just letting it be there. (When we try to change people, places, or circumstances, we see that we are up against the impossible, and the only thing we create is suffering). The minute we just let it be, our experience of it disappears. We move up to a state of painlessness in the presence of pain.

The sensations coming from a painful injury are going on, and who cares about it? The sensations from the amputation are going on, but I do not care about it. It makes no difference. If they are there, they are there, and if they are not there, they are not. That all comes about through the very simple practice in which we are totally indifferent. Most of the pain I have experienced in my own life eventually disappeared of its own. It may take minutes in the case of an acute injury, or it may take months for chronic pain. Other people have reported the same experiences from using this technique.

I had one illness that took well over a year of constantly letting go, constantly releasing, and constantly surrendering before it finally disappeared, so I know that the sensations will eventually disappear, but I am not doing these things to try to achieve that. That would be trying to change it and get rid of it. I do know as a matter of clinical observation that as a person lets go of resisting the pain, there comes a point where they don't care if it is there or not, and then suddenly one morning they wake up and it is gone. We don't let go of resisting it in order to get rid of the pain—that is a happy side effect. When we reach the point where we do not care whether the pain is present or not, then what difference does it make, because at that point, we are immune to the pain.

It is very good to know that our mind has this power and capacity, and that all we need is someone to point it out to us and encourage us to try it so we can see that it works. There is no need to be in a state of suffering over pain of any kind. Pain is one thing; suffering is another. We have to say that over and over to ourself and begin to utilize these techniques. Then we will experience there is a 'me' that is separate from the pain. It is like we are not connected with it anymore, and we are something even greater than and beyond that which is painful.

What is the meaning of life's experiences? The meaning determines how we experience them, how we feel about them. Isn't that so? It does not make any difference at all what happens in the world if we can be with it in a certain way. It is not what is happening out there but how we are with it. People who are quite evolved can be with situations that look dramatically tragic and yet be unaffected by them.

One of the things we can do about pain is to consciously progress in the movement and growth of our own consciousness. Pain proneness comes about as a result of holding a lot of negative thoughts and feelings within ourselves. Spiritual work and evolution have an overall value. The whole process of forgiveness was not really heard about much except within religion, and now it has become almost a social phenomenon. When we go about our social life now and somebody brings up a resentment, the other people will look at the person because they know the next step for them is to learn how to forgive it, or they will be at the painful effect of it.

All pain and suffering come about as a result of what we are already holding in mind. Why are some people so susceptible to pain and suffering, and for others, it is very transitory? The pain and the suffering go through the surface of them but not into their core. They can get extremely upset over something, but who they really are within remains unruffled. Somehow there is a differentiation between who one is and the experience. The true Self is totally unruffled and allows the experience to flow through the self. The upset, such as emotional conflict or whatever it happens to be, may last for hours, but the true inner Self does not even participate in the upset. That is the differential between what is one's real self and what is being experienced. It is the letting go of the habit of identifying that one is the experience. One is that in which the experiencing is happening, but one is not the experience itself.

How can we bring about this evolution and growth in ourselves? That takes us back to the Map of Consciousness to find how we relate to chronic pain in order to transcend it and no longer be in a state of suffering about it.

Near the bottom of the chart is the energy field of Guilt at calibration level 130. Prolonged and excessive guilt, for example, makes us prone to sickness, accident injury, pain, and suffering. The view of the world that comes out of this guiltiness results in a constant habit of sin and suffering and brings about self-hatred. The process in consciousness is one of self-destruction arising from the self-hatred. As a result, one of the belief systems to give up is that guilt and suffering have any particular value. As we go up the energy fields, we can see that those who approach the fields of the saints and the great beings are getting closer to God and farther from guilt, pain, and suffering. As we experience the Ultimate Reality, we go through the doors of a progressive lovingness because love increases and expands as one moves up through joy and ecstasy to a state of peace.

We have to give up worshiping the god of suffering. Christians have to give up solely worshiping the God of the crucifixion, the Christ of the crucifixion, and move on to the Christ of the resurrection. The message was not that of death, sin, and suffering. People who

identify themselves as a body—the strict materialists—
look at the Christ on the cross as a body and come out
with pain, sin, guilt, and suffering. Was that the message? Is that what Christ died for, to teach everybody
that we are a physical body? Or was his message the
direct opposite? His message was that we are not limited.
We have to substitute our confused ideas and begin to
look at moving towards a lovingness and a higher state
of consciousness to learn that the message was the
Christ of the Resurrection.

Now we have to give up the belief that penance,
guilt, sin, and suffering are somehow of enormous spiritual benefit. Frankly, all the thousands of people I have
clinically treated over fifty years who had chronic pain,
guilt, sin, and suffering were the most selfish and self-
centered persons I have ever met. Chronic pain and
suffering does not make people enlightened, loving
beings. It usually makes them cranky, horrible, selfish,
and self-centered, which brings them up to the next
level—that of self-pity. Most people with chronic pain
are into self-pity, grief, 'poor me', and the endless fear
of the continuation of the state, wondering if it is going
to get worse. They continually resist it and have the
constant desire to get away from it.

The bottom area of the Map of Consciousness
reflects the negative energy fields. The people are
very, very angry. The anger of the people in chronic
pain is enormous. They are stuck in it. Some are even
proud of the fact that nobody has been able to help
them. They grimly tell about all the doctors they have
seen, all the treatments they have had, and how all of
those things have not worked.

It is necessary to move up to Courage, which contains the capacity to look at the fact that something can be done about the way we can be with the pain. The way to be with it is by using the simple 'letting go of resisting' and having the willingness to do so. Are we willing to try something? Do we have the courage to try letting go of resisting the pain and ending up at least detached from it in order to move out of this state of suffering? The lower energy fields are all negative states of suffering.

The arrows of the energy fields above 200 all point upwards. This means there is less and less suffering as we move up into Joy. How can we be with that chronic condition? Can we be willing to be with it and let go of resisting it? Can we begin to differentiate and accept that we are that which is with the pain? Can we accept our capacity to be with it in a state of nonsuffering?

When looking at the emotions that go with the energy fields below 200, we can see those that go with chronic pain. There are self-hatred and the feeling of being a victim. The process going on in consciousness is a destructive one of hopelessness. We think nothing can be done about our condition. It is worth remembering the nature of the power of the mind—that what we hold in mind literally creates our experience. The person who says, "My condition is hopeless" then creates a condition that is hopeless and resistive to treatment.

If the person in Grief moves up to Apathy, they are in a constant state of regret, with the feeling of loss and despondency. These are feelings that are only human. They are not feelings that anyone wants to feel guilty about; they are feelings people want to understand. Through understanding, they become resolved.

When I cut my thumb off, I went through all these feelings. First was the feeling that I was somehow being punished or attacked by the forces of retribution or something similar. The pain was acute, and I looked at it and felt hopeless. I felt despair that the thumb could never be replaced, and so on. I went into grief and mourning, as though I had lost a loved one. There was a fear of the consequences and a fear that the pain and suffering were going to continue. I felt myself resisting the desire to get away from the injury, the disability, the pain, the suffering, the surgery, and the rest of it. I was feeling angry—angry at life, at fate, and at myself. These feelings are understandable—they are only very human. Then there was the moving into Pride that I was going to do something about it, and then into Courage to begin to look at the techniques that I knew work in this kind of circumstance. Next arose the willingness to begin utilizing them and let go of resisting, and then using that technique to eventually move up into the acceptance of it so that if it is there, it is okay, and if it is not there, that is okay as well.

Neutral is an interesting energy field, the one in which we say it is okay either way. When we totally release our resistance to the pain, we do not care if it is present or not. There are the willingness to be forgiving and the desire to eventually move into compassion. There is acceptance of the human condition and the human protoplasmic experience without being resentful about it, without going into self-pity, without being angry, without being prideful and going into a 'make wrong', and without attacking ourself. If we do this, then we can move up to an energy field called Love, or even Joy. I can only go back to my personal experience of what is possible. When somebody shares their experience with us, we learn what is possible in human consciousness.

As I moved through this experience, I began to call on the Power greater than myself. I kept surrendering the pain, turning it over to that Power. I remember going to the emergency room and informing them that I could not take anesthesia or analgesia of any kind. The surgeon was somewhat perplexed about how this was going to be handled, and I said, "I have my own ways." He relaxed, feeling that somehow the pain was being handled. I went within myself, detached, and let go of resisting. I called upon the God of my own understanding, that aspect of my greater Self. We can believe there is some energy field greater than the personal self that has unlimited power. So I constantly surrendered to God throughout the procedure. When we are in a situation like that, overwhelmed by excruciating pain and suffering with all the props pulled out, this is when we realize what we really believe in; it is a great opportunity for growth.

As I surrendered and let go of resisting the experience, suddenly it was as though I was lifted out of my body, and I went into a state of profound inner peace, an incredible state of stillness, exquisite inner serenity, and joy. I realized that something other than my personal self was handling the experience and the pain.

What we have learned to do with chronic pain is to surrender it to God, or to whatever one believes in (e.g., angelic beings) to handle the pain for them. When this is done, there is the experience of something greater than the personal self that handles the pain. My personal experience was that some great energy came in and handled it for me. We call it a great energy because we can verify the existence of it. As I said, "God, I can't do it; you do it for me," I surrendered my burden and allowed that which is in the universe to handle it for me.

For those of you to whom this may seem like an outlandish experience, we will look at if from a level that would be understandable. At the level of about 540, healing begins to take place, and there is a release of endorphins within the brain, They are the neurochemicals that are also released by narcotics.

Subsequent to this experience, I was aware that within me something was automatically handling the pain which did not involve my personal self at all. As the intensity of the pain increased, within me was an energy field that expresses itself on the physical plane through the release of endorphins. The power of that field was automatically handling the pain. The pain and suffering were completely and totally released, and in their place was a state of infinite inner serenity and peace.

How can we augment our endeavors in these directions? Certainly, we can do spiritual work, but all those processes, such as forgiveness, take a period of time. In the meantime, what can we do? Are there ancillary procedures, such as acupuncture and hypnosis, that play a part in the alleviation of pain?

We know that acupuncture can be extremely

effective. We said that all forms of illnesses, pain, and suffering are physical, mental, and spiritual. We have just described how they are handled from the spiritual level. Previously, we described how they are handled on the level of consciousness itself through the mind. Certainly, at the same time, we want to do what we can on the physical level. In my personal experience, acupuncture has been extremely effective. I had duodenal ulcers for about twenty-five years that were intractable and incurable. I had received every treatment known to medical science, and it was only a matter of time before it would be necessary to have a subtotal gastrectomy and reparative gastrointestinal surgery, a major procedure. I then tried acupuncture, and by the third treatment, the pain and suffering left, and x-rays revealed that the chronic duodenal ulcers had healed. (They never recurred.) As a result, from personal experience, I would certainly suggest acupuncture for a chronic, intractable condition.

We know that the reliance on analgesics has two negative effects. First, because it is such a magical, short-term solution, one never grows in consciousness. One gives away their power to the pill, the power that is really of one's consciousness. When one gives the power to the pill, personal growth stops. The second negative effect is the progressive dependency on the analgesics or narcotics, which creates and compounds the whole problem with a challenge that may be more severe than the original situation.

Another useful technique is hypnosis. Alternative medicine is now very interested in hypnosis as well as acupuncture. The most useful form of hypnosis is self-hypnosis. It is advisable to learn it for oneself rather than needing to seek it from another, for reasons having to do with the advancement of consciousness. It is a very simple process. One can use the hypnotic state, which is really only a state of high suggestibility, to learn the very things described previously. If one goes into an extremely relaxed state and begins to experiment and experience the truth of what has been presented above, the learning is much faster. In my experience with self and others, the value of self-hypnosis is that it enables one to reach a level of concentration that is not otherwise accessible. In that suggestible state, one is capable of degrees of concentration not available in an ordinary mental state.

There is a simple technique that people who have any chronic physical condition can learn to use. Instead of the word 'hypnosis', which has all kinds of associated beliefs and meanings, we will talk about extreme relaxation in a state of heightened suggestibility and capacity to concentrate. Just sit or lie down in a very comfortable position and start to progressively relax. Picture yourself walking down a series of ten steps and then say, "Level 1." That announces that we are about to do this procedure. Then say, "Level 2" and go deeper into relaxation.

The first step initiates the experience, and the next step allows some time to relax all the muscles in your head. As you do that, you will notice the soreness in your face and jaw muscles reflecting the tension of the day. Your cheeks are actually sore—just poke them and you will find that is true. Why are they sore? It is from the chronic tension of resisted feelings.

Allow yourself several minutes to relax your head. Then say, "Level 3." Now relax your neck. Relax all the tension in your neck and upper shoulders. Then say to yourself, "Level 4," and move and relax your back and chest muscles. As you say "Level 5," just continue to progressively relax, starting with the biggest muscles and then moving to the smallest—the shoulders, the upper arms, the lower arms, the hands, and then the fingers. Say "Level 6" and allow your chest and torso to relax. With "Level 7," move into the lower abdomen, relaxing all the tensions you have been holding there. Say "Level 8," move into the hips and buttocks area, and allow the deep relaxation. At "Level 9," allow that relaxation to flow down your legs. Now say "Level 10" and allow your feet to relax. Next say "I am at level 10." Using that letting go of resistance, allow yourself to let go of all resistance to this profound state of relaxation.

Surprisingly, it will be discovered that no matter how seemingly complete the state of relaxation seems to be, there is yet another, even deeper level. By going through progressively deeper levels, it is discovered that one has never really, really been totally relaxed in their entire lifetime while awake.

In this profound state of relaxation, now tell yourself the things you want to know and then let go of resisting them. Let go of resisting the thought that pain is one thing and suffering is something else. There is no such thing as suffering in pain when that pain is not resisted. In that profoundly relaxed state now, go back to the previous information to deal with chronic pain. Notice that the pain is everywhere, and notice that you can let go of your resistance to that pain. You can open the door and let it happen without its affecting that which you really are. In it, you can begin to move yourself up to a lovingness for yourself and a compassion for your intrinsic beauty as a human being.

At an energy field of about 500 to 540, the lovingness comes forth. We know that it has happened when we become lighthearted about the situation and can laugh at ourself. There is the energy field of humor, which is higher. The fact that humor heals has been reported in books by celebrities who have healed a physical illness through the constant use of laughter. The choosing of laughter and humor and putting ourself in a loving, laughing energy field that is over 500 tends to bring healing out of its own nature. There is the capacity to laugh at the misfortune, which means that the experience is one thing, and that which we are in truth is something else. We are not the experience nor at the effect of it. We are no longer the victim and have stopped struggling with it and resisting it.

In going through Neutral and Willingness to the level of Acceptance, we notice a release from suffering, and what does that mean? When we are resisting and trying to get away from it, we are at a lower energy field and see the process as one of entrapment. As long as we resist the suffering and pain, as long as we are angry, grit our teeth, struggle against it, and try to force our will, we become further enmeshed in it. It's like a quagmire—the more we struggle, the more entrapped we become. To move up to the higher energy field of freedom means to be released from the entrapment and become empowered. The courage to face the issue and do something about it brings empowerment.

Willingness moves us up to a transformation of consciousness and into the willingness to be forgiving, loving, and compassionate. We can transcend this and literally move beyond identification with the body and what has happened to it into a conscious awareness that we are something other than the body.

In another chapter, we will talk about letting go of resistance so completely that there is very little awareness of the body even being present. This also happens with pain in which the thought, memory, and awareness that there is some pain only happens for a few fleeting seconds during the day. I have used the thumb only as an example of the realness of what I am presenting. The pain came to me for only a few seconds throughout the day when it was still present. After about an hour, I suddenly noticed the thumb and said, "Oh, it's like I'm not even aware of its presence." That occurred maybe a few other times during the day. In a twenty-four-hour period, the total amount of suffering I experienced that the world would call painful amounted to maybe five or ten seconds in the morning and maybe a few seconds in the afternoon. The totality of the suffering that came out of this experience, which lasted for only a few months, amounted to probably less than thirty seconds. It is valuable for all of us to do this because through doing it, we realize the truth of who we really are.

Another assist to healing pain or any other distress is to listen to great, beautiful music, which itself releases endorphins in the brain. That beauty provides a healing effect has been known since the days of Hippocrates.

CHAPTER 11

Losing Weight

Is there a way to let go of weight in a way that is practical, easygoing, joyful, and free from any kind of suffering? Can this be done? Yes! All it takes is about an hour or an hour and a half of our attention over a day or two during the time we are doing the things we normally do. The benefits are long lasting for a lifetime! The reward for a couple of hours of just paying attention to a few simple principles is a lifetime of freedom from this challenge. How do I know it works? Because it has worked for everyone who has tried it. It has worked for my patients and for me. I permanently lost fifty pounds by using this very simple technique that emerged out of consciousness research.

The alleviation of a problem should be simple, direct, to the point, long lasting in its effect, and cost nothing. Diets usually do not work in the long run. The usual techniques that people try often bring about feelings of guilt and recrimination. They may work, but only temporarily because they do not really modify the way one is with their body since they do not change those Pavlovian reflexes that drive one's eating despite one's best intentions.

It was discovered that a shift in the state of consciousness occurs in the process of eating, and that a person can easily overcome it so the weight loss becomes permanent. The message is to give up trying will power, give up dieting, and give up resisting eating. Those methods usually do not work; they make us miserable, and we frequently end up the same as we were anyway. There is a much easier way that is truly joyful.

Through an understanding of some very simple concepts that have been presented previously in relation to the Map of Consciousness, we are then put in a place of being able to handle problems that have been baffling and unsuccessful in the past.

Through the use of some techniques based upon the nature of consciousness itself, we can learn how to imagine ourself as slim, energize that image, and then let go of it so that it actually materializes. It is necessary to learn how to come from the heart instead of the head, and to come from love instead of the stomach. The head criticizes us because the stomach wants to eat. The only way to handle this problem is to come from the heart about the whole situation. We are going to be somewhat lighthearted about this subject that many people get quite distressed about. The lightheartedness comes with the eating; the self-recrimination and guilt appear later. We lie in bed and wonder, "Why did I eat all that?" and then begin to attack ourself. There is a way beyond all these problems that will work for all of us.

The medical model commonly followed is really based on the idea of diet and the assumption that the number of calories one eats determines one's weight. There may be some thought about exercise as well. However, the following information is not necessarily going to agree with traditional medical thinking. If traditional medical thinking and counting calories had worked for you, you would not be interested in this information. We are going to present things that we have clinically observed as being true experientially.

Consciousness work has to do with the truth of our inner experience. It does not have anything to do with theory, hypotheses, scientific reasoning, or logic. It has to do with the experiencing of the truth within us.

The first thing to do is to begin to cancel some beliefs about diets and food that have contributed to our problem. To begin with, we have beliefs and thoughts, such as, "Well, being overweight runs in our family—it's in the genes." Or, "It's due to my thyroid," or, "It's due to the fact that as an infant, I was overweight, and that caused too many fat cells." These are all popular medical theories, and if holding those in mind works for you, then that is very good. However, we have found experientially that this really is not so. As an example, two people can eat an identical diet, and one will gain weight and the other will lose it. How can that be explained inasmuch as the activity levels and everything else are about the same? This brings about the questioning of some of the basic medical hypotheses, a few of which are very simple to understand.

First, why assume that the body fully absorbs all the calories it consumes? Why think that the gastrointestinal tracts of two different people are exactly the same? I may eat a 1,000-calorie piece of pie and absorb only 500 calories, with the other 500 running right on through. There are other factors, such as the rate of movement in the gastrointestinal tract. We know that the faster things move through the tract, the less it absorbs. There are factors other than calories to consider, and in doing so, we will arrive at a way of handling this problem that will not involve counting calories.

There are some dietary tricks that are helpful to use in the beginning until the results of working on ourself have adjusted our appestat, which is located in a portion of the brain called the hypothalamus. It takes a day or two to reset the appestat, which controls our feeling of satiety. The adjusted appestat will control our weight. As we hold a certain weight in mind, it begins to materialize on the physical plane. It is helpful to understand the power of mind over body and that what is held in mind creates the body's being what it is, rather than the other way around.

It is necessary to reverse the conventional, so-called 'common sense' of the left-brain logic that says it is the body that creates the mind. Instead, we have to look at the opposite, which is that what is held in mind manifests within the body. Our thoughts and beliefs about weight, activity, calories, and all the phenomena surrounding this have been affecting our weight. For example, the following is known from cases of patients with multiple personalities. One personality appears in the patient and takes over the consciousness named Richard, who does not have any eating or weight problems at all. In fact, he eats very little, is spry and active, and while Richard is in the body, the person is loses weight and becomes slim.

Then the person goes into a trance state or becomes intoxicated, and William comes into the body. William loves to eat, gorging himself on all kinds of things, and the body's weight suddenly increases dramatically. Now we can see that the response of the body is therefore to the mind—the mindset, the mind's belief and attitude, and the way the person holds the relationship to their body in their mind. It is the mind that sets the appestat. It is using consciousness techniques within the mind that release the weight problems, and one can let go of the weight almost automatically.

We will review the nature of consciousness itself and the relationship between body, mind, and spirit, with spirit being the energy field of consciousness that is all pervasive throughout life itself. It is important to understand that the body has no capacity to experience itself. At first this seems amazing because most of us, unless we are enlightened, assume that we are the physical body. We must realize that the body has no way to experience itself. The arm cannot experience the arm nor can the leg experience the leg. Instead, they have to be experienced in something greater than themselves. We experience the body via the senses, which tell us what is going on within it. As the senses of the body have no capacity to experience themselves, they have to be experienced in something greater than what they are, which is in mind itself, so the mind is the place where the sensations in the body are experienced.

Mind itself is incapable of experiencing itself. A thought cannot experience its own thoughtness, nor can a memory experience its own memoryness. A fantasy of the future cannot experience itself, nor can an emotion experience itself. What goes on in the mind has to be experienced in something that is greater than the mind, that is, in consciousness itself. There is the body's experience via sensation. Sensation is

experienced in the mind, and the mind is experienced in consciousness. This can be seen very easily,
for example, when something happens to a portion of
the brain, and the person is unable to experience the
opposite side of the body.

Without mind, the body cannot be experienced.
The whole point of anesthesia illustrates that without
consciousness, one is not aware of what is going on in
mind. If consciousness is deleted via the anesthetic,
there is no knowledge of the experience that is going
on in either mind or body, so consciousness is higher
than both of them. There is a state beyond consciousness itself that is still, unmoving, and allows us to be
aware of what is going on in consciousness; it is called
the state of awareness. The state of awareness is an
aspect of the greater, powerful energy field behind
consciousness, which is the energy of life itself. This
is necessary to know in order to become aware of
where all experience takes place.

All human experience is taking place within consciousness itself. Consequently, we cannot experience
the wall, the floor, or someone else. Instead, what we
experience is within our own consciousness of the
wall, the floor, or another person. This gives an understanding of an area in which we can work that is less
restricted by commonly held belief systems.

If the entire weight problem is a phenomenon
occurring within consciousness, then consciousness
is more powerful than the mind, which is more powerful than the senses, which are more powerful than
the body; therefore, we can bring about a shift in the
body by merely addressing that consciousness. If we

address the problem there, because the body will only do what is held in mind, then we really do not have to bother much with the body; it will just automatically correct itself because the problem is really a problem within the experience within consciousness itself.

The techniques we use have to do with the mind and consciousness, so we do not have to be very concerned with handling the body as such. The body is an effect of what happens in the mind. Consequently, the attempts to solve the weight problem, which are addressed to the body only, are notoriously unsuccessful. Nearly every month, there are headlines on endless magazine covers and in newspapers that are selling a new diet. This lets us know that diets do not work. When there are multiple solutions to a problem and endless articles on the same phenomenon, it is obvious they do not have the answer. If there were an answer to the weight problem, there would not be any articles on diets at all because everyone would have handled it. Addressing it on the physical level alone just does not work. It also does not work for any other problems that involve complicated human behavior.

Problems such as alcoholism and many illnesses, including duodenal ulcers and diverticulitis, are notoriously nonresponsive to being addressed on the physical level only. We have to become more sophisticated and conscious to bring about a resolution of long-standing behavioral problems.

The technique, which I used personally to lose thirty percent of my body weight (fifty pounds) some years ago, enabled me to reach my desired weight. It only takes a matter of minutes over a day or two—collectively, about only sixty to ninety minutes of a person's time and attention. You can actually do this while you are going about your daily activities at home or in the office, and even while driving back and forth to work. It works right into your life and easily fits into your daily routine. You do not have to stop your life in order to use this technique. In order for something to be effective, it has to fit in with your life pattern. We found that any behavioral modification technique works if it fits in with a person's daily life. If you have to change your whole lifestyle, the results are then usually temporary.

With this technique, when the sensation arises that you had previously called hunger, you ignore the thoughts that go with this, especially canceling that thought of hunger. Instead, you go right into the sensation, directly into the inner experience of what you are actually experiencing. You go to where you are experiencing it without labeling it, naming it, or calling it anything. You just experience it and begin to let go of resisting those sensations. You silently go into consciousness itself, into the inner experience of what you are experiencing, and let go of resisting it.

In the beginning we are so controlled by the Pavlovian conditioning that the minute we feel the sensation, we label it 'hunger'. Our behavior goes into immediate action to satisfy it. Like Pavlov's dog that salivated every time the bell rang, we have set up a conditioned reflex that we now want to unset. How can we unset it, how long does this take, and how much effort is required?

Actually it takes very little effort and very little time. When we get this sensation, which was labeled as 'hungry' in the past (I'm 'hungry' now), we let go of labeling and resisting the sensation itself. We just agree and are willing to be with the sensation but to do nothing about it. We let the experience run within us and are willing to be with that inner experience or sensation of whatever it is. Some people may sense it in the stomach, and some may sense it as sort of a physical weakness. Whatever sensation is felt, we stop talking about it in our minds; we stop languaging it and giving it a label. Instead, we go into the inner experience and let go of resisting it. In letting go of the resistance, we can move up to a higher level, if we are willing to choose it, and say to ourselves, "I want more of whatever that is."

The reason for that and the way it becomes acceptable is because there is a limited amount of the sensation that comes up. The mind thinks, "If I don't satisfy this, I'm going to have this hungry feeling continuously." That is not so because the feeling results from resisting it. When we go with it, like in the Tao where the willow tree bends with the wind but does not break, there is no resistance. Instead of being the oak tree that resists the sensation, tries to fight it with will power and then breaks, we can be like the willow tree, going with the sensation and letting go of resisting it. In fact, we welcome it. It is like we are saying, "More." We want more wind, more of this inner experience. As we call forth more of this, sit with the inner feeling, and just be with it, it will run out.

It is a good idea to start this process on a weekend

when at home and we can stop everything and just sit, or better, lie down and focus on it. If we do not let anything distract us from being with the sensation, it will suddenly disappear in a matter of minutes. After it disappears, we can go about our business. After we become used to this technique, we do not have to stop any activities at all. When the experience comes up, we just sit or lie down, concentrate on it, and fix attention on welcoming it. It is like we are opening the barn door and allowing the sensation to come in willingly, being with it but not doing anything about it.

We want to break the cycle of labeling the sensation as 'hunger' when it appears and then satisfying it with food. Doing that just reinforces the cycle, making ourself the victim and at the effect of that behavior pattern. Instead of that, the self stands aside from this sensation and begins to master it so that we are no longer at the effect of it; we becomes the master.

In Zen, there is the famous series of ox-herding pictures. The first picture shows a monk hanging onto a rope that is attached to the ox, and the ox is dragging him across the ground. The monk's knees are bruised, his ears are bleeding, and he is a mess. In the next picture, the monk has the ox tied to a tree with the rope. The monk has caught the ox and identified the problem. In the third picture, the monk is riding on top of the ox. He has become the master. He is no longer the victim at the effect of it. How did he do that? That is what this process is all about. We are going to tether this ox right now by identifying the pattern that has to be handled, and then we are going to be on top of it. The person that we are now stands independently above and beyond and becomes the master of this very simple thing to solve. It is merely the willingness to experience what, in the beginning, may seem like some discomfort, or, in other words, to experience this sensation without satiating it right away. As we do this, the reflex weakens.

But what do we do about our eating during the day? We do what is called 'anticipatory eating'. It means to never eat when we are hungry. The first two days, and probably for the first week or two, we never allow ourself to eat when we are hungry. Instead, we let go of the hungriness by using this radical-truth technique and anticipating the periods of hunger. We know our own hunger patterns, so instead of waiting until we are hungry and then eating, thus reinforcing the pattern, we anticipate the hunger periods. We know that habitually we will be hungry around six o'clock, so instead of waiting until we are hungry and satisfying it, thereby reinforcing our conditioning, we anticipate it. At 4:45 PM, when we are not even hungry yet, we have a cheese sandwich.

The technique is simple—eat when we are not hungry and do not eat when we are, thus substituting this technique for the hunger pattern. How long will it take before we disappear hunger, and what is going to happen? We will no longer experience hunger or appetite; they just seem to disappear. By the second day, we will notice that the pattern is already so weak that we will barely notice it. How many minutes a day will this take? It may take a total of thirty minutes on the first day. You will notice that if you do nothing about the hunger sensation and really let go of resisting it, it will disappear in a matter of minutes. After doing this a number of times, the sensation will disappear in a matter of seconds. We will know that if we sit down and let go of resisting the sensation, it is over in seconds, and we are no longer at the effect of the appetite. We are no longer driven by it and can be absolutely free of it.

In place of this pattern, we may feel a sort of blankness or emptiness. Where there once was hunger and the drive to eat, along with an appetite, enthusiasm about it, and then the satiation, it now seems like nothing is going on in that space in our life. Now we can do some other pleasurable activity, such as rewarding ourself by taking the time to read the book we have been wanting to read and never had the time. Now that we are not out in the kitchen eating all the time, there is time to read for enjoyment instead of feeling guilty because we have more important things to do. We can discover something we really enjoy doing.

One thing to do, for instance, is to take a nap. All the time spent shopping for food, preparing it, eating it, and cleaning up afterward can take up a great part of the day. With this new pattern, it gives us time for a short nap. After a twenty-minute nap, we feel fantastic. After a twenty-minute hunger engorgement, we usually do not feel fantastic; instead, we feel horrible. We just had four Milky Ways, a caramel sundae, and finished off a piece of cheese and now, instead of feeling happy, we feel guilty.

The way off the guilt trip is to really know that there is a very simple technique. It sounds so simple,

but that is why it works. The things that are extraordinarily complicated are generally far from the truth.
The truth is usually amazingly simple. As people at
Alcoholics Anonymous have discovered, they stay
away from one drink one day at a time. It sounds too
simple. The intellect says, "Nonsense! I know that." The
intellect knows this but the self does not know that.
We only know a thing from personal validation
through our own inner experience.

It usually takes exactly one day to get off eating,
hunger, and appetite if we allow ourself to be repro-
grammed. We will notice that as time goes on, we are
beginning to look forward to meals and starting to get
into the habit pattern of getting hungry and satisfying
the feeling. It is very simple to back off and just
release ourself by using this technique a few times. All
we have to do is allow that feeling of hungriness to
come up, be with it, welcome it, and wait till it runs
out, which handles it (usually five minutes or less). We
might have to do it again if we have really gotten into
holiday indulgence for a number of years.

There is another thing that happens as we do this.
There is a center in the hypothalamus at the base of
the brain called the 'appestat'. It sets our degree of
satiety and the amount of satiety that we search for.
The less we eat, the more we turn down the setting
on the appestat. Satiety is something else that is not
really understood by traditional scientific medicine.
Scientific medicine talks about calories as though one
calorie were the same as any other calorie. However,
we know that satiety plays a great role in our hunger
and weight problems. Satiety is more important than

calories; therefore, the diet I follow would make most people who follow diets faint. However, I know what creates a feeling of satiety within myself, such as a hamburger smothered in onions. By the time I finish that, I am totally filled up, satisfied with meat, cheese, and similar foods. Cheese is not on anybody's reducing diet. We know that cheese has a satiety factor, so once one has eaten a certain amount of it, the appetite is satisfied.

We also know that calories are released at different rates. Fats, for instance, are released at one rate and protein at another. We know that it takes a certain number of calories to burn up every gram of protein, so one of the tricks we can use to speed up the process of weight reduction is to go for a high-protein diet. This is not about diet, but I will just throw in a few tricks that I have observed clinically.

Eating sugar on an empty stomach is seriously deleterious to the goals of the program. Why? The body takes sugar in so fast that it is absorbed very rapidly and cannot be metabolized quickly so it just has to be stored as fat within the body. One thing to do for our own sake as part of caring and loving ourselves is to avoid sugar and sweets when introducing this program into our lives. In the beginning, we want to see a fast result. I believe we should have the satisfaction of doing this now and seeing some returns and rewards, including seeing the image that we have been holding of ourself coming into manifestation.

It is best to avoid things that have a high sugar content, especially on an empty stomach, because sugar stimulates the production of insulin, which then brings the blood sugar down rapidly, thus recreating the hunger sensation. In contrast, one-third of the calories of protein are burned up just by the process of metabolizing protein. Therefore, one hundred calories of sugar equal one hundred calories of fat, whereas one hundred calories of excess protein converts to only sixty-six calories' worth of fat. A high-protein diet results in a thirty-three percent discount (not recommended for people with gout). Notice that carnivores are slim. But what about vegetarians? They can also avoid sugar and starch and yet stick to a high-protein diet.

The technique is to let go of resisting and to disappear hunger and appetite. We then live in a world where we are no longer in the cycle. We get used to an eating cycle of overeating, feeling guilty about the overeating, and then trying to control it. Then up comes hunger, and with the hunger come guilt, then appetite, then the expectation of satiation, followed by overindulgence, and guilt again, so there is an endless self-defeating cycle. The only way to beat it is to rise above it, transcend it, and be beyond it. By disappearing it, one will find that appetite and hunger actually disappear, and there is the experience of never being hungry.

The next thing the mind says is, "I don't want to give up the pleasure of eating." Quite the contrary. What happens to the enjoyment of eating once we use this technique is that the appetite arises only out of the act of eating itself rather than anticipatory appetite. I can sit down with no hunger or appetite at all, but the minute I begin to eat, it creates appetite, and the pleasure of eating is greater than it ever was. I enjoy food now more than I ever did. Eating is no longer accompanied by guilt or self-blame. There is no anxiety about eating too many calories or gaining weight from eating. All that is gone, so we do not give up the pleasure of eating at all. We find that when we are not hungry, the food is considerably more enjoyable. We start enjoying the cheese sandwich the minute we take that first bite. We are not even hungry. We pick up the cheese sandwich, bite into it, and the enjoyment is there. There is no loss of enjoyment. I do not believe in letting go of enjoyment and pleasure; on the contrary, I believe in increasing it. So now there is the enjoyment and pleasure of eating as well as the enjoyment, pleasure, and justified pride in having a body that is more appropriate to our aesthetic ambition—how we would like to look.

The first thing to handle is the cycle of eating and getting hungry. We are the victims of a behavioral pattern, a conditioning that has nothing to do with will power or morality. We can condition any kind of animal in this way. What has happened is a sort of Pavlovian-dog conditioning that has nothing to do with our personality or self-worth. It has nothing to do with being self-indulgent, with oral narcissistic needs, or with whatever the psychoanalytic theory might be, such as oral aggression or oral passivity. It merely has to do with a simple, very primary type of conditioning that has been favored in our society.

We picked up those patterns in our social conditioning as children, that is all. We will discuss the part that the child plays in this and arrive at a different way of looking at the whole eating pattern. The mind experiences the body, and consciousness experiences mind; therefore, we really experience within in our consciousness what we formally called 'hunger'. Where is that localized? You will notice that it is only a belief system that is experienced in the stomach. It is actually experienced in a generalized way, sort of everywhere. The thought that it is in the stomach is just a belief system from childhood. As mentioned previously, the body cannot experience anything. What is happening is experienced in a more diffuse, generalized area.

Another technique of letting go of suffering at any time from pain, illness, or physical symptoms, such as hunger, is knowing that it is nothing but a physical symptom. You will notice that it is experienced in a general, diffuse manner, sort of everywhere, because that is where we experience all experience rather than in a localized situation. The localization comes from a strong belief system. We all have these thoughts from childhood. As we let go of resisting the energy of this sensation, it becomes diffuse and finally disappears.

On the Map of Consciousness, we see the lower feelings at the bottom, and when we move up to Desire, which has been running the appetite-hunger-satiation cycle, we notice that it has an energy field that calibrates at 125 and is in a negative direction. In other words, it has a deleterious effect on our lives. The emotions that go with this energy field are wanting, craving, and all the addictions. Therefore, calling a weight problem a food addiction is partially correct in that the characteristics of the negative energy field at 125 are feelings of wantingness, desiringness, and cravingness, and the processing occurring in consciousness is entrapment. The person therefore feels like a victim, and due to the downward direction of the energy field, there are negative feelings about the self having to do with the whole cycle.

As we let go of resisting it and go beyond it, we start moving up the scale to the level of Courage in order to handle the problem of pride in our willingness to look at it. When we move upward and get off this cycle at level 250, we become detached. At that point, the process going on in consciousness is one of being released. Because the energy field now goes upward, we have a good, positive feeling, one that is constructive and makes us feel better. It has a lot of power in it.

How do we experience that detachment? It is the experience similar to if we eat, it is okay, and if we do not, that is okay, too. People ask, "Do you want to eat something now?" I say, "Well, if you are going to fix something, fine." Then they will ask, "What do you want to eat? Do you want to eat fish, or macaroni, or baked beans?" I'll say, "Well, either way." When one reaches this level of handling appetite and hunger, one is no longer really fixed on one particular food or another. One could say, "If we have a steak tonight, that's fine, and if we don't, that's fine." So it is okay either way. This means that one is free.

One characteristic of this attitude is freedom. Freedom from what? There is freedom from being run by a program or a conditioning, and freedom from being a victim of the cycle. There is freedom from the entrapment that made us feel bad about ourselves. As we get detached from these sensations, we begin to feel good about ourselves. In fact, our willingness to do that goes up to level 310, which has an even better feeling about it. We begin to accept that this is nothing other than a phenomenon, just a set of vibrations going on within consciousness. It does not have to do with food or the body. Those are all programs. In essence, physics explains it as just a set of vibrations going on in the field of consciousness that are within our power to alter. Once we do that, we can really begin to love ourselves more than we did before.

There is another very interesting aspect going on in consciousness that will also be very helpful. It is something you can observe within yourself, and something I picked up within myself and saw happening. The cycle in the past was to be run by the hunger, appetite, satiation, and then guilt. All the good intentions I had about dieting and taking off weight suddenly flew out the window and disappeared somewhere. After filling myself up with far more than I knew I needed, suddenly there was a feeling of self-disgust and guilt. People with severe eating problems often experience that. They go into the bathroom, throw all the food back up, and then go into self-hatred, blame, guilt, and even suicidal depression, which can become very severe. What really happens in this type of situation? I observed that when a person sits down to eat, it is only the adult within who wants to take off the weight, and it is really the 'inner child' who is always hungry.

In the past, Dr. Eric Berne, author of *Games People Play* and creator of Transactional Analysis, along with other people in that field, talked about our 'child', 'adult', and 'parent' tapes that are like three voices within us. One is the desirous child; one is the adult who is rational, intelligent, and educated; and one is the parent who tends to be punitive and moralistic. The parent tape is the one that tells us about right and wrong. When we sit down at the table or walk to the refrigerator, the adult within goes unconscious and the child takes over.

What does a child know about diet, weight, and calories? Nothing. The consciousness of the child is, "I want, I satisfy, and I get," so we go to the refrigerator without realizing we are in a different state of consciousness, one in which the child is dominant. So who is poking around in the refrigerator? The child is. Who is ordering a second hot fudge sundae or having a second helping of potatoes and gravy? The child. After we indulge the child without realizing what is going on, when the meal is over, the child leaves. It has had its fill, and then who takes its place? The parent does who then says, "How could you have been so stupid? Why did you have seconds? So did you have a piece of pie? Why did you put ice cream on top of the pie? I mean, think of the calories. You are really stupid and weak; you don't have any will power. You are no good; your self-worth is rotten."

At this point, we are subjected to the inner angry parent who is blaming us. Blaming whom? Blaming the inner child. Where has the adult been all this time? It has been silenced. The adult was not there at mealtime or after mealtime. The child and the parent have taken over the whole eating program, which is natural because that is where the eating patterns get set up in the first place. They get set up with the child, and who is sitting next to the child but the parent? So the child alternates with the parent in running the whole eating pattern.

In order to counteract this, we have to be aware that the pattern is running. Just to be aware of it begins to change it. Now we can make a note to ourself, put it on the table or the refrigerator, and consciously call forth our adult and tell the child, "This is the place for an adult now because my adult is very conscious of its eating." My adult knows about calories, diets, and healthy eating patterns. I consciously call forth my adult to be here at this meal. I say, "The adult me is here now" and consciously reject the presence of the child. Because the overindulgence does not happen, when the meal is finished, my adult stays there. No parent comes in to blame me for what has been done.

It does not take self-control or resisting anything; it just takes being aware. When we sit down, we say hello to our adult and be conscious. Just as we sit down at the dinner table, we watch the kid come up in us. I have watched myself do this. "Oh, look at who is there at the table. Oh, wow! Look at the pile of mashed potatoes! Look at the gravy!" Just watch peoples' faces when they sit down at the table and we see who is 'up' in them. We see the eyes pop open and watch the pupils of the eyes get very large. If that is not a five-year-old kid, then I never saw one.

We may see a serious-looking businessman walk

into a restaurant with his briefcase. He goes through the cafeteria line and then sits down. Now, watch his face as he puts his napkin in front of him. He picks up his napkin—somebody else is already there! There is the kid all ready to have a good time! Of course, after the man gets up to leave, now we instantly see, "Oh, I ate too much." Now who is there? Look at the frown as the man is berating himself as he walks out of the restaurant. In his mind, he is counting all the calories. He just ate 3,850 calories for dinner, and his doctor told him he is supposed to have only 900 calories a day. He figures he cannot eat until next Tuesday now and wonders how is he going to survive.

We can break out of this self-defeating pattern just by being aware. Make a little sign for the refrigerator door that says, "Adults Only." Be conscious; be aware of who is there. We will find that the adult enjoys the eating very much, too, but just does not go crazy so easily.

It is important to avoid a fluctuating blood sugar level as much as possible when first initiating this program because, in the unconscious mind, a drop in blood sugar is often associated with hunger and hungry feelings. For example, if we eat a hot fudge sundae on an empty stomach, the blood sugar shoots up, adrenaline and insulin pour out, and the blood sugar tends to drop rapidly. Behaviorally, in the past, this has been associated with feeling hungry, but we are not actually hungry. The stomach is still full. We have more calories in us than we need, but it is the rapidity and the degree of the drop in this blood sugar from where it was previously that triggers the sensation of hunger again.

It is much easier when initiating this program to stay on a high-protein diet as much as possible because then the blood sugar tends to stay relatively level. We avoid those sudden drops that give the feeling that we want to eat something right away, therefore making it a little easier on ourself. The point is to avoid suffering in all its forms. We do not want to experience suffering in any kind of program because, otherwise, it is not going to work. Counting calories and depriving ourself is setting up a form of suffering. What happens then is unconscious—we get satisfied and the over-indulgence sets up guilt. Then we diet, which is sort of self-punitive, by going on bread and water like a prisoner for a certain period of time. After we have punished ourself sufficiently for all the overindulgence in the past, the guilt disappears and the old habitual eating pattern returns. We want to eliminate the imbalance of extremes of overindulgence, feeling guilty, going into a self-punitive bread-and-water diet—first swinging to the overeating and overindulgence, and then swinging into the guilt and self-punitive deprivation.

Deprivation is not the way to happiness, nor is overindulgence. It is preferable to use consciousness techniques to transcend them and be in the middle of the two so that we are over and above the problem, with the adult there to take over. This makes it easy and enjoyable. It is really delightful to realize that we have just handled and transcended something in just a matter of minutes that has plagued us our whole lifetime.

The first day I tried this, I think I spent about forty-

five minutes sitting down and handling those sensations; the second day, maybe twenty minutes; the third
day, maybe ten minutes; and the fourth day, maybe
four minutes. Since that time, I do not think I have collectively spent an hour using the technique over
many years. One can start a stopwatch, sit down, use
this technique, and hit the stopwatch again when the
hunger feeling is gone. One probably would not col-
lect more than an hour over a ten-year period of time,
so there certainly is not much effort needed or suffering to be experienced.

No will power is involved; willingness is being
used instead because it is a positive, powerful energy
at level 310. Using will power means resistance,
which is a negative energy field with a weak power of
only 125. Instead, we use willingness and acceptance,
which lead to happiness that calibrates closer to 500.
We end up being joyful and feeling great about ourselves. The body becomes pleasing, and we begin to
experience it in a happy way.

Another way to increase the rapidity of the effect
of this is by watching our activities. Exercise is great,
but how many mornings are we going to get up and
do calisthenics? No matter how attractive the person
is on television, we are just going to do this a certain
number of times, and by the fourth day, the enthusiasm wears off; before we know it, we are back into
the same old pattern. Exercise is wonderful. It is good
for that sense of well-being, but weight-reduction
folks know the truth of that one. They have a dozen
exercise machines in the garage.

In contrast, the relatively effortless system just

described actually works so well that you may end up having a problem with being too thin. That is what happened with me. The technique just worked so well that pretty soon the appetite and hunger disappeared, along with all the cycles of eating, indulgence, and feeling guilty. I noticed I forgot to eat breakfast and lunch. I got busy with the activities of the day and totally forgot eating.

Once in a while it comes to us in the beginning, because it is a habit, that it is mealtime. Then we just sit down and let go of resisting that just as we do the sensation, and we will notice that the ideas that "I must eat breakfast," "I must eat lunch," or, "I must eat dinner" are cultural conditions. They do not have any reality to them. It is just as easy to not eat all day. (I have actually gone days without eating and did not even notice it. One time I went from Monday to Thursday. I was so busy with activities, and on Thursday, I suddenly realized, "I don't think I have eaten for the last couple of days." Sure enough, I had not. Then the family began to complain that I was too thin, so then I had to consciously be aware that it was necessary to eat. I had to reprogram myself a little bit to go back into eating. The technique works extremely well and brings a great deal of happiness.

Another consciousness technique, which has a general application, can be used as well. (All the techniques we have discussed have many applications.) You picture the kind of body you want to have and the feeling you want to have about having this kind of body. Then remember sometime in your life when you were feeling joyful and pleased with yourself. Next, picture the body the way you want it to be and reawaken that emotion of joy. For example, if you want to be slim, picture yourself as slim and begin to love that picture of yourself. Love that picture of the body and then let it go, knowing that you have set up a program. You have set up what is going to happen in the future because the mind begins to move in that direction automatically. Just love that picture of yourself. If you like, you can put the number of pounds under it and picture how you want to look, and say, "You know, it's fantastic to be slim and active and feel good about the body. I love myself for that." Research studies confirm that imaging techniques are effective.

We want to stop identifying with the body. We are not the body. We have a body, so how we view our relationship with the body is important. We are that which has a body, just like we are that which has a car or a house to live in. The body becomes like those things, like a pet, which is a great way to look at it. "See, this is my little pet, this is my bicycle, this is my car, this is my pet that carries me around." We can see that it is different from saying, "I am that." If I say I am the body, then I am subject to what goes on with the body. If it gains weight, then it is 'me' who is fat, and I am the one at fault. It does not take too much in the way of meditative self-awareness to realize that we are that which experiences the body, but we are not the body.

At the beginning, we said that the body cannot experience itself; it can only be experienced in mind. Mind can only be experienced by consciousness, and consciousness itself can only be experienced by the field called 'awareness', so we are that which is aware of the body, as well as that which is beyond the body. Our reality is one thing, and the body is another that reflects what we hold in consciousness. Therefore, the problem is not the body at all; the problem is what we hold in consciousness.

The task is really to change the vibrational patterns within consciousness. This body is going to automatically do what it is told to do. It cannot think because it has no mind. That which we are has the mind, and the body follows what the mind tells it to do.

With this imagining technique, the way in which we hold our relationship to the body as pleasurable releases its dominance. As we keep letting go and following these techniques, the body seems to get lighter. The body, having nothing to do with weight, is experienced as progressively weightless. After a while, as we move up the scale of consciousness, we are hardly aware that the body even exists.

In looking at the scale of consciousness differently, we can see how we originate and perpetuate the weight problem by holding it in the form of destructive emotional patterns. It is generally thought that these negative feelings are the 'cause' of the weight problem, but if we look into it, we see this is really not so. We can see that these are the reactions to the weight problem, and sometimes they are the corollary or the parallel.

How have we been holding the weight problem up to this point? Most of us have been down at the bottom of the scale in the area called Guilt, with a very weak energy field of 30. If we try to handle our weight problem or any problem, such as alcohol or relationship, from the level of Guilt, we can see how much energy we have to work with. We have thirty dollars compared to Love, which is five hundred dollars. Thirty dollars is not going to buy us much progress in anything. Not only that, the energy field is negative, meaning we are going to feel negative about the whole thing, along with self-hatred. The process is actually destructive.

People have actually committed suicide over their weight problem and self-indulgence. Even if they do not handle it from Guilt, they move up to Hopelessness. This state at the energy field of 50 is also accompanied by despair. This means, "My case is hopeless. I have tried all the diets; I have tried the milk farms. I have lost the energy with which to even address this problem any more. I'm the victim of it, and I just surrender to it and give up." Therefore, this level is "I am hopeless."

The next one above it is Grief. This is the level of depression and regret about the problem, along with feeling despondent and dispirited. There may be the fear of this problem and its consequences. These are all negative feelings, such as "I'm going to die of a heart attack. This excess weight is going to kill me." This level is full of worry, anxiety, and panic. "It is going to destroy my relationships and my future." Of course, one's self-esteem is deflated, so people with a weight problem often withdraw socially. They compensate in other ways because they feel inadequate due to this energy field. They really are not inadequate people at all. They are just holding that about the situation, and the negativity of it affects their emotions.

We have already discussed Desire at calibration level 125, which includes desiring, wanting, craving, and the entrapment behind all this.

The next field upwards is that of Anger. We know the person is angry about their weight problem. They resent it and are filled with grievances about it. Although energy level 150 is more effective, they may be more successful in utilizing anger rather than guilt or hopelessness. If one is angry enough about their weight problem, they can move up to Pride at level 175. That offers a lot more energy. Through Pride, one can choose to adopt a successful program to follow and then move up to Courage.

Courage provides some tools that really work, and at that level, there is the courage to try them. At 200, there is a lot of power compared to 30 or 50. It enables us to face, cope, and handle, resulting in becoming empowered. The truth is that we have not known how to handle it up to this point. If we had known how, we would have done it.

As we use these letting-go techniques, we become detached from the whole problem. If the weight stays, it stays, and if it does not, it does not make any difference; therefore, we feel good and then move up to the level of Willingness.

Willingness at 310 has a lot of energy when compared to Guilt or Grief. We can see how much power we have now that we are in agreement and aligned with this technique. Our intention is that we are finally going to handle it, and we can accept that it can be handled. We start feeling that we are an adequate person and start becoming confident. A transformation is now occurring because we realize that the power to handle this is within ourselves, and we start moving up into a lovingness. There is the desire to really love ourself and the body now that we do not identify with it as 'me'; this body is not 'me'. If I lose my left leg, I am still 'me'. If I then lose my right leg, I am still 'me'. If I imagine losing my left or right arm, I will still be 'me'. If I lose both ears, I will still be 'me'. We finally realize that only the 'me' is me, and we are not the body. Whether it weighs 200 pounds or 85 pounds, that which we actually are is of a different quality and essence. Therefore, we must learn to love that body now, to begin to really value it and see that it is just an enjoyable little puppet.

The way to relate to the body is to see that it is a happy puppet that just goes about its way. At this level, we can start getting playful with it and experience a sort of joyfulness. As it bounces around, we are just sort of dimly aware of it because we are experiencing our existence from a position of Allness. Once we become conscious about where experience seems to be actually happening, we realize that 'experiencing' is a nonlocal, diffuse, subjective condition. We begin to identify with everywhereness instead of stomachness, bulginess, or ulcerness—all those localized things—and instead realize that what 'I am' is a conscious being.

Consciousness is everywhere, so we then begin to experience existence as being nonspatial. Within this everywhereness and Allness, this happy puppet bounces around, spontaneously doing what it does

and having a good time doing it. Even if we are deliberate, we are only spontaneously being deliberate.
With observation, it will be discovered that all action or
even thinking is actually spontaneously autonomous.
(Confirmed by the neuroscience research of B. Libet, et
al.) By valuing our existence, we come to realize its
intrinsic greatness, bigness, and the joy of aliveness,
and we see the body as a contributor to that fulfillment of something enjoyable. The body is something
to have fun with, experiment with, and play with.

Within a couple of days, once we release this
appetite/hunger cycle, the rest of it is automatic. We
know we do not have to do another thing. If we want
to throw in some common sense and have a diet Coke
instead of a regular Coke to save a hundred calories,
well, that is common sense. That is up to us, which is
different from being at the effect of it. That is different
from being run by the guilt of it because now we
have a choice.

Another trick that works is to never allow ourself
to go over a certain number of pounds. If we choose
132, that means that if by accident we weigh 134,
then we go back to this technique again and get off
that cycle because those old patterns can tend to
recur. However, they are then easy to let go of if they
do. We merely use the technique once or twice. The
first time we feel hungry, we sit down and skip the
eating until the hunger disappears. Then we go out to
the refrigerator if we want to, and remember to have
our adult there. We may put a note inside the refrigerator to see when we open the door, or maybe a picture of ourself as an adult. This helps us to realize that

we have a choice about whose arm is going to reach into the refrigerator. We know to keep the kid out because that kid is going to help himself or herself to whatever is in the refrigerator and not let the adult be there. As a result, it all becomes a very enjoyable experience, one in which we truly begin to love ourself.

The basis of all the self-healing techniques is primarily to learn ways of loving ourself, to begin to value ourself and love that which we are in truth. That which we really are then looks at our little body and begins to get a kick out of it. It says, "Gee, I'm having a good time with you. You are a fun thing." We begin to see that it really almost runs on automatic by itself. We will see that the ego has played a trick on us, too. We think that we make a decision and the body then follows through. Actually, it is doing it by itself because it is on automatic. Once we have released it from a negative pattern, the body will just handle itself very well.

In scientific experiments with young children, if they are allowed to spontaneously select their diets, they will automatically select a balanced diet. One begins to experience a return of faith in nature, allowing the body now to sort of be itself. The nature of that which is natural within the body will automatically handle its nutritional needs. When we get off the social programming, that which is automatically self-healing and healthy within the body takes control. It looks after itself, choosing what it needs and wants to eat, and it does so extremely well.

It could be said that it is wise to have faith in the Divinity within Nature itself, in the body's being part of the beautiful Nature of this planet. It has its own inner wisdom. When we remove the artificial conditioning of our society, the body's innate inner wisdom comes forth and expresses itself in a sense of aliveness, joyfulness, lightness, and in the capacity to feel good at all times, and its weight handles itself automatically.

To achieve this, all that is necessary is just a few minutes of time, with many years of joyful rewards as a result. Have a good time with the body. Love it, be good to it, and give it all the love and attention that it needs. Realize that it belongs to you but is not what you are. It is a lovely possession, so enjoy it while you have it.

"What if I do all the above and it doesn't work? What if I am still overweight despite everything?" If that is the situation, then it is time to shift priorities. Maybe there is a genetic pattern that is familial and even multigenerational. Weight is actually a vanity anyway, is it not, unless it is life threatening. It is better to focus on being a loving and valuable person. Many great people who changed history were probably genetically heavy, such as Winston Churchill, generations of opera stars, William Jennings Bryan, Teddy Roosevelt, and the European monarchs and aristocracy, to name a few. It is better to be hefty and happy and just dismiss the whole issue than to obsess about it. We do not take the body with us when we leave the planet, and aesthetics do not have a priority in heaven.

CHAPTER 12

Depression

The depression and despondency that plague mankind have been prevalent since ancient biblical days. It currently constitutes what is being called a minor epidemic in the form of a rising suicide rate among young people, especially adolescents. Depression affects all our lives. Few of us have managed to live on this planet for any great length of time without experiencing depression. It may be minor, in the form of regret, or major, in the forms of mourning, loss of loved ones, or loss of the things we have valued in our lives because of their meaning to us. We will view depression from the perspective of consciousness and also cover the role of biochemistry and antidepressants. Is the biochemistry the cause or the effect of depression?

At this point, a review of the relationship between body, mind, and spirit is appropriate because we will be talking about the treatment and understanding of depression on all three levels. We need to review again that the body has no way of experiencing itself. The body cannot experience its own bodyness nor can it experience its own sensations. The body is experienced in mind, and mind also has no real capacity to experience itself. All memories, thoughts, feelings, fantasies of the future, and daydreams are registered and experienced in a field that is larger and more diffuse, a field of energy that we call consciousness. It has to be experienced by something greater than mind, which is called awareness. Awareness allows us to know what is going on within consciousness (they are concordant).

Consciousness allows us to know what is going on

in mind, and mind allows us to know what is going on in our feelings and emotions as well as in the sensations from the body. Therefore, all these processes are going on within consciousness itself. It is also important to address issues on the highest level where the most power exists. Therefore, a change in the field of consciousness within mind brings about an alteration within the body.

When talking about depression, the brain, its hormones, neurotransmitters, and physiology are of great interest. What are the real causes of depression? Again, we will refer to the Map of Consciousness, which shows the levels of consciousness from zero all the way up to the highest calibrated levels of joyful states, and then even beyond, up to the state of consciousness the world calls Enlightenment. On the Map we see that within those levels the energy fields have a direction indicated by the arrows, which shows whether we experience something as a positive asset in our lives or as a negative, deleterious event. Near the middle of the Map is the level of Courage, which is the calibrated energy field of 200, the level of Truth. Below 200, the energies are negative, and above 200, the energy field swings upward, indicating a life-supportive energy field.

We are going to review the human experiences, starting at the bottom of the Map, called Guilt, Apathy, and Grief. These fields express themselves in emotions, such as self-hatred, self-recrimination, hopelessness, despair, and despondency. All are accompanied by feelings of regret, loss, and depression.

In these energy fields of depression, our view of the

world is that of a sad and hopeless place of sin and suffering. Our view of God, the God of a world like that,
would be of one who ignores us, who is unfeeling and
uncaring, and from whom we are separated. Out of
guiltiness, worthlessness, and sinfulness, God can be
imagined to have negative (anthropomorphic) human
attributes.

When looking at the process going on in consciousness in the lower energy fields, at the bottom level
(Shame) is a state described as deflated. The one above
(Guilt) is called dispirited, which does not have the
energy of life or the desire to live. In the Apathy state,
the process going on in consciousness is the loss of
energy. Due to the loss of the life energy within, a person no longer attracts energy from the universe. The
process is one of being de-energized, which leads to
the self-hatred of destruction and the lower states that
precede death. From this, there is often a pattern of
passive suicide.

We are going to look at active and passive suicide.
What do they arise from? How can they be handled?
What do they really mean? In what way can we create
an understanding of this whole field of depression, this
plague of mankind? How can we benefit from an
understanding of the nature of consciousness itself?

All the energy fields below the level of Courage
have a negative direction, and seldom does one of
these emotions occur singly. Generally, one negative
emotion tends to pull in others as well to some degree.
In depression, there are also feelings of self-blame, self-
hatred, and worthlessness. These feelings are associated
with the level of hopelessness and despair. There are

regrets about the past and fears about the future, and very often there are also guilt and anger. Frequently it is said that depression is anger turned inward.

Traditional psychotherapy recommends trying to energize and bring up the anger accompanying the depression, and then determine the source of the anger. We will discover that both anger and depression are the result of the same error—having made the same mistake within the mind, and within consciousness itself. What is the error that will be found when looking at the anger, the fear, the grief, the apathy, or the guilt? We will find that the person has placed their survival on something outside themselves.

All the negative energy fields are based on placing the source of our happiness externally. This results in being vulnerable and also being the potential, hopeless victim. Being the victim means perceiving a cause as being outside ourself. Therefore, the vulnerability to depression is present as long as we think the source of our happiness is something outside ourselves.

The common frailty of human consciousness is to make happiness dependent upon externals, such as saying, "Well, when I get that degree, then I'll be successful and happy," or, "When I learn that foreign language; or get to move into that apartment; or get that fur coat or new car; or when I get that advanced college degree; or when I get that relationship; or, if I could just change that person out there; if I could get my aunt to stop drinking; if our company would only come out of the red and go into the black, then I will be successful." It is always 'out there'. Placing the source of our happiness outside ourself is putting us in the position of being vulnerable to depression, anxiety, fear, and a potential loss. It is only by owning ourself as the source of happiness, as the experience of our existence, independent and beyond that which happens within the world, that we become immune to depressive episodes.

Each time we look at the Map of Consciousness, it is from a different perspective with a different emphasis. It alters our understanding of the nature of human consciousness as we approach it from a different context with a broader understanding. The levels of consciousness have either a positive or a negative direction, with a crucial intersection in the middle at the level of Courage, which is crossed over by telling the truth. In this case, the telling of the truth is that "My happiness does not depend on anything outside of me. I, of myself, am the source of my happiness by my own inner decisions, integrity, intentions, and by the way I see myself and my relationships with the events of life."

At the bottom of the Map is maximum victimhood in which the total source of our happiness has been placed outside ourself. The loss of that brings about self-contempt and self-hatred. There is nothing within the self now to love because that which was loved was seen as something outside ourself.

At the stage of Apathy, which we know as hopelessness and despair, there is a state of no energy, so a person in that state is in a severe clinical depression. The person is usually unresponsive and may sit in a chair, staring blankly out the window. They are frequently unresponsive to any communication and are unable to talk. Very often they stop eating and may not be able to sleep or function in the world. These are the severe forms of depression, which also have a biochemical basis in the brain that leads to seeing life as sad, the future as hopeless, and themselves as empty and worthless. The concept of the God of that kind of world is one who ignores and does not care for them. It is a state of total unlovingness and feeling unloved.

Our clinical experience indicates that the three lower states of hopelessness and helplessness, which we collectively call despondence and depression, arise as a consequence of the failure to have handled the energy field above it, which is called Fear. The person is not facing the underlying fear because the depression arises from the loss of meaning. It is not the thing outside of them that the person has placed their happiness on that is the difficulty, but the meaning they have attached to it. It is not the college degree but the meaning of that degree. It is not the relationship but the meaning of the relationship. It is not the position or title of president of the company, or the financial success, or having the right address, but their importance and value. What we project onto a thing, or the way we hold it, depends on the meaning we give to it. In and of itself, it has no meaning; it merely is.

Meaning is a mental construction that we have projected out, thereby assigning value to something. The value arises out of our own mental/emotional values that are being projected onto something outside of us. This results in seeing ourself as separated from the source of happiness. There is 'me', and then there is that 'outside of self' from which we feel separated. There is the fantasy that if we could reunite with that, have that, control that, then that would heal the inner feeling of lack and separation. To feel separated from that which we want is to unconsciously feel separated from God. The view of God in these depressed states is one of being totally separated from the source of our happiness.

The way to get out of a depression is to look at the underlying fear. What is the fear? We have used the actual clinical example of the woman who received a telegram from the Department of Defense that her son was killed in action. She is rocking back and forth in her chair and staring out the window. Several weeks later a telegram arrived stating there had been an error, they regretted the error, and that the son was still alive. When the family told her this, she just kept on rocking back and forth, staring out the window. "Mother, mother," they said as they shook her, "didn't you hear? Joey is not dead. He is alive and fine. He is in an R & R camp in Vietnam." However, she just kept on rocking.

Something had happened. The energy field, the state she had obviously been holding, was that of her son and her relationship to him as a major source of happiness. Being a widow, that relationship was prime in her life. Now something had happened; the energy of the field had brought about a change in the brain chemistry. We can see that in this instance, the shift in the brain chemistry is a consequence. Due to the loss of meaning in her life, the energy field then expressed itself on the level of brain chemistry.

All things are physical, mental, and spiritual. Spiritually, the meaning here was the separation from God; emotionally, it was the significance of this relationship; and on the physical level, it was the brain chemistry. There was a shift and a loss of neurotransmitters. The brain was in a depressive condition. There was a depression of essential neurotransmitters in certain areas of the brain that accompanied the condition. Therefore, it is possible to ameliorate the expression of this symptom on the physical level by the use of antidepressants. In treating all these conditions, we find it most efficacious to treat all levels simultaneously. We address the person in a dialogue where they begin to examine what they had placed meaning and significance on and how they had filled the internal emptiness of their life with things from the outside to give it value. This process thereby created the vulnerability. We have to look at how it is held psychologically and, at the same time, treat it on the physical level.

The antidepressants available these days are very effective. Generally it is safe to treat the depression of the majority of patients pharmacologically with antidepressants as long as there is close clinical supervision, especially in children and adolescents. Pharmacologically, they take the person from the bottom of the Map and lift them up to a higher level so they are then able to respond to psychotherapy or spiritual counseling to try to alleviate the conditions that brought about the vulnerability. The risks of psychopharmacology have to be weighed against the risk of suicide, especially when an apathetic depression becomes agitated (Hawkins, 2005).

Facing the fear that underlies the depression relieves the depression. The fear is that one has lost the meaning of life. They have lost that which is of value, and feel it will never be replaced. Hopelessness means that the expectation of the future is zero. There is no hope that a context of meaning and significance will be recreated that will reenergize and give one's life meaning again. This, of course, is an illusion, but at the time, the hopelessness is based on the perception of oneself and one's relationship to life.

When treating a depressed person, we look to see what the loss is, for example, the loss of a job, the loss of vitality, the loss of youth, or the loss of opportunity. People become depressed at middle age and see life as having passed them by, and now feel they have lost their opportunity. The loss of looks for a person, such as a middle-aged woman for whom her appearance has been very important in her life, affects her sense of self-value and her way of relating to the world. If she has based her power in the world on her looks, then that loss is a great danger to her and not just a superficial thing, such as vanity. It is far more than that; it is her whole sense of self-worth and value. Beauty to her has become valuable and makes her a worthwhile person.

We discover the underlying fear and get the person to be willing to look at the fear. Instead of depression, the person has to handle fear instead because fear has to do with the future. "How am I going to live without what has given my life significance?" This can be seen in the addictions, for example. One might say that anybody who gets depressed has been addicted to placing their survival on something outside themselves.

In the addictions, if we threaten to take away the drug upon which the person has been placing their survival and happiness, we see terror—not just fear, but

absolute terror. The conviction within the addict is that
it will be impossible to live in this world without
access to that substance, so we have the person look at
the fear and then utilize the techniques clinically that
we have found to handle fear; next, we create the willingness to be with it—to stop labeling it and to stop
the thoughts. They focus instead on the exact experience of what is coming up as they look at that which
is feared within mind. The person looks at it and then
goes into the radical truth of what is literally being
experienced within them. They need to be willing to
surrender to that and let go of resisting the fear. As this
happens, the sensations run through the body.

I ask the person, "What are you experiencing in
your body?" They report, "My mouth is so dry, I can
hardly talk. My heart feels like it is fluttering. My stomach feels like it is turning over. I feel cramps in my
abdomen. My knees are so weak, I can hardly stand up."

Then we start with the feelings, one by one. We say,
"All right, tingling in your legs and your knees. Could
you let go of resisting that? Could you just let yourself
experience that and be with that? Stop resisting it.
Don't call it fear. Just sense what you are sensing. What
are you sensing?"

The reply is, "I'm sensing a tingling in my legs."

Then I ask, "Can you handle a tingling in your legs?
You have handled headaches, major surgery, and deaths
in the family. I'm certain you can handle the tingling in
your legs." The person will say they can handle that.

Next I say, "Let go of resisting the tingling in the
legs. Now, how about the cramps in the abdomen?
Could you let go of resisting that? Could you stop call-

ing them 'cramps'? Could you just experience what you are experiencing and let go of resisting that? Right. Let's go up higher. What about the flip-flops in the stomach? Can you handle that?"

"Yes, I can handle that."

"Could you just handle the experience and stop calling it flip-flops in your stomach? How about the beating in your pulse? Could you let go in your mind of resisting that? Just let your pulse beat away if it wants to. How about the dry mouth?"

We get the person to realize, "Yes, I can handle that. I can handle the experience of that, but I cannot handle the fearful thoughts." And we agree that nobody can handle fearful thoughts.

There is no such thing as 'having' fearful thoughts. Fearful thoughts create themselves by the thousands, and as we handle one bank of fearful thoughts, a whole new bank arises. "I'll be late for the plane. I won't get on the plane. I'm afraid of the plane. Something is going to happen to the plane. I might go to the bathroom." The mind will just create an endless series of fears. What it can handle is the dry mouth and the tingling in the legs, and then the willingness to face the underlying fear.

The first thing that benefits the person is relief from depression. They say, "Oh, I see I'm not depressed. I see that I was terrified of the future and that I will never find happiness without what I wished for, longed for, and desired. I was convinced that I had to have that in order to survive and be happy."

People who have been convinced of that and were on sizable doses of alcohol or drugs have been as close to actually needing something to survive as anybody on the planet could be. Yet, after they gave that up and faced the fear of it all, they found that life was joyful, complete, full, and enjoyable for the first time in their lives. We know that fear is based on an illusion; therefore, we have the courage to take the patient with us to look at the fear, just like we take the child by the hand to lead them.

When I was a child, somebody on the block told me about bogeymen. My mother had ridiculed bogeymen, ghosts, and similar things but somehow, because of that older kid's convincingness (and he acted like he knew what he was talking about), I became afraid of bogeymen. My mother took me by the hand and led me down into the dark basement with flashlights and looked all over for bogeymen. None were found there, or in the closets, or behind the curtains, or anywhere else in the house or attic.

It is helpful to have someone with us when looking at the fear because it is our unconscious child that is frightened. Our inner child does not understand the nature of real life in this world, so it comes up and says, "Gee, without that, I won't be able to survive."

As we said before, depression is often aligned with anger turned within. What about that anger? What is the basis of the anger? We will use the example of somebody who bases survival on something outside himself, such as an addict. When we threaten to take away his bottle or supply or flush his drugs down the toilet, he goes into a rage. Now it is very clear to us what the source of the anger is, is it not? The source of the anger is exactly the same fantasy as the source of happiness being something outside of him and which has been placed on some external object—a person, place, or thing. To place the source of our happiness on something outside ourself creates a negative energy field because it is basically a lie. The source of happiness is not something that is outside ourself at all.

Only when we own that we are the source of our happiness does the energy field go in a positive direction. We can move a person out of depression and despondency, get them to face the fear, get them to desire something better for themselves, and turn their anger into anger at being the victim instead of being at the loss of an object.

There are usually endless rationalizations and explanations to try to make their anger sound justified. "They promised me this. They signed a contract. They sent me a check that wasn't any good." The source of that is always outside of oneself, and the explanation, details, and events are only justifications for the anger.

We can use this anger by turning it into anger at the vulnerability. One can say, "Now it is time to be angry at the real cause, which is that I was brought up in a world that taught me to think this way. I was taught that this is the right way to think." That is what we need to be angry about—that we were taught how to think in a way that set us up as potential victims—to think that something or someone outside ourself is the source of happiness. The usual projected fantasy is that 'success' is the source of happiness, is it not? Will success bring us happiness?

I used to live on the East Coast near a community of millionaires, and despite their affluence, occasionally someone committed suicide or took a drug overdose. They were not at all immune to the human vulnerabilities. Therefore, worldly success (e.g., celebrity status) does not bring immunity. What we need to be angry at is what caused us to sell ourselves out and then learn how we do it. Then we can take pride in the fact that we are willing to look at this now and move up to the level of Courage to tell the truth about it. The truth is that something within our consciousness set us up to be vulnerable.

If we start to take responsibility and say, "The way I was looking at this set me up for this depression, frustration, and anger. It set me up for the letdown and this disappointment." The courage to look at that and be willing to tell the truth about it now changes the way we feel about the whole subject. We can now move up to a situation where we can say to ourselves, "Well, it's okay. It's okay if that is how people are taught in this world, and I grew up in this world. I guess I learned the same as everybody else, but I'm willing to look at it in a different way now." We then move up to a willingness to look at it and say, "Yes, I agree to look at this. My intention is up, and I at least see the subject as promising and hopeful. The God of a friendly world is promising and hopeful. In other words, there is going to be a benefit to me, not only in this particular situation, but there is also going to be a benefit to me as a human being that will last my lifetime, because if I solve this one, I have solved it for all time within myself."

The willingness to look at that and accept what is discovered results in a certain confidence that there is a process going on within, and that this depression has arisen to bring something to one's attention. It is as though it is saying, "Something is out; something is wrong within my mind, within my consciousness, and within my spiritual position," because that is what pain means. Pain means, "Please look at me; something is out."

We can treat depression pharmacologically and get the person out of it temporarily, but if the person has not changed in their way of being in the world, in the way they are holding who they are and how they relate to the world and the universe, or in their expectations, their vulnerability remains the same. We know that many people who are treated with just antidepressants will recover from the current episode. We also know that some people are prone to relapses due to genetically determined faulty brain chemistry, and others have additional episodes unless their whole context has changed. Without an understanding of the nature of consciousness itself, the vulnerability remains, and the person who has depressions of psychological origin is subject to repeated bouts of depression within their lifetime.

In looking at this in a holistic way, from the viewpoint of body, mind, and spirit, we want to address the basic understanding to bring about an immunity from further episodes of this debilitating experience of depression. Acceptance means seeing what the internal setup is without blaming oneself or getting into a 'make wrong' scenario. There is nothing wrong with it; it just does not work. We have been trained and set up in our world to think that way by our parents who were also set up to think that way. They just passed it down to us. It has been going on since ancient biblical times, where there are descriptions of very severe depression, so it arises in the inherited collective consciousness, which contains the same program—that somehow happiness and the source of it are outside ourself.

As we move up to level 310, with the willingness to tell the truth and to look at this, we can see the power of the field then goes up to the level of Acceptance at 350. Here the energy field is positive instead of negative because above the level of Courage, the person has stopped projecting the source of their happiness outside themselves. They have begun to re-own their power. At the level of Courage, there is the willingness to tell the truth, face the situation, cope with it, and handle it.

By the time we move up to the energy level of Acceptance, we see a person who is confident and easygoing, which comes from the awareness that one is the source of one's happiness. It means that the person has realized in their emotional, psychological, and spiritual growth that they are the cause of the happiness in their life. If we were to put such a person on a desert island somewhere in the South Pacific, sail away, and return a year later, he would have a coconut factory, he would be making flutes out of bamboo, the children would be learning songs, and he would be teaching French to the natives. He would have found a native girl, built a tree house, and re-created for himself the world around him as an expression of being the source of his own happiness.

The anger was based on placing the source of happiness outside of oneself. On a deeper level, the anger is that of having sold oneself out and having been sold out by being given this program to operate with and then finding out that it does not work. One has to accept that it does not work, be willing to look at it, change, and say, "Okay." It only takes a matter of seconds to find a position from which it will work.

How long does it take to come out of depression? It only takes as long as it takes to become willing to look at the truth of what has happened. The capacity is within ourself to accept what has happened, to realize that we are the source of our own happiness, and to be unwilling to give it out to the world any more. The re-owning of that power suddenly results in a state of confidence. It no longer matters what happens 'out there'. The realization of that truth allows us to experience ourself now in a far more whole and complete way instead of from lack or vulnerability. There is just the realization that we are the source and have the power to create. The self projected the meaning onto this; therefore, they say that one man's meat is another man's poison. The same event that would make one person happy would depress another.

I have watched people resist coming into money, for example, because it was not within their value system. At the time they valued not having money; therefore, it would be a problem if they won the lottery. Thus, winning might make one person joyful and fill the other one with guilt. Why? The difference is meaning.

Who or what created the meaning that gave this thing outside ourself the power and significance? We are the creator of the meaning and the one who chooses what meaning to give to something. Therefore, we have to look at the way in which we have bought into social consciousness. We have to look at the values by which we have unwittingly allowed ourselves to be programmed and say to ourselves, "Do I agree with that? Am I willing to give it that value? Am I willing to set myself up for that vulnerability?"

The realization emerges that we have the power to resource ourselves and to recontextualize our lives by seeing how we are setting ourselves up. It brings a state of inner joy to realize that we alone have the choice and the power. We are the ones who set up the meaning and give these things the power over us; therefore, it really is possible to come out of disappointment, grief, sadness, and anger about the event, to even become indifferent and willing to look into it and re-experience the inner self.

Actually, a depressive episode, even a brief one, has the potential for joy within it because it is something coming up in life, saying, "Look at me! Look at me! Here is a mistake that has been causing you pain and suffering for endless amounts of time and will continue to cause you pain and suffering for endless amounts of time." That inner state of joy and serenity really comes about from a knowingness of our own invulnerability. Therefore, even though the depression is not currently present clinically, the knowledge that we are vulnerable precludes that incredible state called the peace of God, the knowing that we are not separate from the source of anything but are connected with it, and that we are with God.

How does one then experience that which, in body mind, and spirit, is called spirit—that subtle knowingness? It can come from one of life's tragedies, or even from a minor disappointment. All these things have within them the seed of truth that is always present. That which is the spirit and reveals itself as the truth behind consciousness is always present and can therefore be discovered at any moment—in moments of high joy or depression. In Zen, it is said that heaven and hell are only a tenth of an inch apart.

Personally, I have shared what I have experienced, and I have witnessed the truth of what I am talking about. My own inner experience included a time of great, severe, agonizing depression way down in the pits of Hell. In that state of absolute hopelessness in which time stopped, the experience went on for literally eons and eons. (In severe depression, the experience of time is altered and each second seems like an eternity.) In those eons, there was no hope. In fact, there was a sign that said, "All ye who enter here give up all hope." It was like the deepest of the hells in Dante's *Inferno*.

Out of the experience of that infinite suffering and agony, out of that total feeling of abandonment and being separated from love and God, there suddenly came an inner voice that said, "If there is a God, I ask Him for help." From the pits of agony, by a profound, deep surrender, suddenly there was the awareness of an Infinite Presence of Eternal Love and the silent Knowingness of Truth. With the collapse of the ego/self, the mind became silent and disappeared into the Self. The event heralded a major transformation that has been described in other writings.

Self-healing is the willingness to love and forgive ourselves, to look at our vulnerability and call it our humanness. It is the capacity to love our humanness for its weaknesses, errors, and foibles in order to see that within this humanness, as mistaken as it might be, there is a primordial, intrinsic innocence.

The only thing that is certain in the phenomenal aspect of this world and its expression is that all things change. All things change within human experience because human experience is that of change. If all things change and nothing remains the same, then to place the source of our happiness outside ourself on that which changes means it is only a matter of time before the depression ensues. If we place our security on that which is transitory, disappearing, coming and going, or changing, then the vulnerability is ever present.

That simple mistake, which we all make, is common to the whole human condition and arises out of something that is also the same in all of us and which can be rediscovered right in the pain of experience—the intrinsic innocence of consciousness itself, the intrinsic innocence of our own inner self. We can see this in two different ways. First, by reaching that state of compassion ourselves, we attain such a level of consciousness that we literally see into the hearts of others; we just see and know that innocence. The second way is through introspection to see how this arose.

We notice the primordial innocence of the child who is innately trusting. The child has faith in the integrity of adults, and it never dawns in the child's mind to doubt the truth of what is being told. The young child loves its parents and those extensions of parents called teachers, other family members, peers, playmates, television, and commercials. A child looks at a commercial as though it were just as truthful as its parents because of the child's trustingness, openness, lovingness, and lack of paranoia. The innocent, trusting mind is easily programmed, and therefore, out of its innocence, it begins to buy what it hears. The child identifies with those whom it loves as family. As the programs start coming in, the purity of the child becomes programmed because of its intrinsic innocence. Due to that innocence, it buys such statements as, "All of us are allergic," "Heart disease runs in our family," or, "We all have a weight problem in our family."

All the negative programs are bought by the child's innocence. We might say that the child's mind is like the hardware of a computer, which will play any software program that is installed on it. And yet, the nature of the hardware, that which is truly the computer itself, is unchanged. No matter what CD we play, no matter what software programs we play on the computer, the intrinsic innocence, purity, and integrity of the hardware has not been sullied. It has not changed at all. Even if all the programs are erroneous, the hardware remains the same.

Within the adult remains that same childlike consciousness, with its innocence, purity of motive, and capacity to remain pure no matter what the programs may be. It remains essential and unchanged in all of us. It is exactly what is reading these words right now. It is the childlike consciousness, with all its purity and innocence, that is reading this teaching right now—not the person or personality, but that consciousness in all its simple purity.

Even if the person who is reading says, "I don't believe a word of it," where does that statement come from? It comes from another belief system that the child bought out of innocence. The father says, "Don't trust anybody," or some disappointing experience sets up the program within the child's mind. "Don't trust anything you hear." So if we are saying to ourself, "I don't believe anything he says," we are saying that because, out of the childlike innocence, we bought that program. "The way to be secure in this world is to be mistrusting, skeptical, and not believe anything you hear or you will be misled down the primrose path." However, the nature of the innocence that bought that program remains the same because it is trying to listen to the truth and discern that which is truth out of its hopefulness and trustingness. It is hoping to hear that which will be helpful, nurture life, and relieve suffering. The cynic has been programmed to be mistrustful.

When we look within ourself now with the intention of self-healing, we see that intrinsic innocence and understand what program was set up. Now we have to re-own that innocence which is so crucial in all spiritual work as well in personal psychological research and introspection. It is important to always keep within our awareness that whatever we bought was out of the beauty of that which we are. We bought it out of our own love, trustingness, and integrity because we projected our own integrity onto the world and thought it was a place we could trust in and believe anything we heard or read.

We were programmed to believe that sometimes it is very useful to lie, to tell someone that "The check is in the mail." We were programmed with the idea that the only way to survive as a body in this world is to tailor the truth a little bit (called 'creative business ethics'), but did we not buy that out of our own innocence? We thought that was what one had to do in this world to survive, so we guessed we had to do that. Of course, when we do that, we pay the price. Anytime we go below the line at 200, we pay the price, which is the loss of our power within the world.

That is what the anger is all about—"I lost my power. The source of my happiness will never be returned to me because it is outside of myself. I have projected it out there." The healing of it comes from the willingness to look at the truth of it, to say to oneself, "Out of my innocence, like other humans on this planet, like most of us, in fact, I bought a certain way of looking at life in which the source of happiness is, first of all, outside myself, and secondly, it is always in the future."

The separation from the source of happiness is not only in space, but it is also in time, so it is something that is going to come into our life tomorrow, or the next day, or the next week, or the year after, or when we finally graduate, or when we reach middle age, or when we get that big house or Cadillac. Because it is always in the future, we are always separated from the source of our happiness and never feel complete. The realization that we are the source of our happiness, and that we can create it at any second, gives us a sense of completion. The sense of completion runs concomitantly with the experience of life, so it can be cut off at any second yet still feel complete.

If we suddenly stop writing at this moment, it is already complete just as it is. To the best of my ability, I have said exactly what I want to say. At this moment, I am being with the experience of the joy of doing the best I can. Joyfulness accompanies the experience. There is no tomorrow about it because of the sense of completion. If someone enjoys the presentation, so much the better. That is only frosting on the cake because it is not essential.

What one does in the world has to be accompanied by the sense of completion in the doing of the thing itself. The payoff is not something that is an aside, something that is outside or separate from the doingness; it is the experience of it in this moment. The completion is with the experiencing right now, not something separate from it. In that, one is then aware of the lovingness of all experience. That is the way one is with experience. It is the loving of life in all its expressions, including its disappointments. It is the ups and downs, the continual learning process of making the mistake and learning from it, so it is nothing but a mistake.

One might say that depression is nature's way, God's way, and our own psychology's way of saying to us that the way we look at our life is not okay. It is our psychological, biological, and spiritual way; it is our body, mind, and spirit saying, "Look at what is out; look at what needs to be fixed. Please understand me out of your compassion; heal me; heal all of it." The defect is an inner sense of separation that we will not be complete and whole unless we become united with something 'out there' or in the future. The ego moves from incomplete to complete. In contrast, the Self moves from complete to complete. True happiness is always in the 'right now' of this moment. The ego is always anticipating completion and satisfaction in the future 'when' a desire gets fulfilled.

Clinically, there is often a difference between men and women in the precipitating event that leads to suicide or depression. Men experience the Presence of God within them or their connection to God very often in the form of power. The three classical attributes of God are omnipresence, omniscience, and omnipotence, so God is often experienced in the unconscious of men as connection with power. Men seek that power, and frequently the precipitating event leading to their depression is feeling separated from the source of their power. In this case, the power has been out in the world, so it would be the loss of a title, a business, or the status symbols that signify the power; the sense of separation and vulnerability that has not really been healed remains there. Therefore, money, position, and power become the traditional goals of men.

Women commonly experience their connection with God in the unconscious more in the form of relationships. Remember the example of the old woman who sat in the rocking chair, rocking back and forth, staring hopelessly out the window? She had experienced lovingness coming through that relationship with her son and was feeling cut off from it. The interruption of that was the precipitating factor. We see that the basic problem is still the same in the two sexes; it just takes different forms and different expressions.

Depression leads us into the whole subject of suicide. When looking at suicide, we see that what is desired is not really the death of the body but release from suffering. The body did not create the dilemma nor can it experience the dilemma. Therefore, the idea that if one gets rid of the body, one will get rid of the source is fallacious. The body neither created the dilemma nor experienced it. The whole problem is going on in consciousness; therefore, the solution is within consciousness. Looking at the nature of consciousness itself and seeing that is where the problem arose and where it is being experienced, one therefore sees that is also where it has to be solved. The solution is to realize that what is desired is the release from suffering.

The mind identifies itself with the body and thinks it is a body. The loss of the energy of life is because the person is dispirited, which leads to a decrease in energy. Many deaths are really subtle forms of passive suicide. There is loss of the sense of aliveness, excitement, and commitment to life. Passive suicide takes many forms, statistically showing up as an automobile accident or the failure to get out of the way of a bus. For some reason, the person just did not care enough to take the precautions, did not care enough to love their life or value it enough to care for and preserve it. Passive suicide takes the form of the person who ignores their physical disease, such as the diabetic who just does not care to stay on their diet or take the insulin, thus going into insulin reactions, overdoses, and diabetic coma, with three, four, or five times in the hospital in a coma until they succumb.

In the addictions, that is traditionally seen in the form of an overdose. How could it be a miscalculation for a person who has taken multiple drugs for twenty years and then dies of an overdose? They are experts in psychopharmacology who dose themselves thousands of times and then die; it is called an accident. In an automobile accident where the driver was just careless, what we really see is the lack of the desire to live. The failure to heed health advice or to take care of one's health and assets indicates the loss of energy that results in the loss of aliveness coming from entrapment. There are feelings of deflation; then one becomes dispirited and unconsciously seeks a way out so they do not have to feel guilty. One does not have to feel guilty that they died of a diabetic coma. They did not bother to alter their lifestyle to prevent that coronary heart attack.

If we realize that what we want is the release from suffering, that then comes about through an understanding of the nature of consciousness itself and going into the processes that have already been described. We have to have the willingness to experience out all the symptoms that are being experienced and to look at our life using a technique called the 'worst-case scenario'. We sit down, look at life, and ask, "What is the worst possible outcome?" We become aware of the feeling that arises with that and then let go of resisting it, constantly canceling out the thoughts about it and handling the feeling directly. As that progresses, we will notice that the symptoms begin to abate. We come out of the depression willing to look at the fear, at the way it was set up, and how we got it set up. We experience the anger about that and then use the energy of the anger to want something better for ourself, now having the courage to face how it all came about.

It really means that we have to recontextualize our whole life. We have to look at everything in it and say to ourself, "How can I hold this so it will have a value great enough that if it left my life, I would still see that which is worth living for? To what about this can I dedicate my life? What about my job gives it meaning and significance? How can I move to a larger way of holding it? How can I see it in such a way that my value as a human being will not be changed if that should leave my life?"

We have to look at our goals and motives. What are we willing to dedicate our life to? What has significant meaning? Service to others? Even if we lost all capacity to serve our own life, what is the meaning of being of service to others?

There are people with all kinds of disfigurements and losses who go on with their lives. Somehow life still has meaning for them. Does that mean that we are weaker than they are or that they are morally superior? No. It means that they have somehow found some greater meaning in their lives. They have had to let go of a lesser meaning and find a greater meaning. So depression means that we have settled for a smaller meaning, something that is much less than the truth. We have to reexamine and see what was the true meaning of that in our life. What about our life makes it worthwhile, even without that? Correction occurs by asking ourselves very simple questions. Where are our vulnerabilities? They are some aspect of what we think we could not live without, and on which we have based our survival.

The technique is to first find out where the areas of vulnerability lie. We can sit down and picture losing that from our life. We then go through the process of letting go of resisting all the feelings that come up and contact our own inner consciousness—the unconscious, the God within us, our super consciousness, our intuition—to begin an inner questioning search. All of us have to do that. What is the meaning of our life? What is its significance? What is worth dying for? What is worth living for? What do we value that is greater than that which is limited and temporary? By removing all these things one by one, we find that who we are is growing in stature. We are no longer so vulnerable to external events because there are always two things happening.

There is the event going on 'out there' as we see it in ordinary consciousness, and then there is how we feel about it, which depends on our attitude. We can decide how we want to be with it and what our relationship is to that event. For example, I am one thing, and the event is something else. I have power over how I want to hold it, how I want to value that relationship, and how I want to picture it. I have to decide whether I'm willing to give it power over my life. Am I willing to give money enough power over my life so that if I lose it, I no longer desire to live? Am I willing to give possessions, titles, degrees, or cars that power? Think of all the things people value greater than their own lives, and you can see the enormous vulnerability. The high suicide rate is regarded as one of the most important causes of death, especially in adolescents. What does that say about the values that we are teaching them? What are the transitory things we tell them to base their lives on?

We have to reevaluate for ourselves the importance and meaning of our lives and ask what we hold that is of sufficient value to preserve us in the face of any kind of loss. Out of that inner understanding then comes our reevaluation of the relationship between body, mind, and spirit, because it is mind that is setting our goals and purposes.

If we begin to question our values and reevaluate our position with them, whether we like the term or not, we are really doing spiritual work. What is spirit? What is the energy of life itself? We have a decision to make about its form. We can decide what to give meaning and value to. Within that energy field called consciousness, we have great freedom. It is up to our own inner choice. By merely seeing that we have the choice of what we want to give value to, we re-own our power. We move up from victim to source and begin to accept the return of our own power, which we have given away to the world. With that comes an inner state of serenity from experiencing the value of our existence, knowing that we need no proof, and that the world does not have to do anything. We do not need to bring home any trophies to give it value because we see its value within ourselves. We see, treasure, and hold sacred the value of life itself. We accept that which is given to us with thanks. With gratitude we hold the essence of that which we are without asking that the world give us back anything that we have demanded of it.

In doing that, we move into an invulnerable position. We are no longer prone to the disappointment, anger, rage, or turning against ourselves with thoughts of suicide—that hopeless, fallacious idea that by killing the body, we will kill the source of our suffering. By owning that we, ourselves, are the source of our suffering, we transcend it. By transcending it, we bring about that inner healing, which is the purpose of this chapter.

CHAPTER 13

Alcoholism

To understand the nature of alcoholism and addiction, we will approach the subject from the viewpoint of consciousness itself in order to discern the essential nature of the addictive process rather than its symptoms, consequences, or physical correlates. Talking about the nature of consciousness will give us a different context in which to understand the addictive process and its expression as a problematic human behavior.

The Map of Consciousness will again be referenced throughout this chapter, as it has been very useful in our research. It will help to make information understandable that has previously been considered mystical, esoteric, or too 'right brain' for left-brain people to comprehend. On the Map, various levels of consciousness have been calibrated to indicate the relative power of these energy fields and their positive or negative direction. By studying the chart, we will begin to understand a lot of new and useful information about human behavior, and from that, we will come to fully understand addictions.

On the Map, note that Enlightenment, or leaving the world of duality, calibrates at about 600. The energy field of Courage is at 200, and Pride is at 175. We will refer to these numbers later on. It is important to notice that the direction of the arrows shows whether the energy field is negative and not amicable to life or is positive and supportive of life.

In understanding addiction, we need to first understand the nature of consciousness and then see how it applies to the addictive process. We will look at the true nature of addiction and the quality that society missed because its understanding of addiction was nil until the advent of Alcoholics Anonymous (AA). Prior to AA, the recovery rate from addictions was zero, and it was rarely heard that anybody ever recovered from alcoholism. The truth was represented by Dr. Carl Jung who said that science had no answer for this problem, that something above and beyond ordinary human experience had to be sought, and that the answer would be found in spirituality.

We will review the connection between body, mind, and spirit. What is the relationship among the three, and what is spirit, anyway? What is the nature of spirit, and how does it operate in a real way that we can verify through our own clinical experience? We will not be discussing philosophy or theology but instead will be exploring what we can verify for ourselves through our own inner experience. We will look at truth as it can be experienced within ourselves and learn how this can be applied to the understanding of alcoholism, the addictions, and its importance in recovery.

We will emphasize the importance of context, or the overall way in which we hold a thing, and the paradigm from which to understand a subject. Context creates meaning and illuminates the understanding of addiction.

As previously described on the Map of Consciousness, levels below 600 represent the levels of the ego, which is called the 'self', and within the ego are different energy fields, as mentioned previously.

At the bottom of the Map are the energy fields of Guilt, Shame, and Apathy, and to the right of each field is the primary emotion of how we experience that field in daily life. To the right of that is the process going on within consciousness itself. That energy field also determines how we experience and see the world, and how we relate to the understanding of God, which is due to the limitation of the energy field.

The energy field of Shame is at level 20, and Guilt is at level 30. These are states of negativity that are usually experienced in the form of self-hatred. The world is seen as a place of sin and suffering. At this level, God is perceived to be possibly the ultimate threat or destroyer of the soul because He will throw the soul into destruction and hellfire forever. The levels of Guilt and Shame are the lowest energy fields and contain very little power.

When we move up to the energy field of 50, we discover a field of hopelessness and despair. This is like the old lady previously described rocking back and forth in her rocking chair, staring out the window after she got the notice from the Department of Defense that her son was killed in action. Her family shakes her, trying to get her to respond, but she does not respond to anything because, in these energy fields, there are changes in brain chemistry.

Hopelessness, despair, and depression represent the process of the loss of energy that accompanies the lower levels of consciousness. The world is seen as hopeless, and if there were a God, He would have nothing to do with us because our own self-esteem is so low. We call it the worm's view of the nature of

God. If we get the person out of that very low energy field, we can get them up to a higher energy field called Grief.

People in hopelessness cannot help themselves, and we have to pour energy into them to even move them up to the energy field of Grief that calibrates at 75, which has a lot more energy than hopelessness. Grief also has a certain biological purpose, for example, when the child cries to summon its mother. It has the power to pull some kind of response from the world. The emotion that accompanies Grief is regret, a feeling of loss, and despondency. The process going on in consciousness at this level is dispirited. Spirit is that high energy out of which all life manifests. The person in Grief then sees this as a very sad world with an unloving God who does not really care for anyone.

If we go back to the old lady who is rocking back and forth in her rocking chair and not eating or responding, and a telegram arrives from the Department of Defense saying that the previous telegram was a mistake, and her son Joey was not killed but is still alive, the old lady just goes right on rocking back and forth, staring out the window. If we could pour energy into her up to the level of Grief, suddenly she would begin to cry. The expression of that emotion would indicate to us that she is getting better.

Interestingly, these two energy states come out of the failure to face the energy field that lies just above it, which is Fear. The energy field of Fear, at calibration level 100, is still a negative emotion as shown by the direction of the arrow. We can run a long way out of fear, so although the form of the emotion itself is not constructive, the energy out of it can be utilized in a very positive way. All these energy fields have their upside and their downside. The downside affects us negatively; in contrast, the upside can be very constructive in our lives. We generally experience fear in ordinary life as worry, anxiety, and panic, but eventually, it can escalate to become paralyzing terror.

Grief has to do with the past, and fear has to do with the future. The process going on in consciousness is one of deflation. The fearful animal shrinks and hides. For example, when, as child in the third grade, the teacher asked for a response to a question, we can remember how we used to shrink and hide behind the person in front of us. We shrink and become deflated, and the perception of the world that comes out of this energy field is that it is a frightening and threatening place, and that God is very punitive. He is seen as a punisher and much to be feared because of the holding of all the senses of sin, guilt, and low self-esteem in this level of consciousness. This level sees God as the most frightening of all possibilities.

We can move a person out of Fear and up to the next energy field called Desire at level 125, which has a lot of energy. Desire is 'want', so its expression in our ordinary emotions is that of wanting and craving. This can eventually become an obsession or compulsion. We then call it an addiction because the process going on in consciousness is one of entrapment. A person becomes entrapped and is at the effect of that level and run by the desire. It takes on the intensity of craving, which in turn becomes associated with an inner image. To recover from addiction, it is necessary to eliminate an attractive image the moment it emerges in the mind, whether it refers to a sexual image, gambling, or alcohol. If the image is allowed to linger, it gains energy and quickly becomes too strong to resist. Recovery depends on the willingness to eliminate the image immediately and decisively. If delayed, the image becomes too strong to obliterate and its attraction soon wins.

It is the purpose of the marketing industry, of course, to take advantage of our desires by creating wanting and craving to get us entrapped so we will want their products. Once we become entrapped by the desire, whether it is for a fancy car, a certain perfume, or a shampoo that is going to make us lovely, it will run us. We will give up our money and energy to buy their products.

Desiringness, however, leads to the view that the world is very frustrating. The difficulty with wantingness is that all the wantings can run people for an entire lifetime, which leads to the sense of frustration as well as resentment because wantingness does not cure itself by getting; it just leads to additional wantingness. The wantingness, in and of itself, is not satisfied, so this constant frustration leads to a picture of God from whom we are separated. In other words, the God who forever withholds from us what we want easily leads us to anger, which is the next level.

Anger, at level 150, as everyone is aware, has a great deal of energy in it. It is still a negative emotion with a destructive downside, but the energy of anger, if one knows how to use it, can be very useful. We experience the energy of anger in everyday life within the emotions of resentment, within the feelings of hatred and anger at ourself, within grievances and grudges, and in the unwillingness to forgive. The process in consciousness is one of expansion, so as the angry animal swells up with anger, it becomes larger than life. The person who is angry puffs up with the angriness and tries to become imposing on the biological level.

Angriness then leads to competitiveness. The angry person sees a world of competition, conflict, war, and 'me against you'. It is a polarized position of opponents, and therefore the view of God at that level is an angry God. The person sees God as the ultimate angriness, the God of vengeance, and the God who gets even. He is the God who represents the energy of the spleen out of revenge, hatred, and anger. It is as though he now hates that which he created and the humanness of that which he created. He is the God of retaliatory, vengeful angriness.

If we move up out of this angriness to Pride at level 175, we see that pride has a lot of energy and can be a very useful emotion. The difficulty with pride is that its energy field is still in a negative direction. Its downside is denial, and in the addictions, this can be fatal when it takes the form of arrogance and contempt by saying, "Well, those people need it, but not me. I'm different." That comes out of the process of inflation that is going on in consciousness. The ego reflects an inflated sense of self, which is a very dangerous position. Therefore, we see the pridefulness that eventually leads to the destruction of people who get into drugs but who are successful in life. This leads to inflation of the ego and the denial that goes with it, along with the inability to hear the advice of others. Pridefulness thus leads to a very vulnerable defensiveness. It is not a good position to be in, but it is an energy that we can utilize to move from Anger up to Courage and out of the field of Pride.

The person in Pride is very preoccupied with status, ownership, havingness, symbols, and labels, which puts one in a very defensive position. How does that energy field, which comes out of denial, arrogance, contempt, and an inflated energy field, influence one's view of God? The relationship to God will usually be one of two possibilities. Out of the arrogance of the intellect can arise the presumption that the left brain has the capacity to know all of truth, resulting in the position of atheism. Atheism is a denial of the truth of what can be experienced through human experience; or, it can take its opposite in the form of bigotry. It could be in the form of the religionist who takes the position that 'my way' of seeing things is the only way, and because my way is the truth, your way is not. Pride is a condition that polarizes, making the position of everyone else wrong, or 'me against you', or 'us against them', and it is the basis of all the religious wars. Pride has the potential, however, to be a useful energy, as the Marine Corps has discovered, and it is useful to move on through it to the higher energy field called Courage.

Courage is a very crucial level because, as we can see, the arrow on the Map of Consciousness is now neutral, meaning the energy field of that level of consciousness has now shifted to neutral. It is as though the antenna that was tuned to 'negative' is now tuned to 'neutral'. It stops pulling negative experiences to itself. Its energy field is 200, which has a lot of power. Courage has enough energy in it to settle the United States of America, to get mankind to the moon, and to establish a civilization to explore the intellectual frontiers.

Courage at 200 has enough energy to create all the great industrial empires. It is a very powerful energy field, not because it jumped up twenty-five points but because the direction of the field is different. Much of the resistance has dropped off, and for the first time, the person at that level is now emotionally able to face, cope, look at, and handle things. The critical process going on in consciousness is that of the person becoming empowered.

The willingness to tell the truth allowed this huge jump in power. This is crucial in understanding the addictions and the traditional 'twelve steps' because it is the first step—the admission that one is powerless over alcohol and drugs, which make one's life unbearable—that changes this entire energy field and re-empowers the person, putting them in a position of recovery.

When a person starts telling the truth, their view of the world from this energy field of Courage is that of opportunity. It appears to be a world of challenge, a very exciting world in which to grow and experience personal growth. Out of this energy field, a positive view of God opens up to the mind. For the first time, the person really tells the truth from their own experience. They have not really had an experience of what is called God within the universe, so now the mind opens for the first time. The person begins to ask the traditional questions that have always led to the ultimate realization of the truth: "Is there a God? Can He be experienced? Is Divinity a Higher Power that I can verify within myself? Is God something 'out there' or within me? How does a Higher Power express itself? How can I get to know that?"

The whole spiritual exploration then commences at the beginning of self-honesty because that is the first level of integrity of empowerment. The capacity to tell the truth releases the power to face, cope, and handle things, and, for the first time, to be appropriate.

Out of the energy field of Courage arises the strength to look at the facts and admit the truth about them. From here it is possible to let go of resistance and move up to the next energy field called Neutral. We can see that the arrow is now very positively going upwards on the Map. The energy field has jumped to 250, a level that is experienced as being free and unattached. Once we tell the truth about a thing, we may move up to a process that we call 'nonattached' in that one is no longer attached to the outcome. It is then okay, whichever way it goes. A person at this energy level then might say, "If I get the job, it's great, and if I don't get the job, that's okay, too, because I will just find another one." Or, "If this relationship doesn't work out, then I will find another relationship."

There is the experience of the okayness of the world and a sense of God as being the source of freedom. There is the freedom to grow, expand, become conscious, and begin to look into one's self and the nature of human experience. The God of this level looks favorably on the exploration of one's own consciousness. Neutral is a level of comfort.

The upside of Neutral is that it can move up to the state called Willingness, which calibrates at 310. It has a lot more power and energy because, for the first time, positive intention becomes operative and says, "Yes." At the Neutral level, there is a lack of enthusiasm. For example, it is okay to go to the movies, yet actually okay to stay home. There is not much positive energy there yet. However, letting go of the negative creates space for willingness to come in, and there is the beginning of enthusiasm and a very positive energy. We say, "Yes, we are agreeable. We are willing." This willingness takes us out of indifference, flatness, and detachment, and we begin to experience this as a friendly world. The questions of God and life itself become promising and hopeful because now we are saying 'yes' to life. Willingness opens up the opportunity for the next step, which is moving out of Willingness to the level of Acceptance.

Acceptance calibrates at 380, and a person at that level is adequate, confident, and capable. This transformation of consciousness occurs as we begin to re-own our own power. All the fields below Courage are conditions of victimhood in which we have sold out the source of our power and given it away to the world. This will be extremely important as we look at the addiction—the giving away of our power to that which is outside of us, thus bringing about the lower energy fields.

The person who is moving into Acceptance is re-owning that they are the source of happiness in their life. Below that level, people think that the source of happiness lies outside themselves. They think it comes about through 'getting'. These are all conditions of lack in which happiness is dependent on whether one gets that car, title, job, relationship, degree, money, or whatever it is, but it is always outside of oneself. In the addictions, it becomes, "If I get the right dose of that drug . . .." The thought that the source of happiness is outside oneself accompanies all these states of weakness and victimhood.

The person on the level of Acceptance, through willingness and letting go of resistance, has accepted that they are the source of happiness in their life. There then arises the conviction of self-sufficiency and the capacity to create something that is satisfying. As a result, that person is no longer limited by powerlessness or victimhood. That person knows that if they are put on a desert island some place, a year later they will have a coconut factory going, a tree house built, or be teaching French to the natives. The person will have found a relationship and even started a new family.

There is the power to recreate life for oneself. In prison, there is suicide, but on the other hand, there are those who have earned college degrees. People have changed the course of all human history and written powerful and brilliant books while in prison, which demonstrate that the power is not in the prison but instead within the self. The capacity exists to use even the prison experience in a valuable and positive way in order to create a great novel, book, or political treatise. Some of the most influential books ever written were created under extreme conditions.

An aspect of Acceptance is the openness to reason and rationality as guiding principles of life rather than just the emotions that predominate at the lower energy fields. 'Think' gains importance over just 'feel'. Animals are run by emotions, instincts, and feelings, but normal, healthy humans, by virtue of the evolution of the brain's prefrontal cortex, have developed the capacity for intellectual understanding and the comprehension consequent to logic and abstract symbols. The consciousness levels of the 400s thus typify our modern society of education, information, and the critical utilization of intelligence. This leads to learning by means other than just trial and error.

A person in trouble begins to search for answers and solutions, and inquiry eventually leads to the discovery that recovery is possible by means of proven programs, such as AA, whose success is represented by millions of recovered alcoholics worldwide over many decades. The mind is the useful springboard which learns by inquiry that there is a way out of addiction and its accompanying hopelessness and despair.

The acceptance that we are the source of happiness then makes this seem like a harmonious world. As we move upward into the energy field of Love, the vision of God that comes out of this promising, hopeful view is the beginning of the comprehension of the God of mercy and forgiveness. Out of acceptance and owning the power of what we are, and by moving more towards the truth, there arises the willingness to become truly loving. This takes us to the powerful energy field of 500, the field of Love itself.

The level of Love is where true happiness prevails. We can see why more and more gettingness—getting money, sex, power, positions, and all the rest—does not bring happiness. It brings pleasure and only momentary fulfillment. We can see why that if fifty million dollars will not make us happy, then seventy-five million dollars will not either because more millions of dollars are still below level 200; true happiness is associated with the higher level of 500, which is the beginning of the field of Love that leads to Unconditional Love at level 540.

Love is a stable energy field that nurtures and supports life, and out of which come forgiveness and the beginning of revelations into the truth of life. Within the brain at an energy field of 500, and especially at 540, there is the release of endorphins, which is the correlation of love on the physical level within the brain chemistry itself. The view of the world coming out of this lovingness is a loving one, and God is one of unconditional love and forgiveness. This is a very important level for recovery from the addictions as demonstrated by its being the energy field of Alcoholics Anonymous.

The twelve-step groups, which are based on spiritual principles, calibrate at an energy field of 540, a critical level because it is the energy field of healing and unconditional loving. It represents commitment and alignment. Forgivingness becomes automatic because out of revelation, this kind of world is shown, and out of that understanding arises compassion. The capacity and desire to understand become foremost, and what is revealed is what becomes important. If a person has a fractured arm, it is not important whether they were right or wrong. It is just important to fix it. Lovingness then becomes a healingness out of its intention to understand. It heals out of its power of compassion.

This is a different energy field from the one usually called 'love' by the world, which is often attachment and emotionalized sentimentality. When we hear someone say, "Well, I used to love Joey, but I don't love him anymore," what they really mean is that they never really loved Joey. They had a sentimental attachment, a dependency, a back-and-forth control, a lustful attachment, and an ownership in an emotionality. That which is truly loving is a decision, an inner intention, and a commitment that create a stable, unchanging energy field. We see this in the nonjudgmentalism of the twelve-step groups. When a member tells about an unfortunate event, the group is nonjudgmental and supportive. That unconditional love arises because the group is relating to the person's beingness. There is the love of the true self of who that person really is. Thus, there is the moving from the small self up to the large Self. The sustaining, nurturing, healing energy field of the twelve-step groups prevails, regardless of the personalities. AA has a saying: "Just bring the body, and you will get it by osmosis." It places principles above personalities and means that it is the unconditional love of the healing field itself that nurtures, supports, and brings about the miracle of recovery.

The importance of alignment with that energy field is because the feeling of gratitude, which is at about 540, is characteristic of AA. At this level are the

values of laughter, humor, and the capacity for a different way of holding experiences. Instead of self-pity,
fear, or anger and its expression as resentment, there
is now humor about the experience, which at the
time was perhaps tragic. Because of this willingness
to be forgiving and understanding, out of the healing
nature of this energy field arise the joyful states characterized by compassion and the desire to heal
through understanding. This transition marks the
beginning of transfiguration in one's consciousness,
the beginning of seeing the perfection of the world
and experiencing the oneness of all things and all life.

At the consciousness levels of the high 500s, there
emerges an energy field called Ecstasy. It is not the
'jumping up and down' kind of emotionalism but an
inner experience of extreme joy that eventually
evolves into states generically called Bliss. These
blissful states express as feelings of expansive well-
being, of being at one with everything, of generous
lovingness and forgiveness, and of extreme inner
pleasure. This blissful state is important in the understanding of the addictions because the inner experience is the most impressive of all human experiences. It represents the experience of what is possible
within one's Self.

The experience can also come out of meditation.
A person who practices a meditative technique may
suddenly go into an expansive state of Infinite
Oneness and bliss, also called *samadhi,* and become
aware of what is possible. The knowingness of what is
possible creates the desire to return to that state. The
person's life usually changes to a considerable degree

as a result of the experience. Many people leave their current lifestyle and shift to a totally different one that is directed towards spiritual purification and the removal of whatever blocks the experiencing of the state. This is also characteristic of people who have near-death experiences, even when they are declared dead in the operating room. The movie *Revelation* is about such a person and is clinically very accurate in presenting the experiencing of that infinite state of blissfulness. Subsequently, there is a dramatic change in the person's lifestyle that arises from a different knowingness, orientation, and context.

The classic movie *Lost Horizon* depicts the same thing extremely well (Ronald Coleman was in the original version). You may remember that when he falls into Shangri-La (a state of unconditional loving-ness that calibrates at about 600), he experiences that state of consciousness. When he tries to return to the ordinary world, which calibrates around 200, he sees a world of successful doingness and gettingness. He cannot find any satisfaction in this world any longer compared to what he experienced in Shangri-La. This created the desire to return to that state of inner consciousness at any cost (which the movie depicted as a place, but which we know is actually experienced within consciousness). He risks his life in the Himalayas because of the drivenness to return to the state of Shangri-La.

We have to look at where all human experience occurs. As we said, the body is unable to experience itself and is experienced only in mind. It is the mind that experiences the body. Mind itself is experienced by consciousness; otherwise, it would not be aware of what is going on within mind. The experience is taking place within an energy field of consciousness, and it is this inner experience within consciousness of a blissful state that captures people who have never taken drugs.

Now we can understand what happens in the drug or alcohol experience. This powerfully attractive, joyful energy field, the energy field of life itself, is like the sun that is always shining. The lower energy fields are like the clouds that blank out the experience of that which is ever shining. A drug or alcohol blocks off the experience of the lower energy fields and allows the experience of a higher energy field. If we could block off all the energy fields below level 560, we would experience what is left, which is the energy field of Ecstasy. There is even a designer drug called Ecstasy created specifically to block off the experience of the energy fields below 560. With the drug experience, pharmacologically something has blocked off the lower energy fields and allowed the unobstructed experience of a higher one. Thus, at the end of the day, the person who is full of fear, grief, regret, and anxiety stops in for two martinis, and suddenly temporarily jumps over the lower energy fields and moves up to the energy level of about 500, which can be called 'mellow'.

Mellow is that field where we sort of love everybody and are willing to forgive them. We are generous, easygoing, and all the kids love us when we are in that state; we take toys home for the children and flowers for our spouse. This energy state is sought in the drug experience because it blocks off the lower energy levels. As said before, these are addicting experiences because the mind, once having experienced the state, wants to return to it.

When we ask the person who has had an alcohol or addictive problem to look at what they are seeking, to look at the experience that has become habitual and to which they return over and over again no matter what the price is, we find that they are seeking an inner state of consciousness. In reality, they do not even care about the drug itself. The drug is only the mechanics, the only way they know for accessing that state at the time. It is a certain way of experiencing their being, their existence, and it is a pleasurable, highly energized state. This is what they seek, and if a drug does not block off the lower energy fields, thereby preventing them from experiencing that inner state of blissfulness, then the drug is no longer used or valued. We can see that the addiction is not to drugs or alcohol per se but to the 'high' state of consciousness itself.

Many of the psychological explanations of addiction try to present it as though the person is running away from the lower experience of fear or depression. There are some excellent drugs that will handle that; for example, Thorazene eliminates anxiety but does not result in addiction as there is no 'high'. The same is true with antidepressants. An antidepressant will move one out of the depression, but does not result in a 'high'. Therefore, the alleviation of depression, anxiety, fear, or anger, is well handled pharmacologically by traditional medical drugs that are not considered to be addictive substances because they do not block off the energy fields at a sufficient level to allow people to experience the higher state.

We can see that the person is addicted to the energy field within, to that state of consciousness, which creates the desire to return to it. They are willing to pay the price because the mind begins to demand a return to that experience, no matter what the cost. The willingness to pay increases with time so that finally, in the end, it will ask for the body itself. It will say, "If you keep on drinking like that, you are going to be dead within weeks or months." You know what the person does about that—they go across the street to the bartender, their old pal Joe, order a martini and say, "Guess what the doctor told me today?" At that point, the bartender orders him a drink for the good old times, and they kiss the body goodbye. The willingness to let all of it go is absent, and we see the price that people are willing to pay for the so-called addiction to this state of consciousness. It mystifies people who have not accessed that level of consciousness in their drug experience. These people are willing to sacrifice all of it in order to return to this energy field that we call Bliss—the inner Shangri-La.

We see the same thing going on with people who have never taken a drug. By virtue of their destiny or previous spiritual work, they have risen into the energy fields of these higher experiences, and they do the same thing. They have the willingness to give up power, money, position, and titles in the world, and they devote all their time and energy to returning to this state of consciousness. The movie, *Lost Horizon*, really tells us the story of the motive of addiction by showing the willingness to sacrifice all of life for a certain state of consciousness.

There is an innate inner awareness of what is really true, and addiction is a false start to experiencing the truth because it does not work. Thus, the reason for giving up the addiction, alcohol, or drugs is not because it is wrong but because it does not work anymore. It does not work because through drugs and alcohol comes the progressive loss of inner self-respect, along with the adversities and negativities of these energy fields. It is the beginning of experiencing very negative events in one's life. There can be the beginning of the loss of relationships, credit cards, status, physical health, and functioning of body organs, which signifies the downhill course brought about by the denial of the truth. The denial of the truth from level 200 on down is due to putting the power outside oneself. In addiction, the person has given away the source of their happiness and meaning in life by projecting it onto the outer world and giving that power to the drug or alcohol, to some substance outside themselves.

The drug in and of itself has no power at all to create the higher experiences. We tested and researched this for many years with literally hundreds of people clinically and in the classes we gave for people who were fighting or right in the middle of handling their addictive problem. Using the diagnostic method of discerning truth from falsehood, we tested the proposition that "The drug has the power to create this higher experience," and universally, one hundred percent of the people went weak with that statement, proving that it is a lie. The drug has no power whatsoever. Then we presented them with an opposite concept and had everybody in the class hold in mind the thought that "The drug blocks off the energy fields that are coming from the ego self and allows me to experience the joyfulness of that which is my real Self." Instantly, everybody in the class went strong, indicating that the statement is true.

The truth is that the drug has no power whatsoever to create these experiences, but it does have the pharmacological capacity to block off the negative energy fields, allowing a person to at least get into the ballpark. Of course, it is not the real state of Bliss that is experienced by the person who has earned it through their own progressive spiritual work, but at least it is similar to that experience. Feeling the energy that is closer to the truth of one's own being allows us to utilize this knowledge now in understanding recovery from addictions.

When a person seeks treatment for an addiction, they are usually at the bottom of the Map of Consciousness and filled with self-hatred, hopelessness, despair, regret, and despondency. The energy field of apathy, hopelessness, and despair is one in which the person cannot help themselves. Hopeless means just that. For example, the president of a county bar association literally died of starvation while living alone in a rooming house. He was addicted to a combination of Valium and alcohol. He never picked up the phone to call anybody for help. A person of that caliber has many friends, all of whom would have dropped everything to help him, but he felt there was no point in making the phone call because there was no hope. That hopelessness of one's condition often expresses itself as "My case is different; my case is different," meaning "You may well recover from this, but my case is hopeless."

Out of this apathy and hopelessness in which God is dead for the person, all we can do is pour energy into them. The process going on in consciousness is that of the loss of energy. The person is de-energized, as was the woman who was rocking back and forth in her rocking chair, staring blankly out the window. Reason has no effect. We saw that when the telegram arrived from the Department of Defense saying the death of her son was a mistake. Her energy field did not change. She kept right on rocking back and forth, staring out the window. The answer is to pour energy into that person through our concern, lovingness, physical presence, nutrition, and every possible way in order to move them up to the next energy field of Grief.

Grief has to do with the past, and when the person comes out of a blank, shock-like state, they begin to cry and regret the loss that all the addiction has cost them. There is regret, along with a feeling of self-pity and sorrow for the fact that they are in a rehabilitation facility or in the space they are in life. They are sad about life and their addiction and feel completely neglected by God.

At this level there is regret about the past, so we move the person's energy field up to the next level, which is one of Fear. At this point, the person begins to fear the addiction, aided by worry and anxiety.

Fear has to do with the future. The person is no longer in an inflated state of denial; on the contrary, they are deflated. The world looks frightening, and they may feel that God is punishing them for their past sins. They misinterpret the addiction as a punishment and fear more punishment and further loss in the future. But the energy of each thing can move one up to the energy of the next. The person moves out of fear of the addiction into the desire for something better than being a victim or wanting and craving. This moves them up to Anger.

Anger has a lot of useful energy in it, not the form of anger itself but the energy of anger in which the person becomes angry over their predicament in life and being the victim. This anger can be used in a constructive way as a turning point away from defeatism. Better than hopelessness is the pride in doing something about it by taking action and beginning to move up into caring for oneself and one's position, and then moving up to the next energy field of Courage.

The courage to tell the truth is crucial in the addictions. We see the powerful effect of the first of the twelve steps in AA—the admission that one is powerless over alcohol or drugs—which now allows for the capacity to face, cope, handle, and be appropriate. It represents re-empowerment. The world is then seen as an opportunity, and for the first time, there is the benefit of an open mind, and the truth now has a way to enter the mind. Pride can be utilized to move the person up into Courage and to look at the facts. Doing so provides encouragement to move up to the next position, that of letting go of resisting the facts and being released from that resistance in order to begin to view the world as an okay place. This allows one to utilize and experience inner freedom to explore, expand, and then move up to the willingness to say yes, join in the exploration, and agree to align with it. The person thus develops the capacity to see the whole rehabilitative process in a world that is friendly.

Alcoholics Anonymous and other recovery programs are then viewed as promising and hopeful, and the person feels that perhaps they will recover. Acceptance is a very powerful energy field where one realizes the power to make these decisions. Confidence, a feeling of adequacy, and transformation occur through experiencing that the world is harmonious. On the one hand, it has presented the person with a problem, but on the other hand, it has also provided the answer. That which is a merciful God provides the solutions, so although one may have an addiction, there are hundreds of thousands of people around who have found the answers and are only too willing to be helpful.

With surrender, the world begins to look friendly, harmonious, merciful, helpful, and hopeful, and it offers acceptance. With the letting go of the resistance and denial, an energy field of lovingness emerges. The person then commits to an energy field that is healing by joining one of the twelve-step groups whose energy is innately healing. (AA calibrates at 540.) The person's willingness to align with it and accept the healing is essential. Through that willingness then comes acceptance. The truth about this is accepting the necessity to be in an energy field that is nurturing, supportive, understanding, and unconditionally loving. In that field, people know they are in a safe space. To remain aligned with that ensures their survival. With that experience come the joyfulness and the beginning of experiencing an inner serenity and seeing the perfection and oneness of the energy field of which one is now an integral part. It is the willingness to tell the truth that moves one up through this very critical level.

The first step of the twelve-step program is the willingness to admit the truth that one is powerless over alcohol or drugs and that alcohol or drugs are making one's life unmanageable. The second step then becomes very significant in that the 'restoring us to sanity' is by a power greater than oneself. Thereby does the ego surrender to God (as the self surrenders to the power of the Self).

We look at joy and bliss and see that the energy field starts at about 500 and runs all the way up to 600. That field is like a powerful electromagnet pulling one back into wanting to re-experience that experience in consciousness. Therefore, to handle it, something with equal power will be needed to replace it. The second step is really the intuitive knowing that something greater than the ego or the limited small self is going to be needed to handle the attraction of such a powerful energy field.

The third step is the decision that comes out of that, which is the surrendering and willingness to turn one's life over to God, as one understands Him.

Out of willingness itself, the God of one's own understanding is already a friend—a promising, merciful,
and responsive God. The willingness to be trusting
sources the element of faith, so the third step of deep
surrender really moves one into alignment with the
energy field of 540 and above. The rest of the twelve
steps now makes sense from the viewpoint of the
levels of consciousness as we have looked at them.

The fourth step says to honestly look within oneself to discover any defects of character and to take a
fearless moral inventory, which entails the willingness
to look at and own all that was negative in one's life.

Then follows the fifth step, a very healing step by
which to admit to oneself, to God, and to another
human being the exact nature of one's wrongs. That
step changes the energy field and removes the negative charge from it. Taking off the negativity has not
changed the history, but the way it is held has
changed, making inoperative that which previously
had the capacity to corrode and destroy. Bill Wilson,
the founder of AA, used to say that the correct attitude
about the past is a decent regret, which is quite different from self-hatred, shame, or wallowing in guilt.
Instead, one then comes from the heart. Bill used to
say that AA is the language of the heart and from the
heart, which heals with its humor, acceptance, lightness, and willingness to heal the past.

The healing then proceeds out of step five and is
expressed in restitution in steps six through nine,
which are really the reparative steps. In those steps,
the person takes responsibility to actually do something in the world to repair any damage that is

repairable and to mend whatever fences can be mended so it is not just a mental intellectual exercise. It becomes real and relieves the guilt about what one has done in the past. To the best of one's ability, one goes back into the world and tries to repair the damages that have been done to the degree that they are repairable.

Step ten then says that taking responsibility for the content of one's own consciousness and having the willingness to clean it up then becomes a way of life on a daily basis. The daily inventory makes note of what was lacking in integrity, where one could have done better, and where one could have been more loving. Step ten is owning responsibility for the process of spiritual progress and committing to it as a way of life.

Step eleven is interesting because it says if one has thoroughly done steps one through ten, one will reconnect with something that was sought in the first place through drugs and alcohol. It says that prayer and meditation will increase consciousness contact with God as He is understood, asking only for knowledge of His will and the power to carry it out.

Step eleven does not say, "We begin"; it says that conscious contact has already happened. It occurs through internal surrender and honest commitment to lovingness and Self as a lifestyle. One connects with God through the heart because that which is Divine, that which is God, and that which is love are all the same thing. By commitment to lovingness as a lifestyle, as a way of being in the world to the best of our ability, we reconnect with some rock-like, joyful inner experience that was similar to what we sought through alcohol and drugs in the first place.

Step twelve reveals what the whole addictive process is about and what its nature is in the field of consciousness. Step twelve says that having had a spiritual awakening as a result of the steps and becoming conscious is a result of the entire addictive experience. One now has the capacity to carry this message to others and express it in one's entire life. The twelfth step tells us that the whole purpose of the addictive process was to awaken us and move us up from one level of consciousness to another; to go from being asleep and unaware to being awake, conscious, aware, and responsible; to move from being unconscious, irresponsible, and the helpless victim to owning ourselves as being spiritually responsible for the happiness within our life.

This precludes putting the source of happiness outside of oneself. Instead, one realizes that the source of happiness is the same as the source of life and comes from responsibly owning oneself as a spiritually aware person.

There is now a different context within which to hold the whole addictive process of movement, of increasing consciousness and awareness, so that alcoholism and drugs then require a person to become more awake in order to survive. These diseases are progressively fatal, and the only way to recover from them is to become progressively spiritually aware and more conscious. Life itself depends on becoming conscious via major self-confrontation with something that the higher Self has picked that will force one to grow because there is no turning back. The only options are to surrender one's will to God or go insane and die. There is no reprogramming of the brain cells once they are programmed. There is not enough room on the tightrope to turn around and change one's mind. Once one is into the addictive alcoholic process, there is no turning back. There is only confrontation with owning the truth about one's self. Recovery depends on accepting that process, moving joyfully into it, and being grateful.

Now it is understandable why speakers at AA meetings say they are grateful that they are alcoholics. To the newcomer, this indeed sounds like madness. Grateful? How could one be grateful that one has become addicted or an alcoholic? Because that forced one to grow and become conscious. It forced one to become aware and therefore grateful for the process. At first one resents and resists it, but then one actually accepts and agrees with it. One begins to love and experience joy and finally achieves that state called serenity.

There is an inner knowingness that this was one's destiny—the way of doing it, and the way that was chosen—which results in the awareness that one never could have reached this great understanding by any other way. Some people just have to experience it this way. The ego has to hit bottom in order surrender and find God. For those who do, great gratitude comes about, along with a greater understanding of the nature of consciousness itself. Those who surrender to God receive the gifts of God.

CHAPTER 14

Cancer

Thus far, we have been talking about the utilization of basic laws of mind and consciousness when approaching illnesses such as heart disease, depression, alcoholism, and drug addiction. All of these are serious confrontations that require us to change our view of reality and what it really is. This information is addressed especially to patients with cancer, families of people with cancer, people who fear they might have cancer, and people who are in treatment with cancer.

We will present a holistic approach to healing and again will be talking about body, mind, and spirit. We are not saying that the treatment has to be a traditional one or an alternate one, but we are saying that it should include both because true healing requires the larger dimension, which includes physical, mental, and spiritual aspects, with due regard for inherent human limitation.

All the patients or people I have known who have recovered from these chronic, very serious diseases (many of whom were given up as hopeless by their physicians and the medical community) have done so by exploring the greater definition of the truth of reality of that which they are, and by exploring that realm of human knowledge called 'spiritual'.

What is that relationship between body, mind, and spirit? It is not just a catch phrase but something real we can work with in everyday life and see actual results. Those friends walking around who have recovered from all these fatal illnesses are living evi-

dence that we can recover from just about any disease known to mankind.

As shared in earlier chapters, I have had a number
of chronic, intractable illnesses. Although they were
treatable (some of the symptoms were handled), the
diseases did not improve. In fact, they got progressively
worse. Despite traditional medical treatment, I was
merely holding the line on a few and losing it on several
others. It was through exploring the greater dimension
and the field called consciousness and how they related
to self-healing that recovery from all these illnesses
occurred.

One time I had gout and a high uric acid level.
After I learned that the body only does what is held in
mind and began to change what I was holding in
mind, then the body's chemistry literally began to
change. I learned that all the atoms, cells, elements,
electrons, and all of which the body is made are influenced by consciousness. This understanding is very
important in the approaches we use in the treatment
of cancer.

The relationship between body, mind, and spirit is
that the body reflects what is held in mind, which in
turn reflects one's spiritual position. It is necessary to
know where all human experience takes place
because if we address that level, we will be addressing the most powerful level. If the physical is the consequence of the mental, and the mental is the consequence of the spiritual, then we need to address it in
the area called consciousness. Clinically, this is true.
People who address the level of consciousness itself
may even witness transformation in their bodies with-

out even having to address the body directly with any medical approach.

We need to know where experience is experienced and let go of some of the common illusions that people hold in mind because they just have not looked into the matter. We will repeat the basic process: The body itself is incapable of experiencing itself. For example, our hands cannot experience themselves, their existence, their position in space, or even sensations. They have no capacity to do so. This is because of something greater than the physical body, which we call mind. All the physical things that go on with the body, including sensations, are experienced in the greater dimension called mind. It is in mind that the experience of the body takes place.

Curiously enough, however, the mind itself has no capacity to experience itself. A thought is just an energy form and has no capacity to experience its own thoughtness. A feeling has no capacity to experience its own feelingness, and an emotion cannot be experienced other than via mind itself. In turn, it is held within an energy field that is greater than mind, that of consciousness itself, which has no dimension, limitation, or form.

Because of consciousness, we are aware of what goes on in mind. Even consciousness itself is not sufficient. Within the energy field of consciousness is a very high frequency of vibration, analogous to light itself, called awareness. Out of awareness arises a knowingness of what is going on within consciousness, which reports what is going on within mind, and it, in turn, reports what is going on with the physical body. We can see that the physical body itself is several levels removed from that which is the most real and therefore the most powerful. We find that the energy of thought is far more powerful than the energy levels of the physical body.

In previous chapters, we have described a number of techniques that can bring about self-healing. In discussing the nature of consciousness itself, we will create a context for ourselves so that the self-healing modalities to be described later will begin to make sense.

First, we need to learn how to hold and think of the experience of having a life-threatening illness such as cancer. There are two ways to go about it. We can go up or we can go down. Any kind of confrontation, such as a death in the family, any kind of serious illness, or a setback in a person's life presents a choice. We can go down into feeling sorry for ourselves as a victim. We can go down into self-pity, depression, and despair, or we can see it as a challenge and an opportunity.

These confrontations come up repeatedly in our lives until we seize the opportunity and realize they are a springboard to greater awareness. Why is this so? It is because the ordinary events in life do not have the power or the energy. It takes maximum duress for people to stop in their tracks and begin to question the realities of all the things they have believed up to this point. The mind ordinarily will not undertake the expenditure of energy to reorient itself to get a new, different point of view about life and what it yields unless it has to. As a result, this necessary growth will usually only happen when we are up against a major confrontation.

The first thing to understand about cancer or other serious illness is that the purpose of this major confrontation is for us to grow and grow rapidly as fast as we can because we have a certain time limit with terminal illnesses. Things that the mind says are fatal or terminal become fatal and terminal because of the power of the mind. If the mind thinks an illness is fatal and terminal, it will be so, subject, however, to karmic destiny. This illustrates the power of belief systems.

The most important message is that no one needs to succumb to or be the victim of any illness. I count among my friends many people who have conquered nearly every illness known to mankind thus far. The only reason I can write of these things today is because I myself did exactly the same thing in my personal life. If I had not, I would have hemorrhaged to death from a variety of illnesses, all of which went into remission.

The perfection that is held in mind then reflects itself in the progressive perfection of the body and its letting go of disease. We have to understand that the body itself expresses what is held in consciousness. It is merely an expression of the mind and a reflector of what we hold consciously or unconsciously. A person may look back in his mind and say, "Well, I don't remember thinking about such a thing." If one does not remember thinking about something, all one has to do is look to see if it is in one's life. It may have originated from the collective consciousness of mankind or may have been silently programmed by even a television advertisement.

To help create a different context and way of looking at life and experience, we will again refer to the Map of Consciousness from which we can understand all the principles of self-healing. At this point, we may realize that we are not the same person we were when we saw the Map for the first time. Every time we go over it, it is sort of like 'freight-train learning'. We learn it through familiarity. The left brain is linear and logical and learns things sequentially in a piecemeal fashion. The right brain circles over a situation, and by sheer repetitious exposure and familiarity basically understands the whole thing.

We are going to be discussing phenomena that are in the subconscious, somewhere in the periphery of the mind, phenomena that we actually already know about. We are going to pull them together and synchronize them in a useful way.

Referring to the Map of Consciousness, it represents the human ego, the self with a small 's' that people refer to when they say, "I," "me," or "myself." The self is that collection of concepts, impressions, opinions, feelings (conscious and unconscious), the totality of what makes up what a person sees when they say, "I," "me," or "myself."

Shown on the Map are various levels of energy, or consciousness, starting at the very lowest and going up to the very highest. They have all been calibrated through the research we have done. We first found the direction of the energy field. The fields from Courage and below go downward, indicating that they are destructive and do not support life.

The levels from Courage on up show that the energy goes upward. Love is near the top of the scale and, in contrast, Guilt and self-hatred are at the bottom. Understanding the energy fields, their relative powers, and whether they are constructive or destructive, is very helpful. For example, in medical treatment, we hold the medication in our hand and have someone test our muscle strength to see if the medication is good for us or not. If the medication is not beneficial, our arm will go weak; if it is good for us, our arm will go strong. This is a way to find out if a recommended treatment will be helpful.

It is necessary to learn about the energy fields because they are intimately related to cancer and cancer research. All are extremely important because the body, mind, and spirit are all actually expressions of consciousness. Therefore, if it is a negative energy field, it is destructive to all aspects of oneself, right down to the biochemical level. All we have to do is look at the Map to see what emotion is involved in order to know what our energy field is. In looking at self-pity, for example, we can see that we are now in a negative energy field that calibrates at 50, which is very weak compared to Love at 500.

We can see that it is very important to let go of negative energy and negative thoughts. The negative energy of the feeling or thought transmits itself to the body's acupuncture energy system through the twelve meridians and translates itself directly into the body's organs and cells. If we hate someone, the cells of the body get the energy of hate. Anger has the capacity to change the energy field within the body itself as well as the power to actually change the physiological programming within the body.

The mind has enormous power over every aspect of the body's functions, right down to the smallest molecule and atom. It has been discovered that every atom and every molecule within the body is influenced by consciousness levels and beliefs. Every physiological and chemical transaction that goes on in the body is the result of a blueprint of it within consciousness. All of them can be changed by changing consciousness.

The placebo response is illustrative of the power of mind over body. Research over the decades has demonstrated that approximately one-third of patients will improve or recover when they believe that a particular pill is curative. That is why many really inert nostrums (questionable remedies) continue to be sold to the public because at least approximately thirty-three percent of the people will give testimony to experiential benefit. Also easily observed is the 'nocebo' effect whereby a negative belief system can result in ill effects. That is the mechanism whereby about one-third of patients may report side effects from the same medication from which the positive responders report good effects. Plain sugar pills will result in many claims that they resulted in headache, nausea, indigestion, dizziness, insomnia, somnolence, and more. Then there is the one-third of patients who are refractory and report neither benefits nor side effects. Thus arises the old adage in clinical practice that one third gets well, one-third gets worse, and one-third stays the same no matter what the doctor does. As mentioned elsewhere, the power of belief is most dramatically demonstrated with hypnosis by which illnesses or symptoms can easily be brought about merely by suggestion.

The information presented is shared not only from clinical experience but also from the experience of friends and associates, as well as personal experience with my own physical health. I watched my body chemistry literally change as I began to change what I was holding about it within my mind and consciousness. The basic principle essential to healing from all illnesses, no matter what they are, is that *we are primarily only subject to what we hold in mind.*

It is the mind's belief systems that give power to that which subsequently manifests in the physical world. The physical body is an expression of what we have inherited plus what we have been holding in mind, either consciously or unconsciously. People will often say they do not remember holding such a thought; however, there is what Dr. Carl Jung called the 'collective consciousness' that holds the thought form. Unconsciously we buy into it and give energy to a negative belief system without ever remembering it or being consciously aware of it (e.g., via the media).

With cancer, much emotional energy has been given to it by the popular mind—all the fear associated with it, all the negative connotations, and all the thought forms. Therefore, we hold fear itself, which is a negative energy field. If we are holding a lot of unconscious fear, it now opens the door to bring into our mind unconsciously those things that are fearful, including cancer. Without ever having believed that we are susceptible to cancer, we may discover, as it is occurring within the body, that we have unwittingly bought into this collective belief system in terms of thought forms.

In looking further at these energy fields, we can see that the energy field called Guilt is at the bottom of the Map and calibrates at 30. The emotion that goes with Guilt is that of self-hatred. A great deal of research into the psychological and psychosomatic importance of cancer has revealed that there is often a good deal of unconscious self-hatred, self-condemnation, and lack of acceptance of one's humanness at a deep level.

There is a difference between treating, curing, and healing. It is possible to treat an illness and its symptoms in order to bring about an amelioration, or the capacity to live with the illness. As mentioned previously, for many years I had migraine headaches, duodenal ulcers, gout, hypoglycemia, circulatory problems, Raynaud's disease, Grave's disease, diverticulitis, and more, as described elsewhere. All these illnesses came about as the result of belief systems and were also accompanied to some degree by unconscious guilt. We have found that unconscious guilt accompanies all illnesses, no matter what they may be.

If we have a physical illness, we can just presume correctly that there is unconscious guilt. Without the unconscious guilt, the disease cannot actually be present because that which is destructive and accompanied by self-hatred can operate only in a negative energy field. That is the secret of healing.

An analogy is that certain bacteria will only grow in a culture medium under certain conditions, such as a specific temperature, a certain amount of light, and ambient conditions. If the conditions are changed, then the bacteria cannot live in the petri dish any longer and will disappear. Therefore, that which is destructive and which the unconscious needs for its process of destruction can continue only in a negative energy field that allows the negative energy of destruction to take place. That is a clue to healing.

In nature, the rotation of an energy field is decisive. For example, with a drug, the chemical effect of a molecule is dependent on whether it spins to the right or to the left. We will use dextroamphetamine sulfate as an example, 'dextro', meaning 'to the right'. This drug is so-called 'speed', with the effect of weight loss, the feeling of high excitability, grinding one's teeth, and finally, manic attacks. Levoamphetamine ('levo', meaning 'to the left') sulfate has no such effect whatsoever. It is the same molecule, but the rotation is in the opposite direction.

Obviously, all we need to do to heal ourselves is to move from the negative energy field into a positive one. Self-healing is really so simple. It amounts to changing the predominant energy field within our consciousness from negative to positive. The question then arises, how do we do that?

Now that we are aware of the physics, science, metaphysics, and emotional truth of it, along with the medical, psychiatric, and holistic viewpoints, we can understand why we should let go of these emotions. It is not for the purpose of becoming a 'goody goody' person, but because hanging on to them is potentially destructive or even lethal.

We have previously mentioned the muscle-strength testing method. With this process, we can test somebody's strength, which shows that when they hold negative thoughts in mind, they go weak. When they go weak, it means there is an impairment of the acupuncture system, which is connected to the various body organs. There are also changes in the chemical and reproductive patterns of the cells.

The only opportunity to heal anything is to move out of the negative energy field into a positive one. The power of the healing increases with a higher, more positive energy. That is why holistic approaches have worked where medical science has not been able to effect a cure. Without having the benefit of this knowledge, I would have died many years ago of a fatal digestive disease that reversed itself right at the point of death. It is essential to understand that letting go of guilt is crucial to the recovery from any serious disease, especially cancer, where guilt, lack of self-esteem, and the presence of self-hatred and fear have such an overriding influence.

The next energy field above this (which is accompanied by hopelessness and despair) is called Apathy, in the energy field of 50. One has a hopeless view of the world at this level and allows oneself to be overtaken by self-pity and hopelessness. One becomes a victim of the energy field that favors a progression of the cancer.

The field above that is Grief. When people first get a diagnosis, especially if they are younger people, they will naturally ask, "Why me?" They go into regret and a feeling of loss and despondency. The world and life now begin to look sad, and they become the victim of this energy field. 'Energy field' is repeated because it is important to see one's own innocence in this matter. It is because of this innocence that we allow ourselves to be run by this energy field.

The stage above Grief is Fear, which is also very prevalent in patients who develop cancer. Fear, with a very negative energy, has more power now in an energy field of 100. The world and life look frightening from this field, and God begins to look punitive. What kind of God would give us cancer? The process of life itself begins to feel deflated. A person is tempted to become dispirited, de-energized, to give in to the destructiveness, and unconsciously allow the disease to progress.

We have a choice to desire something better for ourselves than being victims. All the people I know who recovered from serious illnesses did not settle for being victims. They all began to desire something better for themselves. They thought there must be a better way, so they began to research and look outside the traditional medical model. They began to say, "Well, Doctor, is that all you have to offer? It is going to take more than that to heal it."

Out of their desire and anger, they began to ask, "Is there something else that can heal me?" This shows that the energy fields of these emotions can be used in a constructive way. The answer to their question is, of course, "Yes." They begin to take pride and now move up to a very decisive point called Courage, which is in the energy field of 200 and has many times more energy than Fear. More importantly, the direction of the energy field has changed from negative to neutral.

The energy field that surrounds the human body is like an antenna, and when it is tuned to the negative, it draws to itself that which is destructive. The body, being right in the way of that destructive energy field, gets hit by it. Because of the negativity and destruction hitting the body and expressing itself through the body, in this case as cancer, we become aware of the fact that some error is involved. It occurs to us to start looking to see where it is. Perhaps the error is in the way we have been holding life and our belief systems, and in the way we think about ourself.

At the level of Courage, we begin to have an open mind. Our view of the world begins to change, and we move up to a world of opportunity where the doors start to open. Before this, the mind is closed. It thinks it knows the answer, but once we have the courage, the mind begins to open and say, "I'll bet there are answers I don't even know about. In fact, I don't even know the right questions to ask." The minute we begin to open ourselves up, we become empowered and have the courage to have an open mind. At level 200, we have the capacity to face the truth and begin to take responsibility for it.

Victims do not take responsibility and instead say, "Well, you know, the reason I got this is because of the bacteria," or, "The reason I got this is the virus," or, "The reason I have this is because of the cancer cells." It is always something outside themselves and their consciousnesses that they become the victims of it. When we open our minds, we can get to own that we may have had something to do with it, and that what is happening in our life is related to something we have been holding in mind, often unconsciously.

The energy field right above Courage is called Neutral. At this level, the arrow goes upward, and the energy field has jumped up to 250. The emotional state is called detached, or nonattached. One experiences the okayness of life and a new and greater freedom, even with serious situations because all events call for the same need to confront the truth within oneself and ascertain what one's position is about that, including fatalism.

Fatalism is an idea we had in the military service during World War II about the bullet—if it was meant for us, it had our name on it, so there was no point in being afraid of bullets because if it didn't have our name on it, it was not going to hit us anyway. That can be expressed as 'karma'. Whatever is going to be is destiny. Karma is the way it is supposed to be, so the fatalistic position gives us a certain peace of mind; we are detached. When the person with cancer reaches that point, they say, "Well, look. If I survive, I survive, and if I don't, I don't. You know what I mean. I'm doing the best I can. If I make it, I make it. If I don't, I don't, and I'm prepared to go either way" (i.e., resignation to God's Will—from dust we arise and then return). We accept the fact that protoplasm is intrinsically temporary.

That is certainly a far more comfortable position than to be in Grief about it, or have self-pity, anger, resentment, arrogance, or denial. People may also deny that they have the cancer. They will come up with a thought that it has been cured without having done the work necessary to bring it about as a reality in their life. It is sort of magical thinking.

When we move above that to a willingness and a friendly view of the world where we see life as challenging and hopeful, we discover, "Yes, there are answers. Yes, there are lots of people walking around who have had terminal, even fatal (hopeless) diseases of all kinds, including cancer."

In this situation, we have introduced the intention to create our power, to prove our power, including accepting the fact that yes, we can let go of this illness, and yes, there are healing modalities. This is a harmonious world in which there are lots of people who have recovered from this illness and are very happy to share with us the truth that they have recovered. This is because they have experienced God as being merciful.

The people in the energy fields at the bottom of the Map of Consciousness frequently conceive of God as punitive, or they do not believe in God. They believe in self-punishment in one form or another, or in pain and suffering.

Feeling adequate and confidant that yes, there is an answer begins the transformation in consciousness. It moves us up to the willingness to become the energy field called Love. This is a crucial level because the energy field of Love is the one that heals, as exemplified by all those organizations that are famous for their capacity to heal, such as Alcoholics Anonymous,

A Course in Miracles, faith-based recovery groups, and others.

There are also spontaneous remissions and recoveries from almost every hopeless, progressive, chronic, intractable disease for which there is no scientific cure, and for which medicine has admitted there is no cure. We know that there are millions of people walking around who have totally recovered from just the illness of alcoholism alone. In fact, their lives were transformed because the affliction was used as a springboard to a greater consciousness, a greater awareness, and as a way to move into a commitment to that which is loving because the nature of it is unconditional love. It is not the conditional love of "I will love you if you will do this or do that." To move into unconditional love begins a process called revelation, which starts the release of certain chemicals called endorphins within the mind and the brain.

All these energy fields have within the mind and the brain concomitant changes in the enzymes. There are neurotransmitter changes, a release and opening of whole banks of neurons. Therefore, the person is moved into the healing energy field of lovingness and has at their fingertips the utilization of millions and millions of neurons that people in a negative emotional state do not have at their disposal. (See the Brain Function and Physiology Chart, Chapter 1.) These are assets. To move into the energy field of Unconditional Love then starts the healing process. We found that healing occurs at an energy field that calibrates at about 540, which is the energy field of the heart.

How do we bring about the self-healing? We have

to let go of a number of things, the first being unconscious guilt. We have to discover how to unearth what
we feel guilty about, so we begin a self-questioning
process. A person is fearful when they do this. They
say, "Well, if I start opening Pandora's Box, I'm going
to be swamped by all the negativity and guilt that I
have depressed, repressed, and pushed out of awareness all my life."

It is obvious that we need some kind of tool, some
kind of practical way to process these things as they
come up. To begin with, we need a context, a way in
which to hold all that comes up in this self-investiga-
tive process that is the realization of what has been
the basis of all our behavior for all our life. Within the
appropriate context for holding the realizations as
they come up, the guilt is automatically wiped out by
a higher understanding that results in forgiveness for
ourself and others

We need to realize that we have committed exactly
one 'sin' throughout our lives, and it is the same 'sin'
over and over again. The 'sin' is that everything we
have ever done (our intentions and purposes) was
consequent to the naïve and basically innocent
thought that it would bring about happiness. It is very
important to know this and to realize that what we
did at the time was because we thought it was necessary for our survival, and that our survival was necessary for our happiness.

Wanting happiness is the basis for all human emotions, is it not? In fact, the basic premise, the basic and
most primitive illusion of all, is that the body is the
source of our happiness. Therefore, the fear of death

is really, "If I lose the body, I will lose the source of happiness. I will lose consciousness itself."

People who are spiritually aware no longer identify their reality as the physical body. If we are awareness, or consciousness itself (out of which comes the knowingness of what is happening with mind and body), then the body is the bottom rung on the ladder. We need to let go of the negative emotions and to stop suppressing and repressing them. The tool for doing that is to let go of resisting them as they come up to our awareness.

It is important to keep our eye on the fact that consciousness within itself is basically innocent. The nature of consciousness is the innocence of the child. How did we begin to believe the things we did as we grew older? We look at the child and see how innocent and trusting it is; it is completely lacking in guile. We know its motivations are pure, at least in our understanding of purity.

This primary innocence becomes the consciousness of the adult because the programs that the child buys into are actually programmable due to the very nature of innocence itself. Because the child is innocent and trusting, it begins to buy and believe everything it hears, including all the thoughts that later express themselves as cancer—all the thoughts having to do with self-condemnation and fear, and all the thoughts of rejecting oneself for the various expressions of the limitations of humanness.

To heal cancer, we need a willingness to heal ourselves by means of compassion, which comes from our greater, higher Self. There is the understanding that, out of innocence, all these weaknesses came out of the belief system that expressed itself in daily life as the thought that if we do this or we have that, then we will be happy. Grief or loss affects us because we thought that something was going to be a source of happiness, and we are regretting what we see as that source. We get angry because some obstacle stands between us and our intentions, what we want, and what we consider to be the source of our happiness. The anger then results in further guilt.

Referring again to the Map of Consciousness, we can ask, "What is the illusion held in consciousness that is now expressing itself in the form of cancer?" All these levels from Courage on down bring about the negative energy field in which the cancer can grow. The illusion is that we all thought the source of happiness is something outside ourselves, that something outside ourselves has the power to make us happy. However, the minute we give away our power and project it outside ourselves, we are in a negative energy field and set ourselves up as victims.

An unconscious purpose of the ego is to prove that we are a victim, and the test of cancer is whether or not we will continue to go along with this and buy into it as do many people in the world. The ego would rather be right, even if it costs us our life, than to give up the position that it is the innocent victim and the perpetrator is something outside itself. (This is the core paradigm of victimology.)

Once we see and own our true innocence, we don't need the pseudoinnocence of victimhood because there is no victim. There was only a belief system in the first place that we picked up out of our innocence.

The thought, for instance, that success brings us happiness is probably the most notorious belief system. As many middle-aged businessmen who have become successful know, what they get out of their success is a daily headache and exhaustion, a number of lawsuits, and some greed and envy from their colleagues. They say to themselves, "Where is all the happiness that success was supposed to bring me? Yes, it has brought me some pleasures, such as a nice car, nice clothes, a nice address, and a nice home." But those things are not happiness.

Worldly success does not bring about happiness. Disillusionment and the feeling of guilt come about as a result of feeling that we have suddenly sold ourselves out, and that we have sold out the truth about ourselves.

To recover from cancer or any other illness, we have to reconnect with our own intrinsic innocence and reaffirm the truth of that which we are within ourselves, which has been totally unaffected by all of life's events. We have to re-own that level of awareness of self that is beyond all worldly events. Something within us remains the same, no matter what is going on in our life experience. Something has remained unchanged. It is the something that wakes us up the first thing in the morning—before we realize where we are, or what day it is, or before we realize what we are supposed to do today.

When we wake up into that state of awareness, we are much closer to the truth of our own higher self.

We realize that it is totally unaffected and beyond all life's events. It is only when our consciousness comes down into the world of concrete thought that we say, "Oh, yes, it's Monday." And, "Oh, yes, I have to go." We are really leaving being close to the truth of that which we truly are, which is beyond all that. We re-own the capacity to decide what our position will be about life's events and all those things that bring about extreme duress. We can become victims of them, or we can see them as a springboard to transcendence.

The first thing to let go of is unconscious guilt. A Course in Miracles is a teaching of love, forgiveness, and the letting go of fear. Many people I know who have recovered from cancer, multiple sclerosis, and other debilitating illnesses have done so as a result of this particular course or others that are similar. All of them are designed to show us how to change our point of view, how to let go of condemnation of self and others, how to let go of guilt and fear, and how to move ourselves into the willingness to be loving, forgiving, and compassionate.

Out of that comes the desire to understand, so in self-healing, we need to almost take ourselves in our own arms and become compassionate and healing because all of us have the healer within us. We begin now to heal our humanness. How do we get rid of the ego? It is not done by making it an enemy, by trying to attack it, or by getting into an adversarial position with it but instead by loving it out of existence. We literally dissolve the ego through compassion, love, and understanding.

When we look within, we can really see that anything we have ever done in our lifetime was done out
of innocence, and when our main intention is to
understand that, it becomes healed out of compassion. When we do this with other people and let go of
the desire to be judgmental towards ourselves and
others, then our own energy field begins to move in a
positive direction. The cancer cannot grow in a positive
energy field, only in a negative one.

In looking at the Map of Consciousness, we can
see that Love at level 500 is available to all of us. There
is a commitment to unconditional love. What is that
kind of love? We are not talking about Hollywood-
style emotionalism, sentimentality, attachment,
dependence, and mutual control back and forth.
Instead, we are talking about an intention, best
described as lovingness, to commit ourselves to nurture and support all life, no matter what its expression.

Life flows equally into the saint and the criminal
alike. Life, truth, and that which is the God within
make no judgment. Life flows equally into all. As it
says in the scriptures, the rain falls equally on all.
Moving out of judgmentalism is the lesson in that
example. Life flows equally into all so we allow our
unconditional love to support the truth of everyone,
including ourselves. Our own capacity for self-healing
depends on accepting that "With God's help, I have
the power to make the decision to go through the
necessary inner work to bring about a healing of this
illness." That is the difference between treating, curing, and healing. Treating is relieving a symptom, curing is overcoming the disease, but healing includes

the whole person.

We set our intention on accomplishing peace of mind because that is the end result of healing. The end result is an inner tranquility, not an indifference to what happens to the body, but a transcendence of the body. No longer do we identify as that physicality. It belongs to us and is part of us, but it is within us because we realize that we are more than the physical body.

The healing of cancer depends on realizing that we are the one who decides that we are greater than the physical body, and that it is within the power of consciousness to call forth the healer within and begin to utilize some of the consciousness techniques that have been presented.

We can ask ourselves, "Can I allow myself to be healed? Is this healable? What within me needs to be healed?" It still does not tell us literally in our own particular case what needs to be healed.

When I had severe diverticulitis that recurred for many years, I ended up in the hospital and had to have emergency blood transfusions. The last time I was there, I almost expired. I followed these general principles and it got better. It did not return for some years, but suddenly, something happened in my life and I had a recurrence. It was the worst attack of diverticulitis I had ever had. The pain was overwhelming; the cramping, bleeding, and all the other symptoms started all over again, this time with greater severity, and I asked, "What is the meaning of this? Why?" I began to question within, and as I did so, a technique came to me of going way, way back to discover the exact, precise meaning that lay within this particular illness (suppressing negative feelings out of guilt about having them in one's 'gut').

For most of us, following the general laws of healing is sufficient to bring about recovery from an illness. For some of us, there is a very particular lesson or message that a given illness offers. The illness will get better, but then something will linger on, or it may recur. The purpose of that is to bring about the awareness that there is a specific hidden message that was missed, and there is more to learn, which is often the consequence of a karmic pattern.

The message for all of us is that these major confrontations of life are something that can lead to major transformation and unseen spiritual benefit. The physical body is temporary, whereas the spirit is not subject to time. The acceptance of that reality then leads to further awareness, which is to transcend the concept of recovery as a gain. This initially seems paradoxical because the hope for recovery is often the initiator of the process of spiritual growth.

When illness is the motivator for spiritual growth, it often starts out from the level of fear and includes anger and guilty regret. With surrender and acceptance, these begin to diminish, and spiritual growth is valued for its own sake. Eventually, with very deep surrender, there even comes a time when resisting the illness is also surrendered and recovery is up to God. This step may also bring to awareness the concepts and understanding of the nature of karma, which itself is a subtle study. What does the term 'karma' mean from a practical viewpoint? Is it just a theory, or is it a verifiable reality?

In its broadest generic sense, karma denotes one's total inheritance—physical, mental, and spiritual. It signifies the contextual significance of inherited humanness itself, with its overall implications and genetic propensities. With consciousness research, it can be affirmed that life itself cannot be extinguished but only made to change from physical expressions to purely energy forms. (This statement calibrates at 1,000.) Thus, human life can be understood to be a valuable opportunity for transcending limitations via the classic undoing of negative karma and the advantages of acquiring positive karma. These are expressed as proclivities in that there is freedom of choice. With deep surrender of the personal will, there is eventually loss of the fear of physical death itself.

If we give the cancer within us our blessing and say, "Thank you because you are giving me the power to transform my consciousness and expand my awareness," then we will be very thankful in the end. Many people who have recovered from these illnesses look back and say, "How grateful I am for that illness arising in my life, for it was the springboard to spiritual awakening." A benefit of a life-threatening illness is that it breaks down the denial of mortality that is necessary to initiate serious spiritual work in most people who are otherwise too busy with the affairs of daily life to embark upon an inner quest.

CHAPTER 15

Death and Dying

Death and dying might be called saying farewell to the body. Hopefully, by the end of this chapter, it will be possible to view the process in a more lighthearted way than usual. I am going to share what I have learned from my clinical experience and research, along with personal experiences, in a way that has not really been shared previously with people. I am just going to share what I have experienced about death and dying and what has come to my own awareness.

Lecture audiences have said it is not possible to do it that way because others are not that sophisticated and are not going to understand it. On the contrary, I have found that people who are involved in spiritual work understand it right away and do not have the slightest problem.

In the process, we will refer to the Map of Consciousness because, in discussing death and dying, we will talk about consciousness and the two things that people really fear. One is the physical experience itself, and the other is what they fantasize to be a loss of awareness, consciousness, and the awareness of existence.

We will refer again to the levels of consciousness that are shown on the Map. The scale represents the human ego, or the self with a small 's', which we commonly refer to as 'me' or 'myself'. In the middle of the scale is the level called Courage. Below Courage, the arrows of all the feeling states are in a negative direction, which are calibrated as to their relative energy and power. For example, Apathy has much less energy than Fear, which is calibrated at 100. Guilt is at level 30; Apathy, or hopelessness, is at 50; Grief and regret are at 75; Fear, in its forms of worry and anxiety, is at 100. Desire, with cravingness and wantingness, is at 125. Anger goes up to 150, and Pride goes up to 175.

By virtue of telling the truth, in this case that life comes only from life (which is a very important statement), we reach level 200, which discerns truth from falsehood. Most of the fears of death are the result of the failure to understand and know that life comes from life and is indestructible. Like matter or energy, it can only change the form of expression (calibrates as true). When we tell the truth, we see that the negative energy field begins to go upward in a positive direction. As we move towards the conscious awareness of the Source of life itself, we move into higher states of Love and Joy. Then we come up to a level at 600 where there is a transition into a different paradigm and the experience of existence in which one no longer identifies with a separate, individual, physical body. We begin to realize the truth of who we are. The expansion of consciousness goes beyond the individual small self.

To the right of these levels of consciousness on the Map are the emotions that correspond with each level. At the bottom of the scale, shame and self-hatred accompany Guilt. The process going on in consciousness is in a destructive direction. Apathy is associated with hopelessness and despair, and the process is the loss of energy. Grief is associated with regret, loss, and despondence. The process is one of becoming dispirited. Fear is associated with worry and anxiety and has to do with the future, which leads to the process of deflation. Generally, when people think of death, they think of grief and fear. They may even move to a higher state called Anger because they are angry and resentful about the whole experience and then include grievances about it.

As we move upwards, we come to the level called Pride, which calibrates at 175. Pride feels a lot better than the lower states, but unfortunately, denial accompanies pride. We have to learn how to overcome some of this denial. It arises out of fear, and once fear is understood, denial drops away and one can then move up to the level of Courage, which has a lot more power at 200.

The energy field of Courage represents the emotional capacity to face, cope, and handle life's events, because telling the truth about a thing empowers a person. A continuing positive attitude can then move us up to the state of Willingness at 310, where we say, "I want to know the truth about the matter for its own sake." The energy field then becomes powerful because now intention is put into it to know more about a goal and the capacity to accept the prevailing conditions around it.

Below consciousness level 200, power is given away, resulting in doubt and lack of confidence. The willingness to look into a matter then results in an open mind that moves us up to level 350, called Acceptance, which is an important capacity for handling the prospect of mortality. At this level we re-own our power and begin to feel adequate and confident. It is the beginning of transformation in consciousness. There is the awareness that "I, myself, am the source of my own happiness, and I have the capacity to find out the truth for myself." Eventually, we can move up to the energy field of Love at 500, where there is the capacity for and dedication to nurturing and supporting life, and the willingness to be forgiving. With that comes a revelation about an energy field called Joy that calibrates at 540 and is associated with healing and gratitude. Joy brings an inner serenity and is characterized by compassion, which is the ability to see into the hearts of others. There is also the willingness to be loving and nonjudgmental of life in all its expressions.

Transformation is then quiet, and we move up to the state called Peace at 600, or the peace of God. The feeling associated with that is eventually bliss and then progressive states of illumination. We may feel as though we are encompassed within a light. As we go into an ineffable state, it is so exquisite that it is difficult to describe. The importance of the body disappears, and it becomes irrelevant. It is forgotten because the body is associated with identification with a personal, separate, limited self. At the more enlightened states, there is an exquisite expansion of consciousness and a loss of identification with the body and the personal self. At the energy fields above the 600s are the states of feeling completeness, wholeness, and oneness with all of life, and a oneness with God.

Humility results in an open mind. An open mind says for the first time, "What is truth? Please, Lord, let me open my mind to know within my own consciousness what is the truth for my own self."

Our expectations of death reflect conceptions about the nature of Divinity. Thus, a person at the level of Neutral at 250 would see the world as okay. They would see all experience, including even death, as okay, and therefore see God as freedom. Lower levels lead to the fear of God, guilt, and expecting God to be the great avenger because of the prevalence of jealousy and hate. The God of hatred is near the bottom of the chart and pictured as an entity that hates man and man's humanness, all of which is a paradox inasmuch as God created us.

When we move up to the levels of truth, we experience life, the world, and all the experiences in the world, including death, and expect them to be positive ones. God now becomes promising and hopeful. We can then look forward to death as some kind of great release into a much larger expansion in consciousness and awareness called Heaven. (The actual reality revealed by consciousness research is that there are multiple regions of Heaven.)

As we move beyond the level of acceptance, which we do by owning back our own power to know, we move into a loving state that is forgiving and understanding, with the beginning of revelations and the experience of all life as loving. We begin to see that love is present everywhere. Therefore, we move on up to a God who is merciful and represents unconditional love. The realization that lovingness is a basic reality leads to an inner state of joy. Out of that comes compassion, the transfiguration of consciousness that reveals the perfection of all creation. There is the realization of the oneness of all life that results in the state of bliss. There are also states of enlightenment and illumination in which one becomes conscious and aware of unity and oneness.

At level 600, we move out of the energy fields of ordinary consciousness and into those that are called nonlinear. In the mid-600s are the more advanced states of awareness and consciousness called 'enlightened' and 'illumined'.

As the foregoing may sound philosophical or theoretical, I am going to share things I have learned clinically through many years of experience plus events that I have personally experienced. As a result, we will have a more practical field of reference about what the death experience really entails. I will be going back to childhood experiences to relate some things that happened to me and how they correlated with other things that happened later.

When I was about twelve years old, I was a paperboy in northern Wisconsin. One night, it was below zero, and I felt like I was practically freezing to death. I dug a hole in the side of a huge snow bank and crawled inside the cubbyhole that I had made. The snow was piled about twenty feet high on the side of the highway, and I crawled into this refuge and curled up in order to just get out of the fierce and relentless wind. Within a few seconds, I began to experience a state of relaxation, and a state of profound warmth began to come over the body. It was a state of exquisite pleasure, and I began to forget about the body. The body just did not seem to exist anymore, and instead, an incredible, blissful state of peace overcame me. I was surrounded by light, but the light had the quality of touching me and being with me as an infinitely loving consciousness that was enveloping and dissolving. I just dissolved and became at one with this infinite field because it had no beginning and no end; it had no dimensions and was outside of time.

The state of the true Self experientially lasted for eons of timelessness. The experience was total, and at every instant, it was all encompassing, timeless, serene, and complete. There was nothing missing, nothing lacking, and nothing further to be accomplished. It was a state of profound Love, Peace, and completeness that is beyond description.

At first, there was an inner feeling of relief, followed by a quiet joy and ecstasy, and then it went beyond ecstasy. It went beyond bliss and became an eternal, infinite state, far beyond ordinary consciousness. Curiously, the Self is more truly personal than the ego self. Sometime later, my father discovered where I was and shook me. He had a very upset, anxious look on his face and said, "Don't ever do that again! Don't you know you could freeze to death?"

I had no context within which to hold this experience or even know what to call it. It was a very profound experience, and in the mind of adolescence, there was really nothing that could be said about it. I could not mention anything about it to my father because he would not have had any way in which to hold it. Additionally, he was frightened at the time, so neither of us knew what the experience meant or signified.

No books on the 'near-death experience' were generally available at the time. The movie *Resurrection* only came out in the last decade. (By the way, that movie was clinically accurate.) All those who have had that kind of experience verify the truth of what the woman in the movie experienced. She was killed in an automobile accident. It is the true story of a person who was declared dead on the operating table. She left the body and experienced that same incredible, infinite state as I have just described it.

My father and I had no context within which to hold this experience or to understand it, and although I mentioned it briefly to him, he did not know what to make of it either. Besides, he was too frightened at the time so the experience was never mentioned again. I did not understand it until I was much older.

Later, when I was in my thirties, I was dying of a very serious and progressive ailment. As I lay in bed in a very moribund condition and grave state, suddenly, much to my surprise, 'I' was about ten feet over the physical body. There I was, in space, in a perfect body that was transparent and ethereal. It was weightless, yet I had all my faculties. I could think, reason, see, and hear. I looked down at the physical body that was lying in the bed about eight to ten feet below me, and it looked like it was about to expire. There I was, outside the physical body, looking down at it, aware that that which I really am is something other than the physical body. (At that time, I had never heard of an out-of-body experience.)

During this very critical illness, I found myself totally out of the body, but it was not time for me to leave, so at a later point, I had to go back into the body. I recovered from that particular episode of the illness and continued to live, but later I relapsed, and the illness got worse again. This time, it was grave indeed, and I was really right at the very door of death itself. I was in a state of deep despair, a state of hell, a state of absolute and total helplessness and hopelessness, and only a couple of seconds away from leaving the body again.

At the time, I had been an agnostic for twenty years. Despite having had these incredible experiences of being something other than the body, I still did not have a context within which to hold it. I was still an agnostic, and I was dying. Suddenly I said, "If there is a God, I ask him to help me," and then I went into oblivion.

When I regained awareness, there had been a major, total transformation. There was no longer any identification with a personal physical body. It walked around and did all the things it was supposed to, but I stood in an energy field that was infinite. The power and dimension of the field were beyond description. It held me in absolute safety; I was like a rock. At the same time, it was exquisitely soft and gentle. Its exquisite gentleness and softness held me in its infinite, loving embrace. The body moved spontaneously as there was no personal will, mind, or entity such as a personal self. I walked around in that state for some months and still did not really have a context within which to hold it. It was not mentioned to anyone as there was nothing I could say about it. It was like going from an absolute blackness, feeling totally cut off from God, into a state in which what had stood between me and God had been removed, and I was now standing in that Infinite Presence.

It is only in recent decades that near-death experiences have become more commonly known. Classic stories written in Victorian times were known only by a very limited number of people, but now there are many books about the subject. Surveys have shown that approximately sixty-five percent of the population has memory of near-death or out-of-body experiences.

Later on, I found out this was a technique that we could learn to do at will. I learned that there are all kinds of people who leave the body spontaneously or at will. Some people are born with this gift while others can sit down to meditate and immediately have this experience.

As a clinician and scientist, I became interested in this phenomenon and discovered a scientifically oriented organization where this was being studied. I read *Journeys out of the Body* by Robert Monroe and then visited the Monroe Institute where I participated in a ten-day training. They have audio tapes with a frequency that entrains the brain to reach a certain altered state of consciousness in which one can leave the body at will. I also learned that people who were not born with the capacity to reach this state or who do not develop it spontaneously could learn to do it. The purpose of that was to learn that we are something other than the body, that we are greater than the physical body, and that the physical body belongs to us but we are not limited to it.

The best-known writings on the subject of death and dying are those of Elisabeth Kubler-Ross *(On Death and Dying)*, which really opened up the subject for the first time for discussion and familiarity with what had previously been a taboo subject. The stages she outlined are now relatively well known.

There is, of course, a prevalence of denial as an initial way of handling the shock, and physical death is a primary biological fear common to sentient beings in general who, over the millennia, have devised innumerable ways to avoid death and stay alive as an individual.

Survival techniques evolved as a function of biological intelligence expressed as learning and memory. While lesser forms of life are subject to biological protoplasmic death, only humankind can consciously anticipate it with foreknowledge. Denial is one of the basic mechanisms of the ego to protect itself from fear. With surrender of denial, the fear arises of ceasing to exist for the ego lacks spiritual awareness due to its identification with the body.

The stage of 'bargaining' is then an attempt by the ego/mind to seek to delay the inevitable, and God is then recognized and entreated to intervene on the ego's behalf. Anger also erupts at the loss of control and the confrontation to the ego's narcissistic core that its infantile will is up against an insurmountable obstacle and cannot have its own way. It does not seem fair that its wishes are being frustrated and denied. This brings up grief and mourning over loss of the previously anticipated future of endless ongoing individual existence.

The basis of all the foregoing reactions is the identification of self and its existence with the physical body as the source of existence. Thus, it is the meaning of the body that brings up the resistance to the prospect of its demise. The prospect of physical death brings up the fear of oblivion, cessation of consciousness and awareness, and its singular characteristic of experiencing.

The processing of the physical stages is greatly facilitated by spiritual alignment and awareness, which progressively becomes the focus of attention, along with one's relationship with God. Hope and faith plus surrender facilitate the strong emergence of progressive reliance on spiritual teachings and allow for a transformation of consciousness to the higher levels, which brings peace. Acceptance is facilitated by the realization that the death process is universal and applies to all living beings now and for all past time. Thus, there is the relief of sharing the common experience of all who are still alive or who have ever lived. This facilitates a certain trust in the process itself by virtue of its universality.

Processing the pain of loss requires relinquishment of the many attachments that the ego has found during a lifetime, especially to loved ones. This is facilitated by the realization that in time, they, too, will face the death process and thus share the same destiny. Love then becomes the means to transcend the ego's limited view of reality and identification with the ever-evolving Reality of Divinity as Love itself. The more we love others, the less the feeling of loss, for love is realized to be the sole value of others. The self separates, whereas the Self unites. Thus death is a fulcrum to illumination.

The greater the amount of spiritual work one has done during their lifetime, the less there is left to do at the prospect of death. A very evolved person is comfortable with the prospect of leaving the body at anytime. One way to accelerate spiritual progress is to entertain the prospect of one's eventual death and process all the attachments and illusions that come up about that eventuality. Paradoxically, the exercise greatly reduces one's fears of life.

At one time in my life, I was studying alternate methods of consciousness-research techniques, including a breathing method. In this experience, gently and softly, there was spontaneously the same experience of suddenly leaving the body and no longer experiencing it. Repeatedly I would go back into the experience I had in the snow bank when I was twelve years old. The re-experiencing, the forgetting about the body—as one leaves it, one forgets everything that went on with it within a couple of seconds, so there is no memory of what happened in that lifetime or even of one's name. All of that becomes irrelevant and has no bearing, significance, or reality. Instead, one begins to experience that which one really is, along with that same experience of incredible peace and lovingness outside of time and space. There is just pure awareness. One is exquisitely aware of the existence of existence as an infinite being.

Returning to the Map of Consciousness, at the bottom of the scale there is great concern with havingness, and status is based on what we own. As we move up into the more powerful levels of courage, capacity, and capability, there is great concern with what we do. As we move toward the top of the scale, there is only the awareness and value of that which we have become and are. Nobody cares any longer about what we have or do. I discovered that when we leave the body, we take with us what we are. What we experi-

ence is that which we have been willing to know and
own about ourself. The truth about ourself, that which
we are, is what we experience, and all that we had is
forgotten. There is no memory of money, possessions,
or power; all that we did is forgotten. In this state, if a
person were asked what they did when they thought
they were a body and moved around in the world,
there would be no recall as to what that was, but that
which they are is overwhelming.

Another interesting personal experience occurred
later in life. My mother and I were not very close
because she lived in Florida, and I lived in New York
and was not able to visit her very often. One day while
out in the woods in New York, suddenly I had an intuitive knowing that I should go down to Florida. 'Out of
the blue', so to speak, I suddenly knew that my mother
was dying. It was like a call to "come down here like
right away." I went back to the house and made a plane
reservation on the first flight I could get for the next
morning. After making the reservation, I called her
house and was told that she was in the hospital. I knew
she was dying.

When I got to the hospital, I had a tremendous feeling of relief for my mother. I suddenly felt a great
release of tension. When I walked into her room, it was
crowded with hospital personnel. I was a 'big-name
specialist' from New York, and this little hospital was
going to make sure that nothing went wrong, that
everything was covered, so practically the whole staff
was there. And there was my mother, with her oxygen
tank and all kinds of tubes sticking in her all over, along
with all kinds of meters and electronic things to make

her heart go. All of a sudden, just as I entered the room, at that moment I knew she had just left the body, and I experienced her absolute ecstasy as she left. She was so glad to get out. It was like an infinite state of joy and ecstasy, and I was psychically at one with her in the experience—I felt exactly what she was feeling. She had waited to leave the body until I got there, and both of our wills joined to know the experience. She had wanted me to experience the experience with her, and so I experienced that ever-expanding, infinite, absolute state of ecstasy as she went into that state. Nobody was ever happier to get out of that body than my mother. For years she had been hoping to get out, and when she did, she was very, very happy.

Of course, the hospital personnel did not know she had died yet, so sort of telepathically, I sent the thought to the cardiologist that "She's dead; you can turn the machine off." He suddenly got the idea and said, "Turn off the machine." The machine that was creating the heartbeat was turned off and the doctor put the stethoscope to her chest and said, "She's dead. Oh." Then the hospital staff looked at me as though they expected me to go into a state of unhappiness or something, and I did not. I was in a state of ecstasy, in the same state my mother was; I was with her. What was there to grieve about? My mother was never happier in her life. There was, however, a nurses' assistant, an LPN, who also 'got it'. She looked at me, broke into a big grin, and said, "Boy, was she ever happy," and I said, "You got it! She sure was!" The two of us grinned at each other, knowing exactly what was going on, but nobody else really understood. They probably thought I did not love my mother and was glad to see her go, or I was going to inherit a lot of money or something. Only God knows what their minds thought about it, but the LPN and I knew what was happening, which took us into the state of joy.

My own experiences, memories, and recalls of leaving the body behind were of two different kinds—the one of infinite lovingness that I had experienced many times, and then those experiences of going out of the body and experiencing nothing. Either way, we do not experience our physical death, but in the 'nothing' experience, the recall would be back in another body.

In this lifetime, at age three, out of oblivion, I was suddenly aware of the body. I can look back at early childhood and remember that moment where there was the realization that "I am. I exist."

Earlier we said that what we hold in mind determines what we experience in the world, and that is what our experience of God is. Many people hold in mind the idea that after death, we go out of the body into oblivion, but I had the experience of the Infinite Presence—an infinite, almost angelic experience. As I was looking at that one day, there came the return of memories of being 'on the other side' with those who were dying. It came back first as an experience on a battlefield, and I remembered being with dying people, looking at their agony, fear, and physical pain. Suddenly, there was this infinite lovingness and infinite state of being with the person who was dying. Before my very eyes, they would become transformed. They would leave the physical body behind, and all the wounds would heal. It was my love united with the love of God, as though I turned the heart over to God, and now the energy field of angelic beings who are absolute love poured through, but my consciousness was there with this dying person. The exquisite love of that energy would then heal all the wounds and the fear. I would see the fear, and the person's eyes would open again. They would look at me, and I could see they were just melting with the experience. All the terror, fear, guilt, and feeling of being separated dissolved, and they would look at me with recognition. Then I saw that they would see that which was significant or divine to them, and that I, myself, was formless. The same experience has also happened in this lifetime.

When we go into higher states of consciousness where we are no longer the physical body, we see that people see what they are projecting there. The dying person would open their eyes and see us as that which would be most significant to them, as we are without any form. Sometimes we are seen as the mother, lover, or a crowd of people with whom the person was dearly in love. Sometimes they would see a divine figure, but this was happening within the phenomenon of mind itself; it was all the phenomenon of mind. The person was experiencing what was most healing to them.

We have come upon a way of overcoming the fear of death. It is the willingness to be that to ourself and to others who are dying. The way to overcome our own fear of death is to picture ourself as being on the other side, like a first-aid receiving station. We open our hearts and ask to be connected with the angelic forces and to become one with them. Now we picture ourselves going to those who are dying. We do it now while we are still in our own physical body, and we send forth that energy of compassion.

Consciousness itself is not limited by bodies. Bodies have to do with the ego and its limited viewpoint. We send forth the energy field of compassion and picture ourselves in our imagination. We can begin it now in our imagination with any person because, in the world at any hour, there are over six billion people on the planet. Thousands and thousands of them are dying every hour. We select somebody that we feel we could be most loving toward—a child in a crib, a teenager just hit by a car, somebody on a battlefield who is riddled with bullets, a mother in childbirth, or a person committing suicide. Then we picture the person for whom we have the most compassion, send ourself forth in our imagination to that person, and see ourself as infinitely loving. In a way, we are now more alone and yet more not alone than ever before because we can fully express all the tenderness and love that we have suppressed during our whole lifetime. Now is our chance to send it forth and be with that person.

We think of the agony and fear of so many people. Then we go to them and begin to heal them by picturing ourself holding them in our arms, pouring forth the love through our heart. It really comes from a high being and radiates out though the heart, suffusing that person with it, and then we begin to see their fear melt away. As many people die, whatever their apprehension was before, we will notice that they go into profound states of serenity as though that compassion coming from the great beings of the world reaches forth to them at their moment of greatest need. When the person says, "O God, help me," because this is a universe of free will, they then open the door to this compassion that is being radiated forth by others and now by us. We are now by their side, and in every way possible, we nurture and heal them. We reach out to them and then lift them out of their body. They are safe; they are home; they are cared for; they are greatly loved by God. They begin to get the inner experience of the truth. We put our personal self aside because it is not needed here. There is no need for the personality, with its likes and dislikes, its aversions and attractions. Just be that energy that flows through the heart.

Through our willingness, that healing energy flows through us and into the being of the other person, and we see the transformation before our very eyes; we literally see it. We see the fear leave their eyes and the painful tension leave their body. We begin to experience that the pain is leaving their body, and they go into that same state of infinite peace, surrounded by the energy of life and love. They are feeling complete, total, and healed. There is no more fear, separation, guilt, or anxiety. The two of us are lifted right out of the body together.

I myself had a similar experience sometime back when I inadvertently sawed off my thumb with a circular saw. At first there was shock, but then in that shock, there was suddenly a sound like a chorus in my mind. It was as though I was surrounded by angelic forces that kept chanting to me as though I had forgotten it, "You are not a body; you are totally free. You are not a body; you are totally free." This chant continued all the way to the hospital.

At the hospital, I had to have an amputation opera-
tion. I cannot take any kind of anesthetic or analgesic,
so the surgery had to be performed without either of
them. The surgeon was a little apprehensive about it,
but I told him, "Well, I know a way of handling this. You
just go right ahead." So I laid back and began to profoundly surrender and did not resist the pain or label it.
The surrender was of the personal will. As I surrendered, I had that same profound experience—it was as
though I was picked up by angelic forces and lifted out
of the body so gently and softly that feathers would
seem rough by comparison. Although the body was
there, I no longer experienced it. Instead, I went into a
state of infinite and profound peace beyond all description; it was an infinite inner joy and happiness that cannot be described. I remember that, in my mind, I was
looking at the thumb or representation of it on a different plane and felt happy at its being removed because
it symbolized something I wished to be rid of. What
could have been an excruciatingly painful experience
was instead ecstatic, and there was an exquisite knowingness that was surrounded by infinite peace. I was
infinitely protected by the love of the universe, by God,
and by the radiance of Divinity.

When we look at the dying experience, we see that
it is a surrendering and letting go. It is a willingness to
open our heart to be love to others. If we are contem-
plating dying, and if we are doing the things I have
talked about, in the morning when we get up, we say
to God, "To those who are dying, I send my consciousness, I send my love and my willingness to be one with

them." It is like the forces of the universe then use the power of our consciousness and literally carries it to the person. At first it will seem like our imagination. It will seem like something that we are doing, but after we do this a few times, we will suddenly realize that we are not doing this any more, and that instead, we are saying yes to its being done through us. Because it is being done through us, we go into a state of high joy and ecstasy.

The fact that our physical body is leaving is no longer important. I have been in those states where I literally felt the Divine energy coming through me, flowing from the heart area, and going to people who were in an automobile accident. I felt this profound energy go through me and out through the heart. This profound sense of loving power bypassed the personal self and went down the highway about a mile or so. As I drove around the bend in the highway, I wondered where this energy was going, and I saw a car upside down. It had just crashed and its wheels were still spinning. People inside the car were severely injured, and I heard them crying out to God. It was as though I were a traveling antenna and God used me as an antenna tower to radiate this energy.

Curiously, that same day, about five miles farther down the highway, it began again; the same powerful energy flowed out through me. The energy spontaneously radiated down the road ahead, and when I drove around the bend, there was a second accident; another car had just turned over. This time a squad car was there, and as I went past, this energy kept flowing backwards to the accident site and continued doing so for several miles. Then it slowly came to a stop as though the person had connected with a more infinite energy field. This has happened over and over again in different locations and circumstances.

During those experiences, I forgot I had a body; whether it was living or dying was so irrelevant because the joy of the experience was overwhelming. There is a willingness to be a servant of God, to forget about the personal self, and instead to allow one's consciousness and energy to be used by angelic forces. Our Infinite Self is everything. It is connected with the angelic realms. When we own that angelic condition within us, and own that we individually have the capacity to join it by our willingness to say yes, to allow ourselves to surrender to that energy, to go to the dead and the dying, we now see that there is no such thing as actual death or dying.

That is why we talked about letting go of the body and saying farewell to it because life goes to life; life never stops. If it leaves our body, we barely notice it because we are so busy being with others that we scarcely notice that the physical body does not even exist any longer. Beyond the experience of the physical body are experiences that are difficult to describe, so we prepare ourselves for an experience of exquisite beauty and peace.

Appendices

APPENDIX A

MAP OF THE SCALE OF CONSCIOUSNESS

God-view	Self-view	Level	Log	Emotion	Process
Self	Is	Enlightenment	700-1,000	Ineffable	Pure Consciousness
All-being	Perfect	Peace	600	Bliss	Illumination
One	Complete	Joy	540	Serenity	Transfiguration
Loving	Benign	Love	500	Reverence	Revelation
Wise	Meaningful	Reason	400	Understanding	Abstraction
Merciful	Harmonious	Acceptance	350	Forgiveness	Transcendence
Inspiring	Hopeful	Willingness	310	Optimism	Intention
Enabling	Satisfactory	Neutrality	250	Trust	Release
Permitting	Feasible	Courage	200	Affirmation	Empowerment

▲

LEVELS OF TRUTH

LEVELS OF FALSEHOOD

▼

Indifferent	Demanding	Pride	175	Scorn	Inflation
Vengeful	Antagonistic	Anger	150	Hate	Aggression
Denying	Disappointing	Desire	125	Craving	Enslavement
Punitive	Frightening	Fear	100	Anxiety	Withdrawal
Uncaring	Tragic	Grief	75	Regret	Despondency
Condemning	Hopeless	Apathy, hatred	50	Despair	Abdication
Vindictive	Evil	Guilt	30	Blame	Destruction
Despising	Hateful	Shame	20	Humiliation	Elimination

APPENDIX B

HOW TO CALIBRATE
THE LEVELS OF CONSCIOUSNESS

General Information

The energy field of consciousness is infinite in dimension. Specific levels correlate with human consciousness and have been calibrated from '1' to '1,000'. (See Appendix A: Map of the Scale of Consciousness.) These energy fields reflect and dominate human consciousness.

Everything in the universe radiates a specific frequency or minute energy field that remains in the field of consciousness permanently. Thus, every person or being that ever lived and anything about them, including any event, thought, deed, feeling, or attitude, is recorded forever and can be retrieved at any time in the present or the future.

Technique

The muscle-testing response is a simple "yes" or "not yes" (no) response to a specific stimulus. It is usually done by the subject holding out an extended arm and the tester pressing down on the wrist of the extended arm, using two fingers and light pressure. Usually the subject holds a substance to be tested over their solar plexus with the other hand. The tester says to the test subject, "Resist," and if the substance being tested is beneficial to the subject, the arm will be strong. If it is not beneficial or it has an adverse effect, the arm will go weak. The response is very quick and brief.

It is important to note that the intention, as well as both the tester and the one being tested, must calibrate over 200 in order to obtain accurate responses.

Experience from online discussion groups has shown that many students obtain inaccurate results. Further research shows that at calibration 200, there is still a thirty-percent chance of error. Additionally, less than twelve percent of the students have consistent accuracy, mainly due to unconsciously held positionalities (Jeffery and Colyer, 2007). The higher the levels of consciousness of the test team, the more accurate are the results. The best attitude is one of clinical detachment, posing a statement with the prefix statement, "In the name of the highest good, _____ calibrates as true. Over 100. Over 200," etc. The contextualization "in the highest good" increases accuracy because it transcends self-serving personal interest and motives.

For many years, the test was thought to be a local response of the body's acupuncture or immune system. Later research, however, has revealed that the response is not a local response to the body at all, but instead is a general response of consciousness itself to the energy of a substance or a statement. That which is true, beneficial, or pro-life gives a positive response that stems from the impersonal field of consciousness, which is present in everyone living. This positive response is indicated by the body's musculature going strong. There is also an associated pupillary response (the eyes dilate with falsity and constrict to truth) as well as alterations in brain function as revealed by magnetic imaging. (For convenience, the deltoid muscle is usually the one best used as an indicator muscle; however, any of the muscles of the body can be used.)

Before a question (in the form of a statement) is presented, it is necessary to qualify 'permission'; that is, state, "I have permission to ask about what I am holding in mind." (Yes/No) Or, "This calibration serves the highest good."

If a statement is false or a substance is injurious, the muscles go weak quickly in response to the command, "Resist." This indicates the stimulus is negative, untrue, anti-life, or the answer is "no." The response is fast and brief in duration. The body will then rapidly recover and return to normal muscle tension.

There are three ways of doing the testing. The one that is used in research and also most generally used requires two people: the tester and the test subject. A quiet setting is preferred, with no background music. The test subject closes their eyes. *The tester must phrase the 'question' to be asked in the form of a statement.* The statement can then be answered as "yes" or "no" by the muscle response. For instance, the *incorrect* form would be to ask, "Is this a healthy horse?" The correct form is to make the statement, "This horse is healthy," or its corollary, "This horse is sick."

After making the statement, the tester says "Resist" to the test subject who is holding the extended arm parallel to the ground. The tester presses down sharply with two fingers on the wrist of the extended arm with mild force. The test subject's arm will either stay strong, indicating a "yes," or go weak, indicating a "not yes" (no). The response is short and immediate.

A second method is the 'O-ring' method, which can be done alone. The thumb and middle finger of the same hand are held tightly in an 'O' configuration, and the hooked forefinger of the opposite hand is used to try to pull them apart. There is a noticeable difference in the strength between a "yes" and a "no" response (Rose, 2001).

The third method is the simplest, yet, like the others, requires some practice. Simply lift a heavy object, such as a large dictionary or merely a couple of bricks, from a table about waist high. Hold in mind an image or true statement to be calibrated and then lift. Then, for contrast, hold in mind that which is known to be false. Note the ease of lifting when truth is held in mind and the greater effort necessary to lift the load when the issue is false (not true). The results can be verified using the other two methods.

Calibration of Specific Levels

The critical point between positive and negative, between true and false, or between that which is constructive or destructive, is at the calibrated level of 200 (see Map in Appendix A). Anything above 200, or true, makes the subject go strong; anything below 200, or false, allows the arm to go weak.

Anything past or present, including images or statements, historical events, or personages, can be tested. They need not be verbalized.

Numerical Calibration

Example: "Ramana Maharshi teachings calibrate over 700." (Y/N). Or, "Hitler calibrated over 200." (Y/N)

"When he was in his 20s." (Y/N) "His 30s." (Y/N) "His 40s." (Y/N) "At the time of his death." (Y/N)

Applications

The muscle test cannot be used to foretell the future; otherwise, there are no limits as to what can be asked. Consciousness has no limits in time or space; however, permission may be denied. All current or historical events are available for questioning. The answers are impersonal and do not depend on the belief systems of either the tester or the test subject. For example, protoplasm recoils from noxious stimuli and flesh bleeds. Those are the qualities of these test materials and are impersonal. Consciousness actually knows only truth because only truth has actual existence. It does not respond to falsehood because falsehood does not have existence in Reality. It will also not respond accurately to nonintegrous or egoistical questions.

Accurately speaking, the test response is either an 'on' response or merely a 'not on' response. Like the electrical switch, we say the electricity is "on," and when we use the term "off," we just mean that it is not there. In reality, there is no such thing as 'off-ness'. This is a subtle statement but crucial to the understanding of the nature of consciousness. Consciousness is capable of recognizing only Truth. It merely fails to respond to falsehood. Similarly, a mirror reflects an image only if there is an object to reflect. If no object is present to the mirror, there is no reflected image.

To Calibrate A Level

Calibrated levels are relative to a specific reference

scale. To arrive at the same figures as in the chart in Appendix A, reference must be made to that table or by a statement such as, "On a scale of human consciousness from 1 to 1,000, where 600 indicates Enlightenment, this _____ calibrates over _____ (a number)." Or, "On a scale of consciousness where 200 is the level of Truth and 500 is the level of Love, this statement calibrates over _____." (State a specific number.)

General Information

People generally want to determine truth from falsehood. Therefore, the statement has to be made very specifically. Avoid using general terms such as a 'good' job to apply for. 'Good' in what way? Pay scale? Working conditions? Promotional opportunities? Fairness of the boss?

Expertise

Familiarity with the test brings progressive expertise. The 'right' questions to ask begin to spring forth and can become almost uncannily accurate. If the same tester and test subject work together for a period of time, one or both of them will develop what can become an amazing accuracy and capability of pinpointing just what specific questions to ask, even though the subject is totally unknown by either one. For instance, the tester has lost an object and begins by saying, "I left it in my office." (Answer: No.) "I left it in the car." (Answer: No.) All of a sudden, the test subject almost 'sees' the object and says, "Ask, 'On the back of the bathroom door.'" The test subject says, "The object is hanging on the back of the bathroom door." (Answer: Yes.) In this actual case, the test subject did not even know that the tester had stopped for gas and left a jacket in the restroom of a gasoline station.

Any information can be obtained about anything anywhere in current or past time or space, depending on receiving prior permission. (Sometimes one gets a "no," perhaps for karmic or other unknown reasons.) By cross-checking, accuracy can be easily confirmed. For anyone who learns the technique, more information is available instantaneously than can be held in all the computers and libraries of the world. The possibilities are therefore obviously unlimited, and the prospects breathtaking.

Limitations

The test is accurate only if the test subjects themselves calibrate over 200 and the intention for the use of the test is integrous and also calibrates over 200. The requirement is one of detached objectivity and alignment with truth rather than subjective opinion. Thus, to try to 'prove a point' negates accuracy. Sometimes married couples, for reasons as yet undiscovered, are unable to use each other as test subjects and may have to find a third person to be a test partner.

A suitable test subject is a person whose arm goes strong when a love object or person is held in mind, and it goes weak if that which is negative (fear, hate, guilt, etc.) is held in mind (e.g., Winston Churchill makes one go strong, and bin Laden makes one go weak).

Occasionally, a suitable test subject gives paradoxical

responses. This can usually be cleared by doing the 'thymic thump'. (With a closed fist, thump three times over the upper breastbone, smile, and say "ha-ha-ha" with each thump and mentally picture someone or something that is loved.) The temporary imbalance will then clear up.

The imbalance may be the result of recently having been with negative people, listening to heavy-metal rock music, watching violent television programs, playing violent video games, etc. Negative music energy has a deleterious effect on the energy system of the body for up to one-half hour after it is turned off. Television commercials or background are also a common source of negative energy.

As previously noted, this method of discerning truth from falsehood and the calibrated levels of truth has strict requirements. Because of the limitations, calibrated levels are supplied for ready reference in prior books, and extensively in *Truth vs. Falsehood*.

Explanation

The muscle-strength test is independent of personal opinion or beliefs and is an impersonal response of the field of consciousness, just as protoplasm is impersonal in its responses. This can be demonstrated by the observation that the test responses are the same whether verbalized or held silently in mind. Thus, the test subject is not influenced by the question as they do not even know what it is. To demonstrate this, do the following exercise:

The tester holds in mind an image unknown to the test subject and states, "The image I am holding in mind is positive" (or "true," or "calibrates over 200," etc.). Upon direction, the test subject then resists the downward pressure on the wrist. If the tester holds a positive image in mind (e.g., Abraham Lincoln, Jesus, Mother Teresa, etc.), the test subject's arm muscle will go strong. If the tester holds a false statement or negative image in mind (e.g., bin Laden, Hitler, etc.), the arm will go weak. Inasmuch as the test subject does not know what the tester has in mind, the results are not influenced by personal beliefs.

Disqualification

Both skepticism (cal. 160) and cynicism, as well as atheism, calibrate below 200 because they reflect negative prejudgment. In contrast, true inquiry requires an open mind and honesty devoid of intellectual vanity. Negative studies of the testing methodology *all* calibrate below 200 (usually at 160), as do the investigators themselves.

That even famous professors can and do calibrate below 200 may seem surprising to the average person. Thus, negative studies are a consequence of negative bias. As an example, Francis Crick's research design that led to the discovery of the double helix pattern of DNA calibrated at 440. His last research design, which was intended to prove that consciousness was just a product of neuronal activity, calibrated at only 135. (He was an atheist.)

The failure of investigators who themselves, or by faulty research design, calibrate below 200 (all calibrate at approximately 160), confirms the truth of the very methodology they claim to disprove. They 'should' get negative results, and so they do, which paradoxically proves the accuracy of the test to detect the difference between unbiased integrity and nonintegrity.

Any new discovery may upset the apple cart and be viewed as a threat to the status quo of prevailing belief systems. That consciousness research validates spiritual Reality is, of course, going to precipitate resistance, as it is actually a direct confrontation to the dominion of the narcissistic core of the ego itself, which is innately presumptuous and opinionated.

Below consciousness level 200, comprehension is limited by the dominance of Lower Mind, which is capable of recognizing facts but not yet able to grasp what is meant by the term 'truth' (it confuses *res interna* with *res externa*), and that truth has physiological accompaniments that are different from falsehood. Additionally, truth is intuited as evidenced by the use of voice analysis, the study of body language, pupillary response, EEG changes in the brain, fluctuations in breathing and blood pressure, galvanic skin response, dowsing, and even the Huna technique of measuring the distance that the aura radiates from the body. Some people have a very simple technique that utilizes the standing body like a pendulum (fall forward with truth and backward with falsehood).

From a more advanced contextualization, the principles that prevail are that Truth cannot be disproved by falsehood any more than light can be disproved by darkness. The nonlinear is not subject to the limitations of the linear. Truth is a paradigm different from logic and thus is not 'provable', as that which is provable calibrates only in the 400s. Consciousness research methodology operates at level 600, which is at the interface of the linear and the nonlinear dimensions.

Discrepancies

Differing calibrations may be obtained over time or by different investigators for a variety of reasons:

1. Situations, people, politics, policies, and attitudes change over time.
2. People tend to use different sensory modalities when they hold something in mind, i.e., visual, sensory, auditory, or feeling. 'Your mother' could therefore be how she looked, felt, sounded, etc., or Henry Ford could be calibrated as a father, as an industrialist, for his impact on America, his anti-Semitism, etc.
3. Accuracy increases with the level of consciousness. (The 400s and above are the most accurate.)

   One can specify context and stick to a prevailing modality. The same team using the same technique will get results that are internally consistent. Expertise develops with practice. There are some people, however, who are incapable of a scientific, detached attitude and are unable to be objective, and for whom the testing method will therefore not be accurate. Dedication and intention to the truth has to be given priority over personal opinions and trying to prove them as being "right."

Note

While it was discovered that the technique does not work for people who calibrate at less than level 200, only quite recently was it further discovered that the technique does not work if the persons doing the

testing are atheists. This may be simply the consequence of the fact that atheism calibrates below level
200, and that negation of the truth or Divinity (omniscience) karmically disqualifies the negator just as hate
negates love.

Also recently discovered was that the capacity for
accuracy of consciousness calibration testing increases
the higher the level of consciousness of the testers.
People in the range of the high 400s and above get the
most reliably accurate test results (Jeffrey and Colyer,
2007).

APPENDIX C

REFERENCES

A Course in Miracles. (1975) 1996. Mill Valley, Calif.: Foundation for Inner Peace.

Benoit, H. 1990. *Zen and the Psychology of Transformation: The Supreme Doctrine.* Rochester, Vermont: Inner Traditions.

Berne, E. 1964. *Games People Play.* New York: Grove Press.

Bristow, D., G. Rees, et al. 2005. "Brain Suppresses Awareness of Blinking." University College, London, Institute of Neurology, published in *Current Biology,* 25 July.

Diamond, J. 1979. *Behavioral Kinesiology.* New York: Harper & Rowe.

—. 1979. *Your Body Doesn't Lie.* New York: Warner Books.

Duffy, William. 1986. *Sugar Blues.* New York: Grand Central Publishing Co.

Great Books of the Western World, The. 1952. Hutching, R. and M. Alden, Eds. Chicago: Encyclopedia Britannica.

Hawkins, D. R. 2008a. *Reality, Spirituality, and Modern Man.* Sedona, AZ: Veritas Publishing.

—. 2008b. *In the World but not of It: Living Spiritually in the Modern World.* (Six CD set) Niles, IL: Nightingale-Conant.

—. 2008c. "Advancing Spiritual Awareness" Lecture Series. Sedona, AZ: Veritas Publishing. (Six 5-hour CD/DVDs.) *Spirituality, Reason, and Faith* (Jan.); *Clear Pathway to Enlightenment* (Mar.); *Belief, Trust, and Credibility* (June); *Overcoming Doubt, Skepticism and Disbelief* (Aug.); *Practical Spirituality* (Oct.); and, *Freedom: Morality and Ethics* (Nov.).

— 2007a. *Discovery of the Presence of God: Devotional Nonduality.* Sedona. AZ: Veritas Publishing.

— 2007b. *The Discovery: Revealing the Presence of God in Your Life.* (Six CD set.) Niles, IL: Nightingale-Conant.

— 2007c. "Spiritual Reality and Modern Man" Lecture Series. Sedona, AZ: Veritas Publishing. (Nine 5-hour CD/DVDs.) *God vs. Science: Limits of the Mind* (Feb.); *Relativism vs. Reality* (April); *What is "Real"?* (June); *What is "Truth"?* (July); *The Human Dilemma* (Aug.); *Review of the Work* (Sept.); *Creation vs. Evolution* (Oct.); *SpiritualSurvival: Realization of Reality* (Nov.); and, *Experiential Reality: The Mystic* (Dec.)

— 2006a. Transcending the Levels of Consciousness. Sedona. AZ: Veritas Publishing.

— 2006b. "Transcending the Levels of Consciousness" Lecture Series. Sedona, AZ: Veritas Publishing. (Six 5-hour CD/DVDs.) *Experiential Reality* (Feb.); *Perception vs. Essence* (April); *Spiritual Truth vs. Spiritual Fantasy* (June); *Reason vs. Truth* (Aug.); *Spiritual Practice and Daily Life* (Oct.); and, *Is the Miraculous Real?* (Dec.)

— 2006c. *Truth vs. Falsehood.* (Six CD Set.) Niles, IL: Nightingale-Conant.

— 2006d. "Paradigm Blindness: Academic vs. Clinical Medicine."*Journal of Orthomolecular Medicine*, 21:4, 4 November.

— 2005a. *Truth vs. Falsehood: How to Tell the Difference.* Toronto: Axial Publishing.

— 2005b. *The Highest Level of Enlightenment.* (Six CD set.) Niles, IL: Nightingale-Conant Corp.

— 2005c. "Devotional Nonduality" Lecture Series. Sedona, AZ: Veritas Publishing. (Eleven 5-hour CD/DVDs.) *Vision* (February); *Alignment* (April); *Intention* (May); *Transcending Barriers* (June); *Conviction* (July); *Serenity* (August); *Transcending Obstacles* (Sept.); *Spiritual Traps* (October); *Valid Teachers/Teachings* (Nov.); and, *God, Religion, & Spirituality* (Dec.)

— 2004a. "The Science of Peace." *Awakened World*, J.A.G.N.T., 6:3.

— 2004b. "*Nonduality: Consciousness Research and the Truth of the Buddha.*" Rourkee, India: Indian Institute of Technology.

— 2004c. "The Impact of Spontaneous Spiritual Experiences in the Life of 'Ordinary' Persons." *Watkins Review*, 7.

— 2004d. "Transcending the Mind "Lecture Series. Sedona, AZ: Veritas Publishing. (Six 5-hour CD/DVDs.) *Thought and Ideation* (Feb.); *Emotions and Sensations* (April); *Perception and Positionality* (June); *Identification and Illusion* (August); *Witnessing and Observing* (Oct.); and *The Ego and the Self* (Dec.).

— 2003a. *I: Reality and Subjectivity.* Sedona, AZ: Veritas Publishing.

— 2003b. "Devotional Nonduality "Lecture Series. Sedona, AZ: Veritas Publishing. (Six 5-hour CD/DVDs.) *Integration of Spirituality and Personal Life* (Feb.); *Spirituality and the World* (April); *Spiritual Community* (June); *Enlightenment* (August); *Realization of the Self as the "I"* (Nov.); and, *Dialogue, Questions and Answers* (Dec.).

— 2002a. *Power versus Force: An Anatomy of Consciousness.* (Rev.). Carlsbad, CA; Brighton-le-Sands, Australia: Hay House.

— 2002b."The Pathway to God" Lecture Series. Sedona, AZ: Veritas Publishing. (Twelve 5-hour CD/DVDs) 1. *Causality: The Ego's Foundation;* 2. *Radical Subjectivity: The I of Self;* 3. *Levels of Consciousness: Subjective and Social Consequences;* 4. *Positionality and Duality: Transcending the Opposites;* 5. *Perception and Illusion: the Distortions of Reality;* 6. *Realizing the Root of Consciousness: Meditative and Contemplative Techniques;* 7. *The Nature of Divinity: Undoing Religious Fallacies;* 8. *Advaita: The Way to God Through Mind;* 9. *Devotion: The Way to God Through the Heart;* 10. *Karma and the Afterlife;* 11. *God Transcendent and Immanent; and,* 12. *Realization of the Self: The Final Moments.*

— 2001. *The Eye of the I: From Which Nothing Is Hidden.* Sedona, AZ: Veritas Publishing.

— 2000a. *Consciousness Workshop.* Prescott, AZ Sedona, AZ: Veritas Publishing. (CD/DVD)

— 2000b. Consciousness and A Course in Miracles. (California.) Sedona, AZ: Veritas Publishing. (CD)

— 2000c. *Consciousness and Spiritual Inquiry: Address to the Tao Fellowship.* Sedona, AZ: Veritas Publishing. (CD)

— 1997. *Research on the Nature of Consciousness.* Sedona, AZ: Veritas Publishing. (The Landsberg 1997 Lecture. University of California School of Medicine, San Francisco, CA)

— 1996."Realization of the Presence of God." *Concepts.* July, 17-18.

— 1995. *Power vs. Force: An Anatomy of Consciousness.* Sedona, AZ: Veritas Publishing.

— 1995. *Quantitative and Qualitative Analysis and Calibration of the Levels of Human Consciousness.* Ann Arbor, Mich.: VMI, Bell and Howell Col.; republished 1996 by Veritas Publishing, Sedona, AZ

— 1995. *Power Versus Force; Consciousness and Addiction; Advanced States of Consciousness: The Realization of the Presence of God; Consciousness: How to Tell the Truth About Anything,* and *Undoing the Barriers to Spiritual Progress.* Sedona, AZ: Veritas Publishing. (CD/DVDs.)

— 1987. Sedona Lecture Series: *Drug Addiction and Alcoholism; A Map of Consciousness; Cancer; AIDS;* and *Death and Dying.* Sedona, AZ: Veritas Publishing. (CDs, DVDs.)

— 1986. *Office Series: Stress; Health; Spiritual First Aid; Sexuality; The Aging Process; Handling Major Crisis; Worry, Fear and Anxiety;*

Pain and Suffering; Losing Weight; Depression; Illness and Self-Healing; and *Alcoholism.* Sedona, AZ: Veritas Publishing. (CDs/DVDs.)

— 1985. "Consciousness and Addiction" in *Beyond Addictions, Beyond Boundaries.* S. Burton and L. Kiley. San Mateo, CA: Brookridge Institute.

Hawkins, D. R., and L. Pauling. 1973. *Orthomolecular Psychiatry.* New York: W. H. Freeman and Co.

Kubler-Ross, E. 1997. *On Death and Dying,* New York: Scribner.

Libet, B., et al. 1999. Article in *Brain* 106, 623-42.

Sadlier, S. 2000. *Looking for God: A Searcher's Guide to Religious and Spiritual Groups of the World.* New York: Perigee Trade.

Stapp, H. 2007. *Mindful Universe: Quantum Mechanics and the Participating Observer.* New York: Springer-Verlag Publishing.

Warren, R. 2002. *The Purpose Driven Life: What on Earth Am I Here For?* Grand Rapids, Mich.: Zondervan.

ABOUT THE AUTHOR

Biographical and Autobiographical Notes

Dr. Hawkins is an internationally known spiritual teacher, author, and speaker on the subject of advanced spiritual states, consciousness research, and the Realization of the Presence of God as Self.

His published works, as well as recorded lectures, have been widely recognized as unique in that a very advanced state of spiritual awareness occurred in an individual with a scientific and clinical background who was later able to verbalize and explain the unusual phenomenon in a manner that is clear and comprehensible.

The transition from the normal ego-state of mind to its elimination by the Presence is described in the trilogy *Power vs. Force* (1995) which won praise even from Mother Teresa, *The Eye of the I* (2001), and *I: Reality and Subjectivity* (2003), which have been translated into the major languages of the world. *Truth vs. Falsehood: How to Tell the Difference* (2005), *Transcending the Levels of Consciousness* (2006), *Discovery of the Presence of God: Devotional Nonduality* (2007), and *Reality, Spirituality and Modern Man* (2008) continue the exploration of the ego's expressions and inherent limitations and how to transcend them.

The trilogy was preceded by research on the Nature of Consciousness and published as the doctoral dissertation, *Qualitative and Quantitative Analysis and Calibration of the Levels of Human Consciousness* (1995), which correlated the seemingly disparate domains of science and spirituality. This was accomplished by the major discovery of a technique that, for the first time in human history, demonstrated a means to discern truth from falsehood.

The importance of the initial work was given recognition by its very favorable and extensive review in *Brain/Mind Bulletin* and at later presentations such as the International Conference on Science and Consciousness. Many presentations were given to a variety of organizations, spiritual conferences, church groups, nuns, and monks, both nationally and in foreign countries, including the Oxford Forum in England. In the Far East, Dr. Hawkins is a recognized "Teacher of the Way to Enlightenment" ("Tae Ryoung Sun Kak Dosa").

In response to his observation that much spiritual truth has been misunderstood over the ages due to lack of explanation, Dr. Hawkins has presented monthly seminars that provide detailed explanations which are too lengthy to describe in book format. Recordings are available that end with questions and answers, thus providing additional clarification.

The overall design of this lifetime work is to recontextualize the human experience in terms of the evolution of consciousness and to integrate a comprehension of both mind and spirit as expressions of the innate Divinity that is the substrate and ongoing source of life and Existence. This dedication is signified by the statement *"Gloria in Excelsis Deo!"* with which his published works begin and end.

Biographic Summary

Dr. Hawkins has practiced psychiatry since 1952 and is a life member of the American Psychiatric Association and numerous other professional organizations. His national television appearance schedule has included *The McNeil/Leher News Hour, The Barbara Walters Show, The Today Show*, science documentaries, and many others. He was also interviewed by Oprah Winfrey.

He is the author of numerous scientific and spiritual publications, books, CDs, DVDs, and lecture series. Nobelist Linus Pauling coauthored his landmark book, *Orthomolecular Psychiatry*. Dr. Hawkins was a consultant for many years to Episcopal and Catholic Dioceses, monastic orders, and other religions orders.

Dr. Hawkins has lectured widely, with appearances at Westminster Abbey, the Universities of Argentina, Notre Dame, and Michigan; Fordham University and Harvard University; and the Oxford Forum in England. He gave the annual Landsberg Lecture at the University of California Medical School at San Francisco. He is also a consultant to foreign governments on international diplomacy and was instrumental in resolving long-standing conflicts that were major threats to world peace.

In recognition of his contributions to humanity, in 1995, Dr. Hawkins became a knight of the Sovereign Order of the Hospitaliers of St. John of Jerusalem, which was founded in 1077.

Autobiographic Note

While the truths reported in this book were scientifically derived and objectively organized, like all truths, they were first experienced personally. A life-long sequence of intense states of awareness beginning at a young age first inspired and then gave direction to the process of subjective realization that has finally taken form in this series of books.

At age three, there occurred a sudden full consciousness of existence, a nonverbal but complete understanding of the meaning of "I Am," followed immediately by the frightening realization that "I" might not have come into existence at all. This was an instant awakening from oblivion into a conscious awareness, and in that moment, the personal self was born and the duality of "Is" and "Is Not" entered my subjective awareness.

Throughout childhood and early adolescence, the paradox of existence and the question of the reality of the self remained a repeated concern. The personal self would sometimes begin slipping back into a greater impersonal Self, and the initial fear of non-existence—the fundamental fear of nothingness—would recur.

In 1939, as a paperboy with a seventeen-mile bicycle route in rural Wisconsin, on a dark winter's night I was caught miles from home in a twenty-below-zero blizzard. The bicycle fell over on the ice and the fierce wind ripped the newspapers out of the handlebar basket, blowing them across the ice-covered, snowy field. There were tears of frustration and exhaustion and my clothes were frozen stiff. To get out of the wind, I broke through the icy crust of a high snow bank, dug out a space, and crawled into it. Soon the shivering stopped and there was a delicious warmth, and then a state of peace beyond all description. This was accompanied by a suffusion of light and a presence of infinite love that had no beginning and no end and was undifferentiated from my own essence. The physical body and surroundings faded as my awareness was fused with this all-present, illuminated state. The mind grew silent; all thought stopped. An infinite Presence was all that was or could be, beyond all time or description.

After that timelessness, there was suddenly an awareness of someone shaking my knee; then my father's anxious face appeared. There was great reluctance to return to the body and all that that entailed, but because of my father's love and anguish, the Spirit nurtured and reactivated the body. There was compassion for his fear of death, although, at the same time, the concept of death seemed absurd.

This subjective experience was not discussed with anyone since there was no context available from which to describe it. It was not common to hear of spiritual experiences other than those reported in the lives of the saints. But after this experience, the accepted reality of the world began to seem only provisional; traditional religious teachings lost significance and, paradoxically, I became an agnostic. Compared to the light of Divinity that had illuminated all existence, the god of traditional religion shone dully indeed; thus spirituality replaced religion.

During World War II, hazardous duty on a minesweeper often brought close brushes with death, but there was no fear of it. It was as though death had lost its authenticity. After the war, fascinated by the complexities of the mind and wanting to study psychiatry, I worked my way through medical school. My training psychoanalyst, a professor at Columbia University, was also an agnostic; we both took a dim view of religion. The analysis went well, as did my career, and success followed.

I did not, however, settle quietly into professional life. I fell ill with a progressive, fatal illness that did not respond to any treatments available. By age thirty-eight, I was *in extremis* and knew I was about to die. I didn't care about the body, but my spirit was in a state of extreme anguish and despair. As the final moment approached, the thought flashed through my mind, "What if there is a God?" So I called out in prayer, "If there is a God, I ask him to help me now." I surrendered to whatever God there might be and went into oblivion. When I awoke, a transformation of such enormity had taken place that I was struck dumb with awe.

The person I had been no longer existed. There was no personal self or ego, only an Infinite Presence of such unlimited power that it was all that was. This Presence had replaced what had been 'me', and the body and its actions were controlled solely by the Infinite Will of the Presence. The world was illuminated by the clarity of an Infinite Oneness that expressed itself as all things revealed in their infinite beauty and perfection.

As life went on, this stillness persisted. There was no personal will; the physical body went about its business under the direction of the infinitely powerful but exquisitely gentle Will of the Presence. In that state, there was no need to think about anything. All truth was self-evident and no conceptualization was necessary or even possible. At the same time, the physical nervous system felt extremely overtaxed, as though it were carrying far more energy than its circuits had been designed for.

It was not possible to function effectively in the world. All ordinary motivations had disappeared, along with all fear and anxiety. There was nothing to seek, as all was perfect. Fame, success, and money were meaningless. Friends urged the pragmatic return to clinical practice, but there was no ordinary motivation to do so.

There was now the ability to perceive the reality that underlay personalities: the origin of emotional sickness lay in people's belief that they *were* their personalities. And so, as though of its own, a clinical practice resumed and eventually became huge.

People came from all over the United States. The practice had two thousand outpatients, which required more than fifty therapists and other employees, a suite of twenty-five offices, and research and electroencephalic laboratories. There were a thousand new patients a year. In addition, there were appearances on radio and network television shows, as previously mentioned. In 1973, the clinical research was documented in a traditional format in the book, *Orthomolecular Psychiatry*. This work was ten years ahead of its time and created something of a stir.

The overall condition of the nervous system improved slowly, and then another phenomenon commenced. There was a sweet, delicious band of energy continuously flowing up the spine and into the brain where it created an intense sensation of continuous pleasure. Everything in life happened by synchronicity, evolving in perfect harmony; the miraculous was commonplace. The origin of what the world would call miracles was the Presence, not the personal self. What remained of the personal 'me' was only a witness to these phenomena. The greater 'I', deeper than my former self or thoughts, determined all that happened.

The states that were present had been reported by others throughout history and led to the investigation of spiritual teachings, including those of the Buddha, enlightened sages, Huang Po, and more recent teachers such as Ramana Maharshi and Nisargadatta Maharaj. It was thus confirmed that these experiences were not unique. The *Bhagavad-Gita* now made complete sense. At times, the same spiritual ecstasy reported by Sri Rama Krishna and the Christian saints occurred.

Everything and everyone in the world was luminous and exquisitely beautiful. All living beings became Radiant and expressed this Radiance in stillness and splendor. It was apparent that all mankind is actually motivated by inner love but has simply become unaware; most lives are lived as though by sleepers unawakened to the awareness of who they really are. People around me looked as though they were asleep and were incredibly beautiful. It was like being in love with everyone.

It was necessary to stop the habitual practice of meditating for an hour in the morning and then again before dinner because it would intensify the bliss to such an extent that it was not possible to function. An experience similar to the one that had occurred in the snow bank as a boy would recur, and it became increasingly difficult to leave that state and return to the world. The incredible beauty of all things shone forth in all their perfection, and where the world saw ugliness, there was only timeless beauty. This spiritual love suffused all perception, and all boundaries between here and there, or then and now, or separation disappeared. During the years spent in inner silence, the strength of the Presence grew. Life was no longer personal; a personal will no longer existed. The personal 'I' had become an instrument of the Infinite Presence and went about and did as it was willed. People felt an extraordinary peace in the aura of that Presence. Seekers sought answers but as there was no longer any such individual as David, they were actually finessing answers from their own Self, which was not different from mine. From each person the same Self shone forth from their eyes.

The miraculous happened, beyond ordinary comprehension. Many chronic maladies from which the body had suffered for years disappeared; eyesight spontaneously normalized, and there was no longer a need for the lifetime bifocals.

Occasionally, an exquisitely blissful energy, an Infinite Love, would suddenly begin to radiate from the heart toward the scene of some calamity. Once, while driving on a highway, this exquisite energy began to beam out of the chest. As the car rounded a bend, there was an auto accident; the wheels of the overturned car were still spinning. The energy passed with great intensity into the occupants of the car and then stopped of its own accord. Another time, while I was walking on the streets of a strange city, the energy started to flow down the block ahead and arrived at the scene of an incipient gang fight. The combatants fell back and began to laugh, and again, the energy stopped.

Profound changes of perception came without warning in improbable circumstances. While dining alone at Rothman's on Long Island, the Presence suddenly intensified until every thing and every person, which had appeared as separate in ordinary perception, melted into a timeless universality and oneness. In the motionless Silence, it became obvious that there are no 'events' or 'things' and that nothing actually 'happens' because past, present, and future are merely artifacts of perception, as is the illusion of a separate 'I' being subject to birth and death. As the limited, false self dissolved into the universal Self of its true origin, there was an ineffable sense of having returned home to a state of absolute peace and relief from all suffering. It is only the illusion of individuality that is the origin of all suffering. When one realizes that one *is* the universe, complete and at one with All That Is, forever without end, then no further suffering is possible.

Patients came from every country in the world, and some were the most hopeless of the hopeless. Grotesque, writhing, wrapped in wet sheets for transport from far-away hospitals they came, hoping for treatment for advanced psychoses and grave, incurable mental disorders. Some were catatonic; many had been mute for years. But in each patient, beneath the crippled appearance, there was the shining essence of love and beauty, perhaps so obscured to ordinary vision that he or she had become totally unloved in this world.

One day a mute catatonic was brought into the hos-

pital in a straitjacket. She had a severe neurological disorder and was unable to stand. Squirming on the floor,
she went into spasms and her eyes rolled back in her
head. Her hair was matted; she had torn all her clothes
and uttered guttural sounds. Her family was fairly
wealthy; as a result, over the years she had been seen
by innumerable physicians and famous specialists from
all over the world. Every treatment had been tried on
her and she had been given up as hopeless by the
medical profession.

A short, nonverbal question arose: "What do you
want done with her, God?" Then came the realization
that she just needed to be loved, that was all. Her inner
self shone through her eyes and the Self connected
with that loving essence. In that second, she was
healed by her own recognition of who she really was;
what happened to her mind or body didn't matter to
her any longer.

This, in essence, occurred with countless patients.
Some recovered in the eyes of the world and some did
not, but whether a clinical recovery ensued didn't matter any longer to the patients. Their inner agony was
over. As they felt loved and at peace within, their pain
stopped. This phenomenon can only be explained by
saying that the Compassion of the Presence recontextualized each patient's reality so that he or she experienced healing on a level that transcended the world
and its appearances. The inner peace of the Self encompassed us beyond time and identity.

It was clear that all pain and suffering arises solely
from the ego and not from God. This truth was silently
communicated to the minds of the patients. This was

the mental block in another mute catatonic who had not spoken in many years. The Self said to him through mind, "You're blaming God for what your ego has done to you." He jumped off the floor and began to speak, much to the shock of the nurse who witnessed the incident.

The work became increasingly taxing and eventually overwhelming. Patients were backed up, waiting for beds to open although the hospital had built an extra ward to house them. There was an enormous frustration in that the human suffering could be countered in only one patient at a time. It was like bailing out the sea. It seemed that there must be some other way to address the causes of the common malaise, the endless stream of spiritual distress and human suffering.

This led to the study of the physiological response (muscle testing) to various stimuli, which revealed an amazing discovery. It was the 'wormhole' between two universes—the physical world and the world of the mind and spirit—an interface between dimensions. In a world full of sleepers lost from their source, here was a tool to recover, and demonstrate for all to see, that lost connection with the higher reality. This led to the testing of every substance, thought, and concept that could be brought to mind. The endeavor was aided by my students and research assistants. Then a major discovery was made: whereas all subjects went weak from negative stimuli, such as fluorescent lights, pesticides, and artificial sweeteners, students of spiritual disciplines who had advanced their levels of awareness did not go weak as did ordinary people. Something important and decisive had shifted in their consciousness. It apparently occurred as they realized they were not at the mercy of the world but rather affected only by what their minds believed. Perhaps the very process of progress toward enlightenment could be shown to increase man's ability to resist the vicissitudes of existence, including illness.

The Self had the capacity to change things in the world by merely envisioning them; Love changed the world each time it replaced non-love. The entire scheme of civilization could be profoundly altered by focusing this power of love at a very specific point. Whenever this happened, history bifurcated down new roads.

It now appeared that these crucial insights could not only be communicated with the world but also visibly and irrefutably demonstrated. It seemed that the great tragedy of human life had always been that the psyche is so easily deceived; discord and strife have been the inevitable consequence of mankind's inability to distinguish the false from the true. But here was an answer to this fundamental dilemma, a way to recontextualize the nature of consciousness itself and make explicable that which otherwise could only be inferred.

It was time to leave life in New York, with its city apartment and home on Long Island, for something more important. It was necessary to perfect 'myself' as an instrument. This necessitated leaving that world and everything in it, replacing it with a reclusive life in a small town where the next seven years were spent in meditation and study.

Overpowering states of bliss returned unsought,

and eventually, there was the need to learn how to be in the Divine Presence and still function in the world. The mind had lost track of what was happening in the world at large. In order to do research and writing, it was necessary to stop all spiritual practice and focus on the world of form. Reading the newspaper and watching television helped to catch up on the story of who was who, the major events, and the nature of the current social dialogue.

Exceptional subjective experiences of truth, which are the province of the mystic who affects all mankind by sending forth spiritual energy into the collective consciousness, are not understandable by the majority of mankind and are therefore of limited meaning except to other spiritual seekers. This led to an effort to be ordinary, because just being ordinary in itself is an expression of Divinity; the truth of one's real self can be discovered through the pathway of everyday life. To live with care and kindness is all that is necessary. The rest reveals itself in due time. The commonplace and God are not distinct.

And so, after a long circular journey of the spirit, there was a return to the most important work, which was to try to bring the Presence at least a little closer to the grasp of as many fellow beings as possible.

———

The Presence is silent and conveys a state of peace that is the space in which and by which all is and has its existence and experience. It is infinitely gentle and yet like a rock. With it, all fear disappears. Spiritual joy occurs on a quiet level of inexplicable ecstasy. Because the experience of time stops, there are no apprehension or regret, no pain or anticipation; the source of joy is unending and ever present. With no beginning or ending, there is no loss or grief or desire. Nothing needs to be done; everything is already perfect and complete.

When time stops, all problems disappear; they are merely artifacts of a point of perception. As the Presence prevails, there is no further identification with the body or mind. When the mind grows silent, the thought "I Am" also disappears, and Pure Awareness shines forth to illuminate what one is, was, and always will be, beyond all worlds and all universes, beyond time, and therefore without beginning or end.

People wonder, "How does one reach this state of awareness," but few follow the steps because they are so simple. First, the desire to reach that state was intense. Then began the discipline to act with constant and universal forgiveness and gentleness, without exception. One has to be compassionate towards everything, including one's own self and thoughts. Next came a willingness to hold desires in abeyance and surrender personal will at every moment. As each thought, feeling, desire, or deed was surrendered to God, the mind became progressively silent. At first, it released whole stories and paragraphs, then ideas and concepts. As one lets go of wanting to own these thoughts, they no longer reach such elaboration and begin to fragment while only half formed. Finally, it was possible to turn over the energy behind thought itself before it even became thought.

The task of constant and unrelenting fixity of focus, allowing not even a moment of distraction from meditation, continued while doing ordinary activities. At first, this seemed very difficult, but as time went on, it became habitual, automatic, requiring less and less effort, and finally, it was effortless. The process is like a rocket leaving the earth. At first, it requires enormous power, then less and less as it leaves the earth's gravitational field, and finally, it moves through space under its own momentum.

Suddenly, without warning, a shift in awareness occurred and the Presence was there, unmistakable and all encompassing. There were a few moments of apprehension as the self died, and then the absoluteness of the Presence inspired a flash of awe. This breakthrough was spectacular, more intense than anything before. It has no counterpart in ordinary experience. The profound shock was cushioned by the love that is with the Presence. Without the support and protection of that love, one would be annihilated.

There followed a moment of terror as the ego clung to its existence, fearing it would become nothingness. Instead, as it died, it was replaced by the Self as Everythingness, the All in which everything is known and obvious in its perfect expression of its own essence. With nonlocality came the awareness that one is all that ever was or can be. One is total and complete, beyond all identities, beyond all gender, beyond even humanness itself. One need never again fear suffering and death.

What happens to the body from this point is immaterial. At certain levels of spiritual awareness, ailments of the body heal or spontaneously disappear. But in the absolute state, such considerations are irrelevant. The body will run its predicted course and then return from whence it came. It is a matter of no importance; one is unaffected. The body appears as an 'it' rather than as a 'me', as another object, like the furniture in a room. It may seem comical that people still address the body as though it were the individual 'you', but there is no way to explain this state of awareness to the unaware. It is best to just go on about one's business and allow Providence to handle the social adjustment. However, as one reaches bliss, it is very difficult to conceal that state of intense ecstasy. The world may be dazzled, and people may come from far and wide to be in the accompanying aura. Spiritual seekers and the spiritually curious may be attracted, as may be the very ill who are seeking miracles. One may become a magnet and a source of joy to them. Commonly, there is a desire at this point to share this state with others and to use it for the benefit of all.

The ecstasy that accompanies this condition is not initially absolutely stable; there are also moments of great agony. The most intense occur when the state fluctuates and suddenly ceases for no apparent reason. These times bring on periods of intense despair and a fear that one has been forsaken by the Presence. These falls make the path arduous, and to surmount these reversals requires great will. It finally becomes obvious that one must transcend this level or constantly suffer excruciating 'descents from grace'. The glory of ecstasy, then, has to be relinquished as one enters upon the arduous task of transcending duality until one is beyond all oppositions and their conflicting pulls. But while it is one thing to happily give up the iron chains of the ego, it is quite another to abandon the golden chains of ecstatic joy. It feels as though one is giving up God, and a new level of fear arises, never before anticipated. This is the final terror of absolute aloneness.

To the ego, the fear of nonexistence was formidable, and it drew back from it repeatedly as it seemed to approach. The purpose of the agonies and the dark nights of the soul then became apparent. They are so intolerable that their exquisite pain spurs one on to the extreme effort required to surmount them. When vacillation between heaven and hell becomes unendurable, the desire for existence itself has to be surrendered. Only once this is done may one finally move beyond the duality of Allness versus Nothingness, beyond existence or nonexistence. This culmination of the inner work is the most difficult phase, the ultimate watershed, where one is starkly aware that the illusion of existence one here transcends is irrevocable. There is no returning from this step, and this specter of irreversibility makes this last barrier appear to be the most formidable choice of all.

But, in fact, in this final apocalypse of the self, the dissolution of the sole remaining duality of existence and nonexistence—identity itself—dissolves in Universal Divinity, and no individual consciousness is left to choose. The last step, then, is taken by God.

—*David R. Hawkins*